The Wills Eye Manual

**Office and Emergency Room
Diagnosis and Treatment of Eye Disease**

Contributors to the Second Edition

Neal H. Atebara, M.D.
Medical Illustrator
Mark C. Austin, M.D.
Jerry R. Blair, M.D.
Benjamin Chang, M.D.
Mary Ellen Cullom, M.D.
R. Douglas Cullom, Jr., M.D.
Jack Dugan, M.D.
Forrest J. Ellis, M.D.
C. Byron Faulkner, M.D.
Mary Elizabeth Gallivan, M.D.
J. William Harbour, M.D.
Paul M. Herring, M.D.
Allen Ho, M.D.
Carol J. Hoffman, M.D.

Thomas I. Margolis, M.D.
Mark L. Mayo, M.D.
Michele A. Miano, M.D.
Wynne A. Morley, M.D.
Timothy J. O'Brien, M.D.
Florentino E. Palmon, M.D.
William B. Phillips, M.D.
Tony Pruthi, M.D.
Carl D. Regillo, M.D.
Scott H. Smith, M.D.
Mark R. Stokes, M.D.
Janine G. Tabas, M.D.
John R. Trible, M.D.
Christopher Williams, M.D.

Contributors to the First Edition

Melissa M. Brown, M.D.
Catharine J. Crockett, M.D.
Bret L. Fisher, M.D.
Patrick M. Flaharty, M.D.
Mark A. Friedberg, M.D.
James T. Handa, M.D.
Victor A. Holmes, M.D.

Bruce J. Keyser, M.D.
Marlon Maus, M.D.
Medical Illustrator
Ronald L. McKey, M.D.
Christopher J. Rapuano, M.D.
Paul A. Raskauskas, M.D.
Eric P. Suan, M.D.

The Wills Eye Manual

Office and Emergency Room
Diagnosis and Treatment of Eye Disease
Second Edition

R. Douglas Cullom, Jr., M.D.
Benjamin Chang, M.D.
Editors for the Second Edition

Mark A. Friedberg, M.D.
Christopher J. Rapuano, M.D.
Founding Editors

J.B. LIPPINCOTT COMPANY Philadelphia

Assistant Editor: Eileen Wolfberg
Indexer: Alexandra Nickerson
Interior Designer: Susan Blaker
Cover Designer: Tom Jackson
Production Manager: Janet Greenwood
Production: P. M. Gordon Associates, Inc.
Compositor: Modern Graphics
Printer/Binder: R. R. Donnelley & Sons

Second Edition

11   10   9   8   7   6   5   4   3

Library of Congress Cataloging-in-Publication Data

The Wills eye manual : office and emergency room diagnosis and treatment of
  eye disease. —2nd ed. / R. Douglas Cullom, Jr., Benjamin Chang.
    p.   cm.
    Rev. ed. of: Wills Eye Hospital office and emergency room diagnosis and
treatment of eye disease. © 1990.
    Includes bibliographical references and index.
    ISBN 0–397–51380–1
    1. Ophthalmologic emergencies—Handbooks, manuals, etc. 2. Eye—Diseases
and defects—Handbooks, manuals, etc. I. Cullom, R. Douglas. II. Chang,
Benjamin. III. Wills Eye Hospital (Philadelphia, Pa.) IV. Wills Eye Hospital
office and emergency room diagnosis and treatment of eye disease.
    [DNLM: 1. Emergencies—outlines. 2. Eye Diseases—therapy—outlines.
3. Eye Diseases—diagnosis—outlines. WW 18 W741 1993]
RE46.W78   1993
617.7—dc20
DNLM/DLC
for Library of Congress   93–39666
                                         CIP

The authors and publisher have exerted every effort to ensure that drug selection
and dosage set forth in this text are in accord with current recommendations and
practice at the time of publication. However, in view of ongoing research, changes
in government regulations, and the constant flow of information relating to drug
therapy and drug reactions, the reader is urged to check the package insert for each
drug for any change in indications and dosage and for added warnings and
precautions. This is particularly important when the recommended agent is a new
or infrequently employed drug.

CONSULTANTS

CORNEA

Major Consultants

Elisabeth J. Cohen, M.D.
Christopher J. Rapuano, M.D.

Consultants

Peter R. Laibson, M.D.
Michael A. Naidoff, M.D.
Irving M. Raber, M.D.

GLAUCOMA

Consultants

L. Jay Katz, M.D.
Marlene R. Moster, M.D.
George L. Spaeth, M.D.
Richard P. Wilson, M.D.

NEURO-OPHTHALMOLOGY

Major Consultants

Peter J. Savino, M.D.
Robert C. Sergott, M.D.

OCULO-PLASTICS

Consultants

Edward H. Bedrossian, Jr., M.D.
Marc S. Cohen, M.D.
Joseph C. Flanagan, M.D.
Ignatius S. Hneleski, Jr., M.D.
Thaddeus S. Nowinski, M.D.
Robert Penne, M.D.
Mary A. Stefanyszyn, M.D.

ONCOLOGY

Consultants

James J. Augsburger, M.D.
Jerry A. Shields, M.D.

PEDIATRICS

Consultants

Joseph H. Calhoun, M.D.
Leonard B. Nelson, M.D.
Robert D. Reinecke, M.D.

RETINA

Major Consultant

William Tasman, M.D.

Consultants

William H. Annesley, Jr., M.D.
Jonathan B. Belmont, M.D.
William E. Benson, M.D.
Gary C. Brown, M.D.
Jay L. Federman, M.D.
David H. Fischer, M.D.
Alfred C. Lucier, M.D.
J. Arch McNamara, M.D.
Hermann D. Schubert, M.D.
Lov K. Sarin, M.D.

GENERAL

Consultants

Edward A. Jaeger, M.D.
John B. Jeffers, M.D.
Stephen B. Lichtenstein, M.D.

FOREWORD

When the first edition of this book was published in 1990, I pointed out that it was the product of a group effort by the second year resident class at the Wills Eye Hospital. Basically, the same is true with the second edition. In that regard it remains a unique enterprise. I am pleased that this totally new group of residents has felt dedicated to revising the first edition at a time when the uncertainties in medicine are even more scary than they were in 1990. Once again, the authors have kept the volume concise and have used as a basis for updating the book the large and diversified number of patients that Wills residents have the opportunity to see.

Finally, I am pleased that, while the bulk of the work was shared by the second year class, the effort has involved residents from each of the three years of training.

William Tasman, M.D.

PREFACE

The first edition of *The Wills Eye Hospital Office and Emergency Room Diagnosis and Treatment of Eye Disease* was an overwhelming success. The authors hope that the second edition will also be well received. Several changes have been made, including altering the title to *The Wills Eye Manual,* as the book has been popularly referred to by its audience. As with the first edition, our goal has been to provide a quick reference containing crisp and concise answers to diagnostic and therapeutic problems that span most of ophthalmology.

The Wills Eye Manual should continue to appeal to residents, comprehensive ophthalmologists, and even subspecialists who encounter problems outside their field of interest. In addition, emergency room physicians, family practitioners, and medical students will find that this book remains a useful resource when administering primary care and triaging patients with eye disorders.

The changes in ophthalmology over the last several years have been manifold. New diagnostic tests have been developed. There are many new ocular medications, as well as new indications for already established drugs. Antibiotic recommendations from corneal ulcers to endophthalmitis have changed. Results of important collaborative clinical ophthalmic research trials, such as the *Optic Neuritis Treatment Trial* and the *Macular Photocoagulation Study,* have altered the way we treat common ophthalmic disorders. The ocular complications of AIDS are more widespread and the appropriate treatments more complex. Thus, in the second edition of *The Wills Eye Manual* we have thoroughly and critically reviewed recent clinical data for inclusion in our diagnostic and treatment protocols. We have added simplified charts and illustrations, consolidated some chapters, and, when necessary, expanded others. At the same time we have resisted unnecessarily expanding a manual that has been valued for its concise and accessible nature.

Once again, as residents, we have consulted with our many mentors at the Wills Eye Hospital. They have assisted us in interpreting the changes in ophthalmology and in determining which data have led to modification of treatment regimens.

We hope this book continues to provide a quick and useful source of information for the diagnosis and treatment of eye disease. If so, then our goal will have been achieved.

R. Douglas Cullom, Jr., M.D.
Benjamin Chang, M.D.

PREFACE TO THE FIRST EDITION

Our goal has been to produce a concise book, providing essential diagnostic tips and specific therapeutic information pertaining to eye disease. We realized the need for this book while managing emergency room patients at one of the largest and busiest eye hospitals in the country. Until now, reliable information could only be obtained in unwieldy textbooks or inaccessible journals.

As residents at Wills Eye Hospital we have benefited from the input of some of the world-renowned ophthalmic experts in writing this book. More importantly, we are aware of the questions that the ophthalmology resident, the attending ophthalmologist, and the emergency room physician (not trained in ophthalmology) want answered immediately.

The book is written for the eye care provider who, in the midst of evaluating an eye problem, needs quick access to additional information. We try to be as specific as possible, describing the therapeutic modalities used at our institution. Many of these recommendations are, therefore, not the only manner in which to treat a particular disorder, but indicate personal preference. They are guidelines, not rules.

Because of the forever changing wealth of ophthalmic knowledge, omissions and errors are possible, particularly with regard to management. Drug dosages have been checked carefully, but the physician is urged to check the *Physicians Desk Reference* or *Facts and Comparisons* when prescribing unfamiliar medications. Not all contraindications and side effects are described.

We feel this book will make a welcome companion to the many physicians involved with treating eye problems. It is everything you wanted to know and nothing more.

Christopher J. Rapuano, M.D.
Mark A. Friedberg, M.D.

ACKNOWLEDGMENTS

We would like to thank the numerous residents from several residency classes who assisted us in updating this edition of *The Wills Eye Manual.* We are particularly grateful to the many Wills Eye Hospital attendings, without whose support and guidance this book would not have been possible.

CONTENTS

5 CONJUNCTIVA/SCLERA/EXTERNAL DISEASE 109

6 EYELID 133

7 ORBIT 153

11 NEURO-OPHTHALMOLOGY   241

12 RETINA   293

13 UVEITIS   351

14 SYSTEMIC DISORDERS   389

DIFFERENTIAL DIAGNOSIS OF OCULAR SYMPTOMS

Burning

More common Blepharitis, dry eye syndrome, conjunctivitis (discharge or eyelid sticking additionally).

Less common Corneal problem (fluoresccin staining of the cornea usually), inflamed pterygium/pinguecula, episcleritis, superior limbic keratoconjunctivitis.

Crossed Eyes in Children

See "Esodeviations in Children" (eyes turned in), Section 9.3, or "Exodeviations in Children" (eyes turned out), Section 9.4.

Decreased Vision

I. Transient visual loss (Vision returns to normal within 24 hours, usually within 1 hour.)

More common Few seconds (usually bilateral): Papilledema.

Few minutes: Amaurosis fugax (TIA) (unilateral), vertebrobasilar artery insufficiency (bilateral).

10–60 minutes: Migraine (with or without a subsequent headache).

Less common Impending central retinal vein occlusion, ischemic optic neuropathy, ocular ischemic syndrome (carotid occlusive disease), glau

The Wills Eye Manual: Office and Emergency Room Diagnosis and Treatment of Eye Disease, Second Edition, edited by R. Douglas Cullom, M.D. and Benjamin Chang, M.D. © 1994 J. B. Lippincott Company.

coma, sudden change in blood pressure, central nervous system (CNS) lesion, optic disc drusen, giant cell arteritis.

II. Visual loss lasting longer than 24 hours
   A. Sudden, painless loss
      More common   Retinal artery or vein occlusion, ischemic optic neuropathy, vitreous hemorrhage, retinal detachment, optic neuritis (usually pain with eye movements).
      Less common   Other retinal or CNS disease.
   B. Gradual, painless loss (over weeks, months, or years)
      More common   Cataract, refractive error, open-angle glaucoma, chronic retinal disease [e.g., age-related macular degeneration (ARMD), diabetic retinopathy].
      Less common   Chronic corneal disease (e.g., corneal dystrophy), optic neuropathy/atrophy (e.g., CNS tumor).
   C. Painful loss: Acute-angle closure glaucoma, optic neuritis (pain with eye movements), uveitis, corneal hydrops (keratoconus).

❖ **Note** *Always remember nonphysiologic visual loss.*

Discharge

See "Red Eye" in this chapter.

Distortion (of Vision)

More common   Refractive error, macular disease (e.g., central serous chorioretinopathy or ARMD), corneal irregularity.
Less common   Cataract, topical eye drops (miotics), retinal detachment, migraine (transient), CNS abnormality.

Double Vision

I. Monocular   (The double vision remains when the uninvolved eye is occluded.)
   More common   Refractive error, corneal opacity or irregularity, cataract.
   Less common   Dislocated natural lens or lens implant, extra pupillary openings, macular disease, retinal detachment, nonphysiologic.
II. Binocular   (The double vision is eliminated when either eye is occluded.)
   A. Typically intermittent: Myasthenia gravis, intermittent decompensation of an existing phoria.
   B. Constant: Isolated sixth-, third-, or fourth-nerve palsy; orbital disease (e.g., thyroid eye disease, orbital inflammatory pseudotumor, tumor); cavernous sinus/superior orbital fissure syndrome; status post ocular surgery (e.g., residual anesthesia, displaced muscle); status posttrauma

(e.g., orbital wall fracture with extraocular muscle entrapment, orbital edema); internuclear ophthalmoplegia, vertebrobasilar artery insufficiency, other CNS lesions, spectacle problem.

Dry Eyes

See Section 4.2.

Eyelid Crusting

More common   Blepharitis, meibomianitis, conjunctivitis.
Less common   Canaliculitis, nasolacrimal duct obstruction, dacryocystitis.

Eyelid Droop

See "Ptosis" and "Pseudoptosis" in Chapter 2.

Eyelid Swelling

A. Associated with inflammation (usually erythematous)
   More common   Hordeolum, blepharitis, conjunctivitis, preseptal or orbital cellulitis, trauma, contact dermatitis.
   Less common   Ectropion, corneal abnormality, urticaria/angioedema, insect bite, dacryoadenitis, erysipelas, eyelid or lacrimal gland mass.
B. Noninflammatory: Chalazion; prolapse of orbital fat (retropulsion of the globe increases the prolapse); laxity of the eyelid skin; cardiac, renal, or thyroid disease; eyelid or lacrimal gland mass.

Eyelid Twitch

Fatigue, lack of sleep, excess caffeine, habit, corneal or conjunctival irritation (especially from an eyelash or cyst), dry eye, blepharospasm (bilateral), hemifacial spasm, albinism (photosensitivity), a serum electrolyte abnormality or anemia (rarely).

Flashes of Light

More common   Retinal break or detachment, posterior vitreous detachment, migraine, rapid eye movements (particularly in darkness).
Less common   CNS (particularly occipital lobe) disorders, retinitis.

Floaters

See "Spots in Front of the Eyes" in this chapter.

Foreign-Body Sensation

Dry eye syndrome, blepharitis, conjunctivitis, trichiasis, corneal abnormality (e.g., corneal abrasion or foreign body, recurrent erosion, superficial punctate keratitis), contact lens–related problem, episcleritis, pterygium or pinguecula.

Halos Around Lights

Cataract, acute-angle closure glaucoma or corneal edema from another cause (e.g., corneal endothelial dystrophy, aphakic/pseudophakic bullous keratopathy), corneal haziness or mucus, drugs (e.g., digitalis, chloroquine).

Headache

See Section 15.3.

Itchy Eye

Conjunctivitis (especially viral, vernal, and allergic), blepharitis, dry eye syndrome, topical drug allergy or contact dermatitis, giant papillary conjunctivitis or another contact lens–related problem.

Light Sensitivity

See "Photophobia" in this chapter.

Night Blindness

More common   Refractive error (especially undercorrected myopia), advanced glaucoma, small pupil (especially from miotic drops), retinitis pigmentosa, congenital stationary night blindness, drugs (e.g., phenothiazines, chloroquine, quinine).

Less common   Vitamin A deficiency, gyrate atrophy, choroideremia.

Pain (Ocular)

A. Typically mild to moderate: Dry eye syndrome, blepharitis, conjunctivitis, episcleritis, inflamed pinguecula or pterygium, foreign body (corneal or conjunctival), corneal disorder (e.g., superficial punctate keratitis), others.

B. Typically moderate to severe: Corneal disorder (abrasion, erosion, infiltrate/ ulcer), anterior uveitis, scleritis, acute-angle closure glaucoma.

Photophobia

More common   Corneal abnormality (e.g., abrasion) or anterior uveitis.
Less common   Conjunctivitis (mild photophobia), posterior uveitis, albinism, total color blindness, aniridia.
With normal eye examination   Migraine, meningitis, retrobulbar optic neuritis, subarachnoid hemorrhage, trigeminal neuralgia, or a lightly pigmented eye.

Proptosis

See "Orbital Disease," Section 7.1.

Ptosis

See "Ptosis" and "Pseudoptosis" in Chapter 2.

Red Eye

I. Discharge present
   More common   Conjunctivitis, ophthalmia neonatorum in infants, blepharitis.
   Less common   Acute allergic reaction, dacryocystitis, canaliculitis.
II. No discharge present
   A. Pain present: See "Pain" in this chapter.
   B. Minimal or no pain present
      More common   Subconjunctival hemorrhage, injected pterygium/pinguecula, blepharitis, dry eye syndrome.
      Less common   Conjunctival tumor.

Spots in Front of the Eyes

A. Transient: Migraine.
B. Permanent or long-standing
   More common   Posterior vitreous detachment, posterior uveitis, vitreous hemorrhage, vitreous condensations/debris.
   Less common   Retinal detachment, corneal opacity.

❖ **Note** *Some patients are referring to a blind spot in their visual field caused by a retinal, optic nerve, or CNS disorder.*

Tearing

I. Adults
   A. Pain present: Corneal abnormality (e.g., abrasion, foreign body/rust ring, recurrent erosion), anterior uveitis, eyelash (trichiasis, entropion), cyst or foreign body rubbing against the cornea, conjunctival abnormality (e.g., foreign body, laceration).
   B. Minimal or no pain present: Dry eye syndrome, nasolacrimal duct obstruction, punctal occlusion or other tear drainage abnormality, ectropion, conjunctivitis (especially allergic and toxic), lacrimal sac mass or inflammation.
II. Children: Nasolacrimal duct obstruction, congenital glaucoma, corneal or conjunctival foreign body or other irritative disorder.

Watery Eyes

See "Tearing" in this chapter.

White Pupil

See "Leukocoria," Section 9.1.

DIFFERENTIAL DIAGNOSIS OF OCULAR SIGNS

Anterior Chamber/Anterior Chamber Angle

Blood in Schlemm's Canal on Gonioscopy

Compression of episcleral vessels by a gonioprism (iatrogenic), Sturge-Weber syndrome, arteriovenous fistula (e.g., carotid-cavernous sinus fistula), superior vena cava obstruction, hypotony.

Hyphema

Following trauma or intraocular surgery, bleeding from iris or corneal wound neovascularization, herpes simplex or zoster iritis, blood dyscrasia or clotting disorder (e.g., hemophilia), intraocular tumor (e.g., juvenile xanthogranuloma, retinoblastoma, leukemia).

Hypopyon

Infectious corneal ulcer, endophthalmitis, severe iritis, reaction to an intraocular lens or retained lens protein following cataract surgery, intraocular tumor necrosis [e.g., retinoblastoma (a pseudohypopyon)], a tight contact lens.

Cornea/Conjunctival Findings

Band Keratopathy

See Section 4.11.

The Wills Eye Manual: Office and Emergency Room Diagnosis and Treatment of Eye Diseases, Second Edition, edited by R. Douglas Cullom, Jr., M.D., and Benjamin Chang, M.D. © 1994 J. B. Lippincott Company.

Corneal Crystals

Schnyder's crystalline dystrophy, multiple myeloma, cystinosis, gout, uremia, hypergammaglobulinemia, drugs (e.g., indomethacin, chloroquine), infectious crystalline keratopathy.

Corneal Edema

A. Congenital: Congenital glaucoma, congenital hereditary endothelial dystrophy, posterior polymorphous dystrophy (PPMD), birth trauma (forceps injury).

B. Acquired: Early postoperative, aphakic or pseudophakic bullous keratopathy, Fuchs' endothelial dystrophy, contact lens overwear, trauma, acute-angle closure glaucoma and other causes of acute elevation in intraocular pressure, corneal hydrops (acute keratoconus), herpes simplex or zoster keratitis, iritis, failed corneal graft, iridocorneal endothelial (ICE) syndrome, PPMD.

Corneal Filaments

See "Filamentary Keratopathy," Section 4.3.

Dilated Episcleral Vessels (in the Absence of Ocular Irritation or Pain)

Underlying uveal melanoma, arteriovenous fistula (e.g., carotid-cavernous fistula), polycythemia vera, leukemia, ophthalmic vein or cavernous sinus thrombosis.

Enlarged Corneal Nerves

Most important   Multiple endocrine neoplasia type IIb (medullary carcinoma of the thyroid gland, pheochromocytoma, mucosal neuromas; may have marfanoid habitus).

Others   Keratoconus, keratitis, neurofibromatosis, Fuchs' endothelial dystrophy, Refsum's syndrome, trauma, congenital glaucoma, failed corneal graft, leprosy.

Membranous Conjunctivitis

(Removal of the membrane is difficult and causes bleeding). Streptococci; pneumococci; chemical burn; ligneous conjunctivitis; corynebacterium diphtheria; rarely, adenovirus or herpes simplex virus. See also "Pseudomembranous Conjunctivitis" in this chapter.

Opacification of the Cornea in Infancy

Congenital glaucoma, birth trauma (forceps injury), congenital hereditary endothelial or stromal dystrophy (bilateral), PPMD, developmental abnormality of the anterior segment (especially Peter's anomaly), metabolic abnormalities (bilateral) (e.g., mucopolysaccharidoses, mucolipidoses), interstitial keratitis, herpes simplex virus, corneal ulcer, corneal dermoid, sclerocornea.

Pannus (Superficial Vascular Invasion of the Cornea)

Rosacea, tight contact lens or contact lens overwear, phlyctenule, chlamydia (trachoma and inclusion conjunctivitis), superior limbic keratoconjunctivitis (micropannus only), staphylococcal hypersensitivity, vernal keratoconjunctivitis, herpes simplex virus, chemical burn, aniridia.

Large Papillae on the Superior Tarsus

Vernal or atopic conjunctivitis, giant papillary conjunctivitis, exposed suture, prosthesis-induced trachoma, superior limbic keratoconjunctivitis (fine papillae).

Pigmentation of the Conjunctiva

Racial pigmentation (perilimbal), nevus, primary acquired melanosis, melanoma, ocular and oculodermal melanocytosis (congenital, blue, episcleral, not conjunctival), Addison's disease, mascara, pregnancy, radiation, drug (e.g., chlorpromazine) or metal (e.g., argyrosis from silver).

Pseudomembranous Conjunctivitis

(Removal of the membrane is easy, and no bleeding results). All of the causes of membranous conjunctivitis, as well as ocular cicatricial pemphigoid, Stevens-Johnson syndrome, superior limbic keratoconjunctivitis, gonococci, staphylococci, chlamydia in newborns, and others.

Symblepharon [Fusion of the Eyelid (Palpebral) Conjunctiva with the Conjunctiva Covering the Globe (Bulbar Conjunctiva)]

Ocular cicatricial pemphigoid, Stevens-Johnson syndrome, chemical burn, trauma, drugs, long-standing inflammation, epidemic keratoconjunctivitis, atopic conjunctivitis, radiation.

Whorl-like Opacity in the Corneal Epithelium

Amiodarone, chloroquine, Fabry's disease and carrier state, phenothiazines, indomethacin.

Eyelid Abnormalities

Eyelid Edema or Swelling

More common   Orbital fat herniation from aging, conjunctivitis, allergy, chalazion, orbital disease.

Less common   Cardiac disease, renal disease, urticaria/angioneurotic edema, dacryoadenitis, hypothyroidism, superior vena cava syndrome.

Eyelid Lesion
See "Malignant Tumors of the Eyelid," Section 6.11.

Pseudoptosis
Dermatochalasis (laxity of the eyelid skin from old age), brow ptosis, enophthalmos (e.g., from a traumatic blow-out fracture), phthisis bulbi, microphthalmia (small eye), chalazion or other eyelid tumor, eyelid edema, hypotropia (e.g., in double-elevator palsy) and retraction of the contralateral eyelid.

Ptosis
More common   Aging (e.g., levator dehiscence), following intraocular surgery or trauma, congenital.
Less common   Myasthenia gravis, Horner's syndrome, third-nerve palsy, chronic progressive external ophthalmoplegia, corneal or anterior segment disease (e.g., corneal abrasion), prolonged use of topical steroids, botulinum toxin or subtenons steroid injection.

Fundus Findings

Bone Spicules (Widespread Pigment Clumping)
More common   Retinitis pigmentosa and associated syndromes, disseminated chorioretinitis (especially old syphilis), trauma, pigmentary changes of aging.
Less common   Following spontaneous reattachment of a retinal detachment (e.g., toxemia of pregnancy, Harada's disease), Kearns-Sayre syndrome, abetalipoproteinemia, vitamin A deficiency, viral infections (e.g., rubella), drugs (e.g., thioridazine and other phenothiazines), retinopathy of prematurity (when seen years later as an adult), cystinosis, old vascular occlusions.

Bull's-Eye Macular Lesion
Age-related macular degeneration (ARMD), Stargardt's disease, cone dystrophy, chloroquine retinopathy, Spielmeyer-Vogt syndrome.

Choroidal Folds
Orbital or choroidal tumor, thyroid orbitopathy, orbital inflammatory pseudotumor, posterior scleritis, hypotony, retinal detachment, marked hyperopia, scleral laceration, papilledema.

Choroidal Neovascularization (Gray-Green Membrane or Blood Seen Deep to the Retina)
More common   ARMD, ocular histoplasmosis syndrome, high myopia, angioid streaks, choroidal rupture (trauma).
Less common   Drusen of the optic nerve head, tumors, following retinal laser photocoagulation, idiopathic.

Cotton-Wool Spots, without Other Abnormalities (White Fluffy Lesions with Feathered Edges, Often Obscuring Retinal Vessels)

More common   AIDS retinopathy, hypertension, diabetes, collagen-vascular disease (e.g., systemic lupus erythematosus), retinal artery/arteriole occlusion.

Less common   Retinal vein occlusion, cardiac valvular disease, carotid artery obstruction, chest trauma (Purtscher's retinopathy), anemia, leukemia, lymphoma.

Embolus

See "Amaurosis Fugax," Section 12.6; "Branch Retinal Artery Occlusion," Section 12.2; or "Central Retinal Artery Occlusion," Section 12.1.

- Platelet-fibrin   [Dull gray and elongated (as opposed to round): Carotid disease. NOTE   Similar-appearing fibrin emboli may also arise from the heart.]
- Cholesterol   (Sparkling yellow, usually at an arterial bifurcation: Carotid disease.)
- Calcium   (Dull white, typically around or on the disc: Cardiac disease.)
- Cardiac myxoma   (Common in young patients, particularly in the left eye. Often occludes the ophthalmic or central retinal artery behind the globe and is not seen.)
- Talc and cornstarch   (Small yellow-white glistening particles in macular arterioles. May produce peripheral retinal neovascularization: IV drug abuse.)
- Lipid or air   [Cotton-wool spots, not emboli, are often seen. Results from chest trauma (Purtscher's retinopathy) and fracture of long bones.]
- Others   (Tumors, parasites, other foreign bodies.)

Macular Exudates

More common   Diabetes, choroidal (subretinal) neovascular membrane, hypertension.

Less common   Macroaneurysm, Coats' disease (children), peripheral retinal capillary hemangioma, retinal vein occlusion, papilledema, radiation.

Normal Fundus in the Presence of Decreased Vision

Retrobulbar optic neuritis, cone degenerations, Stargardt's disease/fundus flavimaculatus, other optic neuropathy (e.g., tumor, alcohol/tobacco), rod monochromatism, amblyopia, nonphysiologic visual loss.

Optociliary Shunt Vessels on the Disc

Orbital or intracranial tumor (especially meningioma), status post central retinal vein occlusion, chronic papilledema (e.g., pseudotumor cerebri), chronic open-angle glaucoma, optic nerve glioma.

Retinal Neovascularization

A. Posterior pole: Diabetes, following central retinal vein occlusion.

B. Peripheral: Sickle cell retinopathy, following branch retinal vein occlusion, diabetes, sarcoidosis, retinopathy of prematurity, embolization from IV drug abuse, chronic uveitis, others (e.g., leukemia, anemia, Eales' disease).

Roth's Spots (Hemorrhages with White Centers)

More common   Leukemia, septic chorioretinitis (e.g., secondary to subacute bacterial endocarditis), diabetes.

Less common   Pernicious anemia (and rarely other forms of anemia), sickle cell disease, scurvy, systemic lupus erythematosus. other collagen-vascular diseases.

Sheathing of Retinal Veins (Periphlebitis)

More common   Syphilis, sarcoidosis, pars planitis, sickle cell disease.

Less common   Tuberculosis, multiple sclerosis, Eales' disease, viral retinitis (e.g., HIV, herpes), Behçet's disease, fungal retinitis, septicemia or bacteremia.

Tumor

See "Malignant Melanoma of the Choroid," Section 8.3.

Glaucoma

Acute Rise in Intraocular Pressure

Acute-angle closure glaucoma, glaucomatocyclitic crisis (Posner-Schlossman syndrome), inflammatory open-angle glaucoma, malignant glaucoma, postoperative glaucoma, suprachoroidal hemorrhage, retrobulbar hemorrhage.

Iris

Iris Heterochromia (Irides of Different Colors)

A. Involved iris is lighter than normal: Congenital Horner's syndrome, Fuchs' heterochromic iridocyclitis (most), chronic uveitis, juvenile xanthogranuloma, metastatic carcinoma, Waardenburg's syndrome (white forelock, decreased hearing, telecanthus).

B. Involved iris is darker than normal: Ocular melanocytosis or oculodermal melanocytosis, hemosiderosis, siderosis, retained intraocular foreign body, ocular malignant melanoma, diffuse iris nevus, retinoblastoma, leukemia, lymphoma, ICE syndrome, Fuchs' heterochromic iridocyclitis (some).

Iris Lesion

A. Melanotic (brown): Nevus, melanoma, adenoma or adenocarcinoma of the iris pigment epithelium. NOTE   In heavily pigmented irides, cysts, foreign bodies, neurofibromas, and other lesions may appear pigmented.)

B. Amelanotic (white, yellow, or orange): Amelanotic melanoma, inflammatory nodule or granuloma (sarcoidosis, tuberculosis, leprosy, other granulomatous disease), neurofibroma, patchy hyperemia of syphilis, juvenile xanthogranuloma, foreign body, cyst, leiomyoma, seeding from a posterior segment tumor.

Neovascularization of the Iris

Diabetic retinopathy, central retinal vein or artery occlusion, branch retinal vein occlusion, ocular ischemic syndrome (carotid occlusive disease), chronic uveitis, chronic retinal detachment, intraocular tumor (e.g., retinoblastoma), other retinal vascular disease.

Lens

Iridescent Lens Particles

Drugs, hypocalcemia, myotonic dystrophy, familial, idiopathic.

Lenticonus

A. Anterior (marked convexity of the anterior lens): Rule out Alport's syndrome (hereditary nephritis).

B. Posterior (marked concavity of the posterior lens surface): Usually idiopathic—may be associated with persistent hyperplastic primary vitreous.

Neuro-ophthalmic Abnormalities

Afferent Pupillary Defect

A. Severe (2–3 +): Optic nerve disease (e.g., ischemic optic neuropathy, optic neuritis, tumor, glaucoma); central retinal artery or vein occlusion; less commonly, a lesion of the optic chiasm/tract.

B. Mild (1 +): Any of the above, amblyopia, vitreous hemorrhage, macular degeneration, branch retinal vein or artery occlusion, retinal detachment, or other retinal disease.

Anisocoria (Pupils of Different Sizes)

See Section 11.1.

Limitation of Ocular Motility

A. With exophthalmos and resistance to retropulsion: See "Orbital Disease," Section 7.1.

B. Without exophthalmos and resistance to retropulsion: Isolated third-, fourth-, or sixth-nerve palsy; multiple ocular motor nerve palsies (see "Cavernous Sinus/Superior Orbital Fissure Syndrome," Section 11.8); myasthenia gravis; chronic progressive external ophthalmoplegia; orbital blow-out fracture with muscle entrapment; ophthalmoplegic migraine; Duane's syndrome; other CNS disorders.

Optic Disc Atrophy
More common   Glaucoma; status post central retinal vein or artery occlusion; ischemic optic neuropathy; chronic optic neuritis; chronic papilledema; compression of the optic nerve, chiasm, or tract by a tumor or aneurysm; traumatic optic neuropathy.

Less common   Syphilis, retinal degeneration (e.g., retinitis pigmentosa), toxic/metabolic optic neuropathy, Leber's optic atrophy, Leber's congenital amaurosis, retinal storage disease (e.g., Tay-Sachs), radiation neuropathy, other forms of congenital or hereditary optic atrophy (nystagmus almost always present in the congenital forms).

Optic Disc Swelling (Edema)
See "Papilledema," Section 11.12.

Optociliary Shunt Vessels
See "Fundus Findings" in this chapter.

Paradoxical Pupillary Reaction (Pupil Dilates in Light and Constricts in Darkness)
Congenital stationary night blindness, cone dystrophy, optic neuritis, dominant optic atrophy. Rarely, amblyopia and strabismus.

Orbit

Extraocular Muscle Thickening on CT Scan
More common   Thyroid orbitopathy, orbital inflammatory pseudotumor.

Less common   Tumor (especially lymphoma, metastasis, or spread of lacrimal gland tumor to muscle), carotid-cavernous fistula, cavernous hemangioma (usually appears in the muscle cone without muscle thickening), rhabdomyosarcoma (children).

Lacrimal Gland Lesions
See "Lacrimal Gland Mass/Chronic Dacryoadenitis," Section 7.7.

Optic Nerve Lesion (Isolated)
More common   Optic nerve glioma (especially children), optic nerve meningioma (especially adults).

Less common   Metastasis, leukemia, orbital inflammatory pseudotumor, sarcoidosis, increased intracranial pressure with secondary optic nerve swelling.

Orbital Lesions/Proptosis
See "Orbital Disease," Section 7.1.

Pediatrics

Leukocoria (White Pupillary Reflex)
See Section 9.1.

Nystagmus in Infancy
Congenital nystagmus, albinism, Leber's congenital amaurosis, thalamic injury, spasmus nutans, optic nerve or chiasmal glioma, optic nerve hypoplasia, congenital cataracts, aniridia, congenital corneal opacities.

Postoperative Problems

Shallow Anterior Chamber
A. Accompanied by increased intraocular pressure: Pupillary block glaucoma, suprachoroidal hemorrhage, malignant glaucoma.
B. Accompanied by decreased intraocular pressure: Wound leak, choroidal detachment.

Hypotony
Wound leak, choroidal detachment, cyclodialysis cleft, retinal detachment, ciliary body shutdown, aqueous suppression caused by medication.

Refractive Problems

Progressive Hyperopia
Orbital tumor pressing on the posterior surface of the eye, serous elevation of the retina (e.g., central serous chorioretinopathy), posterior scleritis, presbyopia, hypoglycemia, cataracts.

Progressive Myopia
High (pathologic) myopia, diabetes, cataract, use of miotic drops, staphyloma and elongation of the globe, medications (e.g., sulfa drugs, tetracycline), childhood (physiologic).

Visual Field Abnormalities

Altitudinal Field Defect
More common   Ischemic optic neuropathy, hemibranch artery or vein occlusion.
Less common   Glaucoma, optic nerve or chiasmal lesion, optic nerve coloboma.

Arcuate Scotoma
More common   Glaucoma.
Less common   Ischemic optic neuropathy (especially nonarteritic), optic disc drusen, high myopia.

Binasal Field Defect
More common   Glaucoma, bitemporal retinal disease (e.g., retinitis pigmentosa).
Rare   Bilateral occipital disease, tumor or aneurysm compressing both optic nerves or chiasm.

Bitemporal Hemianopsia
More common   Chiasmal lesion (e.g., pituitary adenoma, meningioma, craniopharyngioma, aneurysm, glioma).
Less common   Tilted optic discs.
Rare   Nasal retinitis pigmentosa.

Blind Spot Enlargement
Papilledema, glaucoma, optic nerve drusen, optic nerve coloboma, medullated nerve fibers off the disc, drugs, myopic disc with a crescent, others.

Central Scotoma
Macular disease; optic neuritis; ischemic optic neuropathy (more typically produces an altitudinal field defect); optic atrophy (e.g., from tumor compressing the nerve, toxic/metabolic disease); rarely, an occipital cortex lesion.

Homonymous Hemianopsia
Optic tract or lateral geniculate body lesion; temporal, parietal, or occipital lobe lesion of the brain (stroke and tumor more common; aneurysm and trauma less common). Migraine may cause a transient homonymous hemianopsia.

Constriction of the Peripheral Fields Leaving Only a Small Residual Central Field
Glaucoma; retinitis pigmentosa or some other peripheral retinal disorder; chronic papilledema; status post panretinal photocoagulation; central retinal artery occlusion with cilioretinal artery sparing; bilateral occipital lobe infarc-

tion with macular sparing; nonphysiologic visual loss; carcinoma-associated retinopathy; rarely, drugs.

Vitreous

Vitreous Opacities

Asteroid hyalosis; synchysis scintillans; vitreous hemorrhage; inflammatory cells in vitritis or posterior uveitis; snowball opacities of pars planitis or sarcoidosis; normal vitreous strands from age-related vitreous degeneration; tumor cells; rarely, amyloidosis or Whipple's disease.

TRAUMA

3.1 CHEMICAL BURN

Treatment should be instituted IMMEDIATELY, even before making vision tests.

❖ **Note** *This includes alkali (e.g., lye, cements, plasters), acids, solvents, detergents, and irritants (e.g., mace).*

Emergent Treatment
1. Copious irrigation of the eyes, preferably with saline or Ringer's lactated solution, for at least 30 minutes. However, if nonsterile water is the only liquid available, it should be used. Do *not* use acidic solutions to neutralize alkalies or vice versa. It is helpful to place an eyelid speculum and topical anesthetic (e.g., proparacaine) in the eye prior to irrigation. Pull down the lower eyelid and evert the upper eyelid, if possible, to irrigate the fornices. Manual use of IV tubing connected to an irrigation solution facilitates the irrigation process.
2. Five minutes after ceasing irrigation to allow for equilibration, litmus paper should to touched to the inferior cul-de-sac. If the pH is not neutral (i.e., 7), irrigation should be continued until neutral pH is reached.

A. Mild-to-Moderate Burns

Critical Signs
   Corneal epithelial defects range from scattered superficial punctate keratitis (SPK) to focal epithelial loss to sloughing of the entire epithelium. *No signifi-*

The Wills Eye Manual: Office and Emergency Room Diagnosis and Treatment of Eye Diseases, Second Edition, edited by R. Douglas Cullom, Jr., M.D., and Benjamin Chang, M.D. © 1994 J. B. Lippincott Company.

cant areas of perilimbal ischemia are seen (no sign of interrupted blood flow through the conjunctival or episcleral vessels).

Other Signs

Focal areas of conjunctival chemosis, hyperemia, and/or hemorrhages; mild eyelid edema; mild anterior-chamber reaction; first- and second-degree burns of the periocular skin.

Work-up

1. History: Time of injury? Chemical to which the patient was exposed? Duration of the exposure until irrigation was started? Duration of the irrigation?
2. Slit-lamp examination with fluorescein staining. Evert the eyelids to search for foreign bodies. Check the intraocular pressure (IOP).

❖ **Note** *In the presence of a distorted cornea, IOP may be most accurately measured with a McKay-Marg tonometer or Tono-Pen.*

Treatment After Irrigation

1. Fornices should be thoroughly searched, including a sweep with a moistened cotton-tipped applicator or glass rod to remove any sequestered particles of caustic material and necrotic conjunctiva which may contain residual chemicals. Calcium hydroxide particles may be more easily removed with a cotton-tipped applicator soaked in sodium EDTA.
2. Cycloplegic (e.g., scopolamine 0.25%). Avoid phenylephrine because of its vasoconstrictive properties.
3. Topical antibiotic ointment (e.g., erythromycin).
4. Pressure patch for 24 hours.
5. Oral pain medication (e.g., acetaminophen with or without codeine) as needed.
   - If IOP is elevated, acetazolamide (e.g., Diamox) 250 mg po qid or 500 mg sequel po bid, or methazolamide (e.g., Neptazane) 25–50 mg po 2–3 times per day may be given. Add a topical beta-blocker (e.g., timolol 0.5% bid or levobunolol 0.5% bid) if additional IOP control is required.

Follow-up

Recheck and repatch with antibiotic ointment plus a cycloplegic drop every day until the corneal defect is healed. Watch for corneal ulceration and infection.

❖ **Note** *Rapid-setting super glues harden quickly on contact with moisture. If the eyelids are glued together, they can be separated with gentle traction. Misdirected lashes or hardened glue mechanically rubbing the cornea, as* *well as glue adherent to the cornea, should be carefully removed. Resulting epithelial defects are treated as corneal abrasions, (see Section 3.2).*

B. Moderate-to-Severe Burns

Critical Signs

Pronounced chemosis and perilimbal blanching; corneal edema and opacification, sometimes with little-to-no view of the anterior chamber, iris, or lens; a moderate-to-severe anterior-chamber reaction (may not be appreciated if the cornea is opaque).

Other Signs

Increased IOP, second- and third-degree burns of the surrounding skin, and local necrotic retinopathy as a result of direct penetration of alkali through the sclera.

❖ **Note** *If you suspect an epithelial defect but do not see one on fluorescein staining, repeat the fluorescein application to the eye. Sometimes the defect is slow to take up the dye. Occasionally, the whole epithelium may slough off, leaving only Bowman's membrane, which takes up fluorescein poorly.*

Work-up

Same as for mild-to-moderate burns (A).

Treatment After Irrigation

1. Admission to the hospital may be necessary for close monitoring of IOP and corneal healing.
2. Debride necrotic tissue containing foreign matter.
3. Topical antibiotic [e.g., trimethoprim/polymyxin (e.g., Polytrim) drops 4 times per day, erythromycin ointment 2–4 times per day].
4. Cycloplegic (e.g., scopolamine 0.25% or atropine 1% 3–4 times per day). Avoid topical phenylephrine as it is a vasoconstrictor.
5. Topical steroid (e.g., prednisolone acetate 1% or dexamethasone 0.1% 4–9 times per day) if significant inflammation of the anterior chamber or cornea is present.
6. Pressure patch between drops/ointment.
7. Antiglaucoma medications if the IOP is elevated or cannot be determined. See the antiglaucoma recommendations above.
8. Lysis of conjunctival adhesions using a glass rod or end of a thermometer covered with an antibiotic ointment, sweeping the fornices bid. If symblepharons begin to form despite attempted lysis, consider using a scleral shell or ring to maintain the fornices.
   - Consider a therapeutic soft contact lens, collagen shield, or tarsorrhaphy. (Usually used if healing is delayed beyond 2 weeks.)

- If any melting of the cornea occurs, collagenase inhibitors may be used [e.g., acetylcysteine 10–20% (e.g., Mucomyst) q 4 h.]
- If the melting progresses (or the cornea perforates) consider cyanocrylate adhesive. An emergent patch graft or corneal transplant may be necessary; however, the prognosis is better if this procedure is performed 12–18 months after the injury.

Follow-up

These patients need to be followed closely, either in the hospital or daily as outpatients. Topical steroids must be tapered after 7 days because they can promote corneal melting. Long-term use of artificial tears and lubricating ointment (e.g., Refresh drops q 1–6 h and Refresh PM ointment 1–4 times per day) may be required. A severely dry eye may require a tarsorrhaphy, conjunctival flap, or mucous membrane graft. A conjunctival transplant may be performed in unilateral injuries that fail to heal within several weeks to several months.

3.2 CORNEAL ABRASION

Symptoms

Pain, photophobia, foreign-body sensation, tearing, history of scratching the eye.

Critical Sign

Epithelial staining defect with fluorescein.

Other Signs

Conjunctival injection, swollen eyelid, mild anterior-chamber reaction.

Work-up

1. Slit-lamp examination: Use fluorescein, measure the size of the abrasion, diagram its location, and evaluate for an anterior-chamber reaction.
2. Evert the eyelids to make certain no foreign body is present.

Treatment

A. Non–contact lens wearer
   1. Cycloplegic (e.g., cyclopentolate 2%).
   2. Antibiotic ointment (e.g., erythromycin).
   3. Pressure patch for 24 hours.

❖ **Note** *A pressure patch is generally not applied when the abrasion is at significant risk for infection (e.g., scratches from a tree branch or a false fingernail).*

B. Contact lens wearer
   1. Cycloplegic (e.g., cyclopentolate 2%).
   2. Tobramycin drops 4–6 times per day. Can add tobramycin ointment qhs if the patient is significantly uncomfortable.
   3. No eye patch.

Follow-up
   A. Non–contact lens wearer with a small, noncentral abrasion
      1. Patient removes the patch after 24 hours.
      2. Topical antibiotic for 4 days [e.g., erythromycin ointment 2–3 times per day or trimethoprim/polymyxin (e.g., Polytrim) drops 4 times per day], after the patch is removed.
      3. Have the patient return if the symptoms persist or worsen.
   B. Non–contact lens wearer with a central or large corneal abrasion
      1. Return the next day to determine if the epithelial defect is improving.
      2. If the abrasion has resolved or only superficial punctate keratitis (SPK) remains, then treat with topical antibiotics for 4 more days [e.g., erythromycin ointment 2–3 times per day or trimethoprim/polymyxin (e.g, Polytrim) drops 4 times per day].
      3. If the injury is healing and the remaining abrasion is small and noncentral, then treat with topical antibiotics for 4 days as above.
      4. If the abrasion remains large or a central area of staining persists, then repeat the cycloplegic, antibiotic ointment, and pressure patch as described previously, and have the patient return the following day.
   C. Contact lens wearer
      Have the patient return every day until the epithelial defect resolves, then treat with topical tobramycin drops for 1–2 additional days. The patient may resume contact lens wear after the eye feels perfectly normal for 3–4 days (after having had the lens examined for tears, scratches, protein build-up, and other defects by their contact lens specialist).

❖ **Note** *If at any time a corneal infiltrate is observed, appropriate smears and cultures should be obtained and more aggressive therapy instituted (see Section 4.12).*

3.3 CORNEAL FOREIGN BODY/RUST RING

Symptoms
   Foreign-body sensation, tearing, blurred vision, photophobia; commonly, a history of a foreign body in the eye.

Critical Sign

Corneal foreign body, rust ring, or both.

Other Signs

Conjunctival injection, eyelid edema, mild anterior-chamber reaction, and superficial punctate keratitis (SPK). A small infiltrate may surround the foreign body, especially if the foreign body has been present in the eye for more than 24 hours. This infiltrate is usually sterile.

Work-up

1. History: Was the patient wearing safety goggles? Did the foreign body arise from metal striking metal (which may suggest an intraocular foreign body)?
2. Document visual acuity before any procedure is performed. One or two drops of topical anesthesia may be necessary to control blepharospasms and pain.
3. Slit-lamp examination: Locate the foreign body. Evert the eyelids and inspect the fornices for additional foreign bodies, especially in the presence of linear SPK. Measure the dimensions of the infiltrate, if present, and the degree of any anterior-chamber reaction.
4. Dilate the eye and examine the vitreous and retina when a history of hammering or forcibly striking metal is provided (or a possible intraocular foreign body from another cause is considered).

Treatment

1. Remove the corneal foreign body with a foreign-body spud or a 25-gauge needle using magnification, usually at a slit lamp. Apply a topical anesthetic (e.g., proparacaine)—2 drops prior to removal.

❖ **Note** *Multiple superficial foreign bodies may be more easily removed by irrigation.*

2. Remove the rust ring. Occasionally, it can be shelled out in one piece with a foreign-body spud, but usually, it is most easily removed with an ophthalmoscopic rust-ring drill after topical anesthesia as above.

❖ **Note** *It is sometimes safer to leave a rust ring centered in the visual axis (especially when it is deep) to allow time for the rust to migrate to the corneal surface, at which point it can be more easily extracted.*

3. Measure the size of the resultant corneal epithelial defect.
4. Cycloplegic (e.g., cyclopentolate 2%).
5. Antibiotic ointment (e.g., erythromycin).
6. Pressure patch for 24 hours.

Follow-up

A. Small (< 1–2 mm in diameter), clean, noncentral epithelial defect present after foreign-body removal: The patient may remove the patch after 24 hours and take topical antibiotics for 3–4 days (e.g., trimethoprim/polymyxin drops qid or erythromycin ointment 2–3 times per day). Follow-up as needed.

B. Central or large epithelial defect, mucopurulent discharge, infiltrate, residual rust in cornea, or moderate anterior-chamber reaction: Follow-up in 24 hours to reevaluate.

❖ **Note** *An infiltrate accompanied by a significant anterior-chamber reaction, purulent discharge, or extreme redness and pain should be cultured to rule out an infection and treated with antibiotics more aggressively (see Section 4.12).*

3.4 CONJUNCTIVAL/SUBCONJUNCTIVAL FOREIGN BODY

Symptoms

Ocular irritation or pain, foreign-body sensation, tearing, red eye; often, a history of trauma to or a foreign body in the eye.

Signs

Linear, vertically oriented corneal scratches may be observed when a foreign body is under the upper eyelid. A conjunctival laceration is observed when a subconjunctival foreign body is present. A conjunctival or subconjunctival hemorrhage may also be present.

Differential Diagnosis

See "Foreign-Body Sensation" in Chapter 1.

Work-up

1. History: Determine whether an intraocular or intraorbital foreign body may be present and whether the globe may be ruptured. Be especially suspicious when a history of hammering or grinding metal is present.

2. Ocular examination including an intraocular pressure (IOP) measurement and a thorough slit-lamp evaluation. To evaluate the superior fornix, double evert the eyelid over an instrument such as a Desmarres eyelid retractor.

Careful inspection in the area of a conjunctival laceration is always required to definitively rule out a scleral laceration and an intraocular foreign body.

3. Dilated retinal examination is needed if a subconjunctival foreign body exists or the eye has had significant trauma. Carefully examine the area under the conjunctival lesion; look for retinal damage and possibly an intraocular foreign body.

4. Consider a B-scan ultrasound to rule out an intraocular foreign body.

5. Consider a CT scan of the orbit (axial and coronal views) to rule out an intraocular or intraorbital foreign body and a ruptured globe.

Treatment

1. Remove the foreign body under topical anesthesia (e.g., proparacaine).
   a. Multiple loose foreign bodies can often be removed with saline irrigation.
   b. A foreign body on the conjunctival surface can be removed with a cotton-tipped applicator soaked in topical anesthetic or a foreign-body spud.
   c. A foreign body embedded in the conjunctiva or beneath the conjunctiva can be removed with fine forceps.

❖ **Note** *In the presence of multiple small foreign bodies, remove as many as possible. Small, relatively inaccessible subconjunctival foreign bodies may sometimes be left in the eye without harm. Occasionally they will surface with time, at which point they can be removed more easily.*

2. Sweep the conjunctival fornices with a glass rod or sterile cotton-tipped applicator soaked with a topical anesthetic to catch small pieces of loose material that may have been missed on examination.

See Section 3.5 if there is a significant conjunctival laceration. If no laceration is noted:

3. A topical antibiotic [e.g., erythromycin ointment bid or trimethoprim/poly-myxin (e.g., Polytrim) drops qid] may be used if SPK or a corneal or conjunctival abrasion is present.

4. Artificial tears (e.g., Refresh qid for 2 days) may be given for a mildly irritated eye.

Follow-up

As needed, unless residual foreign bodies were left in or under the conjunctiva. A patient with residual foreign material should be reexamined within 1 week.

3.5 CONJUNCTIVAL LACERATION

Symptoms

Mild pain, red eye, foreign-body sensation; usually, a history of ocular trauma.

Signs

Flourescein staining of the conjunctiva, noted after instillation of fluorescein dye, and examination of the eye with the blue light of the slit lamp. With the white light, the conjunctiva can be seen to be torn and rolled up on itself; the exposed white sclera may be noted. Conjunctival and subconjunctival hemorrhages are often present.

Work-up

1. History: Determine the nature of the trauma and whether a ruptured globe or intraocular or intraorbital foreign body may be present.
2. Complete ocular examination, including a careful exploration of the sclera [after topical anesthesia (e.g., proparacaine)] in the region of the conjunctival laceration to rule out a scleral laceration or a subconjunctival foreign body. The entire area of sclera under the conjunctival laceration must be inspected. The fundus, especially the area underlying the conjunctival injury, must be carefully evaluated by indirect ophthalmoscopy.
3. Consider a CT scan of the orbit (axial and coronal views) to rule out an intraocular or intraorbital foreign body or a ruptured globe. A B-scan ultrasound may additionally be helpful.
4. Exploration of the site in the operating room under general anesthesia may be necessary when a ruptured globe is suspected.

Treatment

In case of ruptured globe or penetrating ocular injury, see Section 3.15.

1. Antibiotic ointment (e.g., erythromycin) tid for 4–7 days. A pressure patch can be used for the first 24 hours.
2. Large lacerations (e.g., > 1–1.5 cm) may be sutured (e.g., with 8-0 Vicryl), but most lacerations heal without surgical repair. When suturing, it is important not to bury folds of conjunctiva (e.g., by not correctly suturing the edges of the conjunctiva) nor to incorporate the tenons capsule in the wound. Additionally, avoid suturing the plica semilunaris or caruncle to the conjunctiva.

Follow-up

If there is no concomitant ocular damage, patients with large conjunctival lacerations are reexamined within 1 week; patients with small injuries are seen only as needed.

3.6 EYELID LACERATION

All patients receive a complete ocular examination, including a dilated retinal examination, prior to laceration repair. A CT scan (axial and coronal views) of the orbit and brain should be obtained prior to repair in cases of significant orbital trauma or when an orbital foreign body or a ruptured globe are suspected.

Treatment

All patients should be considered for tetanus prophylaxis (see Appendix 11 for indications).

A. Eyelid lacerations repaired in the operating room or requiring complicated surgical repair:
- Those associated with ocular trauma requiring surgery (e.g., ruptured globe).
- Those involving the lacrimal drainage apparatus (i.e., punctum, canaliculus, common duct, or lacrimal sac).
- Those involving the levator aponeurosis of the upper eyelid (producing ptosis) or the superior rectus muscle; orbital fat is often exposed.
- Those in which the medial canthal tendon is avulsed (exhibits a displaced medial canthus or abnormal laxity of the medial canthus).
- Those associated with an intraorbital foreign body that may require removal.
- Those that cause extensive tissue loss (especially more than one third of the eyelid) or severe distortion of anatomy.

The treatment of these lacerations is beyond the scope of this book.

B. Delayed repair is beneficial in some eyelid lacerations:
- Wounds at significant risk for contamination.
- Wounds from human bites (controversial).

These lacerations are treated as follows:
1. Clean the area of injury and surrounding skin (e.g., Betadine).
2. Irrigate the wound thoroughly with saline in a syringe.
3. Search the wound for foreign bodies, and remove them if present. Debride any severely infected or necrotic tissue. In general, minimal debridement of the eyelid is performed because of its vascular nature.
4. Leave the wound open and treat with a topical antibiotic (e.g., bacitracin tid).
5. Apply a sterile dressing to keep the wound clean.
6. Systemic antibiotics as described below.
7. Surgical debridement and repair 3–4 days later.

❖ **Note** *Some feel that the excellent blood supply in the eyelid area allows for primary repair of dirty injuries, including animal and human bites. These wounds require thorough cleaning and irrigation combined with prophylactic antibiotics.*

C. Eyelid lacerations reparable in the office or emergency room:
1. Clean the area of injury and surrounding skin (e.g., Betadine).
2. Local subcutaneous anesthetic (e.g., 2% lidocaine with epinephrine).
3. Irrigate the wound thoroughly with saline in a syringe.
4. Search the wound carefully for foreign bodies, and remove them if present.
5. Isolate the surgical field with a sterile eye drape.
6. Place a drop of topical anesthetic (e.g., proparacaine) into the eye and a protective eye shell over the eye before suturing.
7. Repair the laceration using one of many methods (Fig. 3.1):
    a. *Lacerations involving the eyelid margin:* The eyelid margin is closed with three sutures prior to closing the part of the laceration extending into the eyelid.

    Suture #1 (5-0 silk): Place through the gray line just anterior to the meibomian orifices of one wound edge, approximately 2 mm from the laceration margin and 2 mm deep, and then through the gray line of the other wound edge to arise just anterior to the meibomian orifices of the opposite wound edge. Cut the suture long and do not tie it yet.

    Suture #2 (6-0 silk): Pass suture #2 posterior and parallel to suture #1 in the same manner, through the tarsus of one wound edge and then through the tarsus of the other wound edge. Avoid passing the suture through the palpebral conjunctiva. Cut the suture long and do not tie it yet.

    Suture #3 (6-0 silk): Pass suture #3 anterior and parallel to suture #1 in the same manner as suture #2, just posterior to the eyelash line, through both wound edges.

    Tie all three sutures, leaving the suture ends long. Stretch the eyelid by pulling on the three suture arms and clamp the sutures with a hemostat to maintain the eyelid in a stretched position. The suture arms will be incorporated into the knot of the skin suture closest to the eyelid margin at the end of the repair.
    b. *Lacerations of the eyelid:* If the laceration is deep, a two-layer closure is required.

    Interrupted 6-0 absorbable (e.g., Vicryl) sutures are used to close the tarsus (the deep layer) without passing through the palpebral

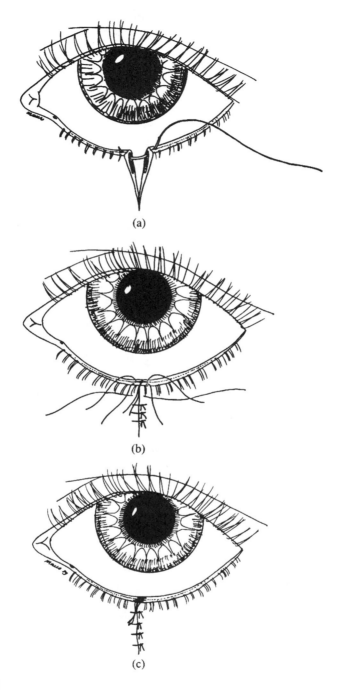

(a)

(b)

(c)

Figure 3.1
Eyelid margin repair. (a) Suture #1 (see text). (b) and (c) At the conclusion of the repair, the eyelid margin sutures are tied under the knot of the skin suture closest to the eyelid margin.

conjunctiva (the posterior aspect of the eyelid). These sutures are cut close to the knot.

The skin and orbicularis (the superficial layers) are closed with interrupted 6-0 or 7-0 nonabsorbable sutures (e.g., nylon).

If the eyelid margin was repaired, the long ends of the three eyelid margin sutures are released from the hemostat and tied under the knot of the skin suture closest to the eyelid margin, to prevent these arms from rubbing against the cornea. The portions of the three arms extending beyond this skin suture are then cut.

The protective eye shell is removed.

8. Antibiotic ointment is applied to the wound bid (e.g., bacitracin).
9. A systemic antibiotic is given if contamination is suspected [e.g., dicloxacillin 250–500 mg po qid (adults); 25–50 mg/kg/day divided into 4 doses for 2 days (children); alternative treatment is cephalexin given at the same dose as dicloxacillin; for human or animal bites, consider penicillin V (same dose as dicloxacillin)].

❖ **Notes**
1. *Do not shave the eyebrow if it has been lacerated; in some cases the hair will not grow back or will do so irregularly.*
2. *Absorbable sutures (e.g., Vicryl) may be used to close the skin when the patient is a child or cannot be counted upon to return.*
3. *In animal bites (especially dog bites), rabies must be considered.*

Follow-up
Eyelid margin sutures are left in place for 10–14 days. All other superficial sutures are removed in 4–6 days.

3.7 TRAUMATIC IRITIS

Symptoms
Pain, photophobia, tearing, history of ocular trauma within the preceding few days.

Critical Signs
White blood cells and flare in the anterior chamber (seen under high-power magnification by focusing into the anterior chamber with a small, bright beam from the slit lamp).

Other Signs

Pain in the traumatized eye when a light is shined in either the nontraumatized or traumatized eye; lower (although sometimes higher) intraocular pressure (IOP), smaller pupil (which dilates poorly) in the traumatized eye; perilimbal conjunctival injection; sometimes, decreased vision.

Differential Diagnosis

- Traumatic corneal abrasion   (Corneal epithelial defect which stains with fluorescein. May have an accompanying anterior-chamber reaction.)
- Traumatic microhyphema   (*Red* blood cells [RBCs] suspended in the anterior chamber. Often accompanied by iritis.)
- Traumatic retinal detachment   (May produce an anterior-chamber reaction. May also see pigment in the anterior vitreous. A detachment is seen on dilated fundus examination.)

Work-up

Complete ophthalmic examination, including IOP measurement and dilated fundus examination.

Treatment

Cycloplegic agent (e.g., cyclopentolate 2% qid or scopolamine 0.25% tid).

❖ **Note** *Some physicians additionally give a steroid drop (e.g., prednisolone acetate 0.125%–1% qid); initially, we do not.*

Follow-up

- Recheck in a few days to 1 week (usually 1 week unless the iritis is severe.)
- If there is no improvement after 5–7 days, a steroid drop (e.g., prednisolone acetate 1% qid) may be given in addition to the cycloplegic agent.
- If resolved, the cycloplegic agent is discontinued.
- Examination of the anterior-chamber angle in both eyes by gonioscopy and the ora serrata by indirect ophthalmoscopy with scleral depression are performed 1 month after the trauma to look for angle recession (which predisposes the eye to glaucoma) and retinal breaks or detachment.

3.8 HYPHEMA AND MICROHYPHEMA

Symptoms

Pain, blurred vision, history of trauma.

Critical Sign

Blood in the anterior chamber:

- Hyphema: Layering and/or clot.
- Microhyphema: Suspended RBCs only.

Work-up
1. History: Type of injury; exact time of injury; exact time of visual loss, if any.
2. Complete ocular examination, first ruling out a ruptured globe (see Section 3.15). Quantitate (percent or millimeters) and/or draw the extent of layering of RBCs and the presence of any clot; measure the intraocular pressure (IOP), and perform a dilated retinal evaluation, if possible. Do not perform gonioscopy or scleral depression.
3. External and periocular examinations, evaluating for other traumatic injuries (e.g., orbital fracture).
4. Black patients should be screened for sickle cell disease (e.g., Sickle Dex) and, when admitted to the hospital, also have a hemoglobin electrophoresis test.
5. Consider B-scan ultrasound if a retinal detachment cannot be ruled out because of a poor view of the fundus.
6. CT scan (axial *and* coronal views) or the orbits and brain, when indicated.

Treatment
A. Hyphema and unreliable microhyphema patients
1. Hospitalize the patient; confine to bed rest with the head of the bed elevated 30 degrees, allowing him or her to rise only to use the bathroom.
2. Shield the involved eye at all times (no eye patch unless corneal pathology is present, because a patch prevents recognition of sudden visual loss in the event of rebleed).
3. Atropine 1% drops 3–4 times per day.
4. Aminocaproic acid (e.g., Amicar) 50 mg/kg po q 4 h (maximum: 30 g/day), liquid form (inform the patient of potential postural hypotension, particularly during the first 24 hours).[1]
5. No aspirin-containing products.
6. Mild analgesics only [e.g., acetaminophen with or without codeine].
7. Antiemetic [e.g., prochlorperazine (Compazine) 10 mg IM q 8 h or 25 mg pr q 12 h prn. Under 12 years old, use trimethobenzamide (e.g., Tigan) suppositories 100 mg pr q 6 h prn.]
8. If IOP is elevated (e.g., >24 mm Hg in a sickle cell or sickle trait–positive patient or >30 mm Hg in other patients), treat with a topical beta-blocker (e.g., levobunolol 0.5% bid or timolol 0.5% bid). If IOP is still elevated, consider adding acetazolamide (e.g., Diamox) 500 mg po q 12 h [methazolamide (e.g., Neptazane) 50 mg po q 8 h should be substituted if the patient is sickle trait–positive]. For further control of IOP, add IV mannitol once in a 24 hour period (1–2 g/kg IV over 45 minutes. A 500-cc bag of mannitol 20% contains 100 grams of mannitol.

---

[1]Aminocaproic acid should not be used in pregnant patients or those with coagulopathies, renal failure, or hematuria of renal origin, and it should be used with caution in patients with hepatic, cardiovascular, or cerebrovascular disease.

❖ **Note** *IOP may be transiently elevated following trauma (as a result of trabecular meshwork overload) and may resolve spontaneously within a few hours with bed rest and head elevation.*

      9. To prevent heavy, fibrinous anterior-chamber reaction, or if the eye becomes photophobic, consider a topical steroid (e.g., prednisolone acetate 1% 4–8 times per day).

    B. Compliant microhyphema patients

      1. To be seen on a *daily* basis as an outpatient for 4 additional days.

      2. Bed rest with the head elevated as much as possible. No strenuous activities.

      3. No aspirin-containing products.

      4. Mild analgesics only (e.g., acetaminophen).

      5. Atropine 1% drops 3–4 times per day.

      6. Shield the involved eye at all times (no patch).

      7. The patient should be instructed to return immediately for reevaluation if he or she notes a sudden increase in pain or decrease in vision.

❖ **Note** *A sickle cell or sickle trait–positive patient with microhyphema and IOP > 24 mm Hg should be admitted for aminocaproic acid administration and control of IOP as described above.*

Follow-up

    A. Hyphema and unreliable microhyphema patients: Check visual acuity and IOP, and perform a slit-lamp examination bid. Look for new bleeding, increased IOP, corneal blood staining, and other intraocular pathology as the blood clears (e.g., iridodialysis).

      • If the IOP rises (e.g., to > 24 mm Hg in a sickle cell or sickle trait–positive patient or > 30 mm Hg in other patients), treat as described above.

      • If a rebleed does not occur, the dose of Amicar may be halved on posttrauma (or post-rebleed) day 3, and stopped on posttrauma (or post-rebleed) day 4. Observe the patient for one additional day before discharge.

      • If there is a rebleed, continue the above treatment for an additional 4 days, observing closely for elevated IOP and corneal blood staining. Check coagulation profile and Amicar dose. (Patients rarely rebleed on the appropriate dosage of Amicar.)

      • Surgical evacuation of hyphema may be indicated if vision deteriorates significantly, corneal stromal blood staining occurs, the entire anterior chamber becomes filled with blood, a substantial clot persists for 7 days, or the IOP cannot be lowered to a safe level despite maximum medical therapy.

    If no complications arise, the patient may be discharged on posttrauma day 5.

Discharge instructions:

1. Atropine 1% drops 1–4 times per day (dosage depends on the amount of anterior-chamber reaction).
2. Topical steroid (e.g., prednisolone acetate 1%) 3–4 times per day if an inflammatory element results in patient discomfort.
3. Antiglaucoma medication if required to control increased IOP.
4. Glasses or eye shield during the day and eye shield at night for 2 weeks posttrauma, after which the patient should be advised to wear protective eyewear (polycarbonate lenses) any time the potential of an eye injury exists.
5. Have the patient refrain from strenuous physical activities for 2 weeks from the date of the initial injury and then *gradually* resume activities. The patient cannot resume all normal activities until 4 weeks from the date of the original injury.

Outpatient examinations following discharge:

1. 2–3 days later.
2. 3–4 weeks later for gonioscopy and dilated fundus examination with scleral depression (scleral depression and gonioscopy should not be performed until this time if it can be avoided).
3. Yearly (because of the potential of developing angle-recession glaucoma).

If any complications arise, more frequent follow-up examinations are required.

B. Compliant microhyphema patients: Vision, IOP, and the anterior segment are evaluated daily until the fourth posttrauma day and then 1 week later. Gonioscopy and dilated fundus examination with scleral depression are performed 2 weeks posttrauma.
- If a rebleed or an intractable IOP rise occurs, the patient should be hospitalized and treated as above.

❖ Notes
1. *A spontaneous hyphema may be caused by blood-clotting disturbances, rubeosis iridis, or other iris vascular abnormalities. Gonioscopy and careful slit-lamp examination of the iris should be performed, along with a complete blood count, platelet count, prothrombin time, partial thromboplastin time, and bleeding time. Consider IV fluorescein angiography of the iris.*
2. *A spontaneous hyphema in a child should make the physician suspect juvenile xanthogranuloma, child abuse, leukemia, or possibly retinoblastoma.*
3. *Postoperative hyphemas generally resolve spontaneously, usually requiring*

simple observation. The IOP must be monitored closely. Gonioscopy should be performed to rule out a bleeding vessel from a corneal wound.

3.9 COMMOTIO RETINAE

Symptoms
Decreased vision or asymptomatic; history of recent ocular trauma.

Critical Sign
Confluent area of retinal whitening.

Other Signs
The retinal blood vessels are seen distinctly and are undisturbed in the area of retinal whitening. Other signs of ocular trauma may be noted.

Differential Diagnosis
- Retinal detachment   (Retinal vessels can be seen to rise upward with the detached retina. A retinal break or dialysis may be seen. Anterior vitreous pigment and an anterior-chamber reaction are common. See Section 12.19.)
- Branch retinal artery occlusion   (Rarely follows trauma. Whitening of the retina with edema occurs along the distribution of an artery; cotton-wool spots, narrowed arterioles, and dilated veins with sludging of blood in the affected vessels may be seen. See Section 12.2.)
- White without pressure   (A common retinal anomaly unrelated to trauma. A prominent vitreous base is seen in the peripheral retina, often in several locations, including the unaffected eye.)

Work-up
Complete ophthalmic examination, including dilated fundus examination with scleral depression.

❖ **Note** *Scleral depression is not performed when a hyphema, microhyphema, or iritis is present.*

Treatment
No treatment is required, as this condition usually clears without therapy.

Follow-up
A dilated fundus examination is repeated in 1–2 weeks. Patients are instructed to return sooner if decreased vision, floaters, or flashing lights are experienced, or if a curtain appears to drop over part of the visual field.

3.10 TRAUMATIC CHOROIDAL RUPTURE

Symptoms

Decreased vision or asymptomatic; history of ocular trauma.

Critical Signs

A yellow or white crescent-shaped subretinal streak, usually concentric to the optic disc. It may be single or multiple. Often, the rupture cannot be seen until several days or weeks posttrauma, as it may be obscured by overlying blood.

Other Signs

Rarely, the rupture may be radially oriented. A choroidal neovascular membrane (CNVM) may later develop.

Differential Diagnosis

- Lacquer cracks of high myopia   (Often bilateral. A tilted disc, a scleral crescent adjacent to the disc, or a posterior staphyloma also may be seen. A CNVM also may develop in this condition.)
- Angioid streaks   (Bilateral reddish brown or gray subretinal streaks that radiate out from the optic disc, sometimes associated with a CNVM. See Section 12.13.)

Work-up

1. Complete ocular examination, including dilated fundus evaluation to detect a traumatic choroidal rupture. A CNVM is best seen with a slit lamp and either a fundus contact or 60 or 90 diopter lens.
2. Consider fluorescein angiography to confirm the presence of a choroidal rupture or to delineate a CNVM.

Treatment

Laser therapy is instituted when a CNVM >200 μm from the center of the fovea is discovered within the macula and there is no foveolar hemorrhage or exudate. Treatment should be applied within 72 hours of obtaining the fluorescein angiogram.

Follow-up

Following ocular trauma, patients with hemorrhage obscuring the underlying choroid are revaluated every 1–2 weeks until the choroid can be well visualized. If a choroidal rupture is present, patients are instructed in the use of an Amsler grid and asked to test themselves daily and return immediately if a change in the appearance of the grid is noted (see Appendix 3). Fundus examinations are performed every 3–6 months. Patients treated for a CNVM need to be followed closely after treatment; watch for a persistent or new CNVM (see Section 12.10 for further follow-up guidelines).

3.11 ORBITAL BLOW-OUT FRACTURE

Symptoms

Pain (especially on attempted vertical eye movement), local tenderness, binocular double vision (the double vision disappears when one eye is covered), eyelid swelling after nose blowing, recent history of trauma.

Critical Signs

Restricted eye movement (especially in upward and/or lateral gaze), subcutaneous or conjunctival emphysema, hypesthesia in the distribution of the infraorbital nerve (ipsilateral cheek and upper lip), palpable step-off along the orbital rim, point tenderness, enophthalmos (may initially be masked by orbital edema).

Other Signs

Nosebleed, eyelid edema and ecchymosis, superior rim and orbital roof fractures may show hypesthesia in the distribution of the supratrochlear or supraorbital nerve (ipsilateral forehead), ptosis, point tenderness.

Differential Diagnosis

- Orbital edema and hemorrhage without a blow-out fracture   (May have limitation of ocular movement, periorbital swelling, and ecchymosis, but these resolve over 7–10 days.)
- Cranial-nerve palsy   (Limitation of ocular movement, but no restriction on forced-duction testing.)

Work-up

1. Complete ophthalmologic examination, including measurement of extraocular movements and globe displacement. Compare the sensation of the ipsilateral cheek with that on the contralateral side; palpate the eyelids for crepitus (subcutaneous emphysema); and evaluate the globe carefully for a rupture, hyphema or microhyphema, traumatic iritis, and retinal or choroidal damage. Intraocular pressure should be measured.
2. Forced-duction testing is performed if restriction of eye movement persists beyond 1 week (see Appendix 5).
3. CT scan of the orbits and brain (axial and coronal views) is obtained if

the diagnosis is uncertain, if surgical repair is being considered, or if an orbital roof fracture is suspected.

Treatment

1. Nasal decongestants (e.g., Afrin nasal spray bid) for 10–14 days.
2. Broad-spectrum oral antibiotics [e.g., cephalexin (e.g., Keflex) 250–500 mg po qid or erythromycin 250–500 mg po qid] for 10–14 days.
3. Instruct the patient not to blow his or her nose.
4. Ice packs to the orbit for the first 24–48 hours.
5. Surgical repair at 7–14 days posttrauma is undertaken if the patient has persistent diplopia when looking straight ahead or attempting to read, if he or she has cosmetically unacceptable enophthalmos, or if a large fracture is present.
6. Neurosurgical consultation is recommended for most orbital roof fractures.

❖ **Note** *Some physicians use oral steroids initially to decrease the inflammatory reaction; generally, we do not.*

Follow-up

Patients should be seen at 1 and 2 weeks posttrauma and evaluated for persistent diplopia or enophthalmos after the acute orbital edema has subsided. The presence of these findings may indicate entrapment of the orbital contents and the need for surgical repair. Patients should also be monitored for the development of associated ocular injuries (e.g, orbital cellulitis, angle-recession glaucoma, and retinal detachment). Gonioscopy of the anterior-chamber angle and dilated retinal examination with scleral depression is performed 3–4 weeks posttrauma. Warning symptoms of retinal detachment and orbital cellulitis are explained to the patient.

3.12 TRAUMATIC RETROBULBAR HEMORRHAGE

Symptoms

Pain, decreased vision, recent history of trauma to the eye or orbit.

Critical Signs

Proptosis with resistance to retropulsion, diffuse subconjunctival hemorrhage extending posteriorly.

Other Signs

Eyelid ecchymosis, chemosis, congested conjunctival vessels, elevated intra-ocular pressure (IOP); sometimes, limited extraocular motility in any or all fields of gaze.

Differential Diagnosis

- Orbital cellulitis   (Fever, proptosis, chemosis, limitation of eye movements with pain on motion; also may follow trauma, but generally not as acute. See Section 7.4.)
- Orbital fracture (blow-out, medial wall, or tripod fracture)   (Limited extraocular motility, infraorbital hypesthesia, and crepitus. Enophthalmos, not proptosis, may be present. See Section 3.11.)
- Ruptured globe   (Subconjunctival edema and hemorrhage may mask a ruptured globe. A deep anterior chamber, a hyphema, and limitation of ocular motility are often present. IOP is commonly low, and there is usually no proptosis. See Section 3.15.)
- Carotid-cavernous fistula (may follow trauma)   (Pulsating exophthalmos, ocular bruit, corkscrew-arterialized conjunctival vessels, chemosis. IOP may be elevated. Often bilateral involvement because of venous communications. See Section 11.9.)

Work-up

1. Complete ophthalmic examination; check specifically for an afferent pupillary defect, loss of color vision (color plates), elevated or decreased IOP, pulsations of the central retinal artery, and choroidal folds (signs that vision is threatened). (Pulsations of the central retinal artery often precede a central retinal artery occlusion.)
2. CT scan of the orbit (axial and coronal views). The CT scan should be delayed until treatment has been instituted in cases in which vision is threatened.

Treatment

If IOP is elevated (e.g., >30 mm Hg in a patient with a normal optic nerve or >20 mm Hg in a patient whose optic cup is very large and who normally has a lower IOP), any or all of the following methods are employed to lower the IOP. When vision is threatened, all of them are instituted immediately.

1. Carbonic anhydrase inhibitor (e.g., acetazolamide 250 mg po × 2 simultaneously).
2. Topical beta-blocker (e.g., timolol 0.5% q 30 min × 2).
3. Hyperosmotic agent (e.g., mannitol 20% 1–2 g/kg IV over 45 minutes. NOTE   A 500-cc bag of mannitol 20% contains 100 g of mannitol.)
4. Lateral canthotomy and cantholysis (see Fig. 3.2)   [A hemostat is placed horizontally over the lateral canthus and clamped for one minute to compress the tissues and reduce bleeding. (a) The clamp is released and sterile scissors are used to make a horizontal incision approximately 1 cm into the tissue compressed by the hemostat. (b) The skin and conjunctiva in the area of the incision are separated, and the scissors are placed between them to cut the inferior arm of the lateral canthal tendon. (c) Hemostasis

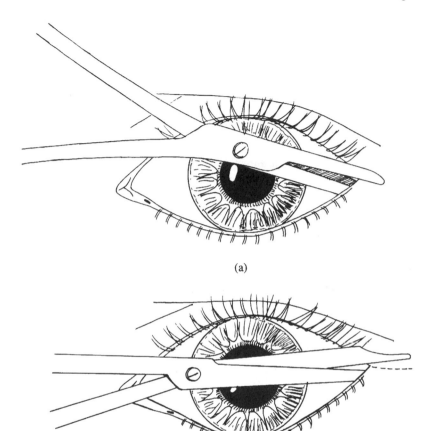

(a)

(b)

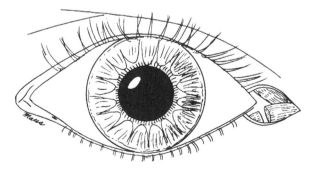

(c)

Figure 3.2
Lateral canthotomy and cantholysis. See text.

is generally achieved with pressure. A sterile dressing is place over the wound.)

If IOP is not lowered or if vision is still threatened after the above treatment, hospitalization is indicated. Emergent orbital decompression surgery may be required if the optic nerve becomes compromised, visual acuity decreases, or color vision is lost.

Follow-up

In cases in which vision is threatened, follow the patient daily until stable. After the acute episode has resolved, reexamination should be performed every few weeks at first; watch for infection and abscess formation. Fibrosis may develop later, limiting extraocular motility.

3.13 INTRAORBITAL FOREIGN BODY

Symptoms

Decreased vision, pain, double vision, or may be asymptomatic; usually, a history of trauma (days to years prior to presentation).

Critical Signs

Orbital foreign body identified by x-ray, CT scan, and/or orbital ultrasound.

Other Signs

A palpable orbital mass; limitation of ocular motility; proptosis; erythema, edema, or ecchymosis of eyelids; an eyelid or conjunctival laceration with or without hemorrhage. An inert orbital foreign body may not produce any signs. The presence of an afferent pupillary defect may be the result of a traumatic optic neuropathy.

Types of Foreign Bodies

A. Poorly tolerated (often lead to inflammation)   Organic (e.g., wood and vegetable matter) and sometimes copper foreign bodies.
B. Fairly well tolerated (typically produce a chronic low-grade inflammatory reaction)   Copper alloys < 85% copper (e.g., brass, bronze).
C. Well tolerated (inert)   Stone, glass, plastic, iron, lead, steel, aluminum, and most other metals.

❖ **Note** *BBs and shotgun pellets are typically made of 80–90% lead and 10–20% iron.*

Work-up

1. History: Determine the composition of the foreign body, the time since the original injury, and the degree of symptoms.
2. Complete ocular and periorbital examination, with special attention to pupillary reaction, intraocular pressure (IOP), and retinal evaluation (determining whether an afferent pupillary defect and decreased vision can be accounted for by the retinal findings). Examine carefully for an entry wound.
3. CT scan of the orbit and brain (axial and coronal views). Rule out a ruptured globe, determine the location of the intraorbital foreign body, and rule out optic-nerve or CNS involvement. MRI is contraindicated if a metal foreign body is suspected or cannot be ruled out.
4. B-scan orbital ultrasound if a foreign body is suspected but not detected by CT scan.
5. Culture any drainage sites.

Indications for Surgical Treatment

The following may be indications for surgical exploration and attempted extraction of the foreign body.

1. Signs of infection (e.g., fever, proptosis, restricted motility, severe chemosis, a palpable orbital mass, an abscess on CT scan).
2. Fistula formation.
3. Signs of optic-nerve compression.
4. The presence of a poorly tolerated intraorbital foreign body (see previous) when it can be well localized.
5. A large or sharp-edged foreign body (independent of composition) that can be easily extracted.

Treatment

1. Hospitalization.
2. Systemic antibiotics (e.g., cefazolin 1 g IV q 8 h for "clean" inert objects. May be treated as orbital cellulitis if contaminated material is involved (see Section 7.4).
3. Tetanus toxoid prn (see Appendix 10 for indications).
4. Surgical exploration and removal of the foreign body when indicated. No food or drink prior to surgery (NPO).
5. Patients with small, nonorganic foreign bodies not requiring surgical intervention may be discharged without hospitalization on oral antibiotics with daily follow-up (see below).

Follow-up

Daily, check vision, assess the degree (if any) of an afferent pupillary defect, measure IOP, and evaluate motility, proptosis, and eye discomfort. If no complications develop and a decision to leave the foreign body within the orbit is made, the patient is discharged from the hospital after 4–10 days. Oral antibiotics (e.g., amoxicillin/clavulanate (e.g., Augmentin) 250–500 mg po q 8 h) are given to complete a 10–14 day course of antibiotic therapy. The patient is told to return in 1 week for a checkup, sooner if the condition worsens.

See "Ruptured Globe and Penetrating Ocular Injury" and "Traumatic Optic Neuropathy," in this chapter, and "Orbital Cellulitis," Section 7.4.

3.14 CORNEAL LACERATION

A. Partial-Thickness Laceration

The anterior chamber is not entered and, therefore, the cornea is not perforated.

Work-up
1. Complete ocular examination; use a slit lamp to carefully rule out ocular penetration. Carefully inspect the cornea, conjunctiva, and sclera. Make sure the anterior chamber is deep and does not contain blood. Measure the intraocular pressure (IOP) by applanation tonometry only if the laceration site can be avoided (otherwise, gently assess IOP with your fingers).
2. Seidel test (see Appendix 4). If Seidel's test is positive, and a full-thickness laceration is present, then see (B).

Treatment
1. A cycloplegic (e.g., scopolamine 0.25%), and antibiotic (e.g., erythromycin ointment or gentamicin drop), and a pressure patch.
2. Occasionally, a bandage soft contact lens is used with an antibiotic drop (e.g., gentamicin qid) after cycloplegia, as described previously.

❖ **Note** *When a moderate-to-deep corneal laceration is accompanied by wound gape, it is often best to suture the wound closed in the operating room.*

Follow-up
Reevaluate daily as described previously until the epithelium heals.

B. Full-Thickness Laceration

See Section 3.15.

3.15 RUPTURED GLOBE AND PENETRATING OCULAR INJURY

Symptoms

Pain, decreased vision, history of trauma.

Critical Signs

A. Ruptured globe: Severe subconjunctival hemorrhage (often involves 360 degrees of bulbar conjunctiva), a deep or shallow anterior chamber compared with the contralateral eye, hyphema (often with clotted blood), limitation of extraocular motility (greatest in the direction of rupture), intraocular contents may be outside of the globe.

B. Penetrating injury: Full-thickness scleral or corneal laceration accompanying signs of a ruptured globe, history of a sharp object entering the globe.

Other Signs

Low intraocular pressure (IOP) (although it may be normal or elevated), irregular pupil, iridodialysis, cyclodialysis, periorbital ecchymosis, dislocated or subluxed lens, commotio retinae, choroidal rupture, retinal breaks, vitreous hemorrhage, traumatic optic neuropathy.

Work-up/Treatment

Once the diagnosis of a ruptured globe or penetrating ocular injury is made by penlight (or slit-lamp examination if necessary), further examination should be deferred until the time of surgical repair in the operating room (to avoid placing any pressure on the globe and risking extrusion of the intraocular contents). The following measures should be taken:

1. Protect the eye with a shield.
2. NPO.
3. Systemic antibiotics [e.g., cefazolin 1 g IV q 8 h and gentamicin 2.0 mg/kg IV load, then gentamicin 1 mg/kg IV q 8 h (adults); cefazolin 25–50 mg/kg/day IV in three divided doses and gentamicin 2 mg/kg IV q 8 h (children)].[2]
4. Tetanus toxoid prn (see Appendix 10).
5. Antiemetic [e.g., prochlorperazine (e.g., Compazine) 10 mg IM q 8 h] prn.

---

[2]Antibiotic doses may need to be reduced if renal function is impaired. Gentamicin peak and trough levels are obtained one-half hour before and after the fifth dose, and blood urea nitrogen and creatinine levels are evaluated every other day.

6. Bed rest with bathroom privileges.
7. Determine when the patient had his last meal. The timing of surgical repair may be influenced by this information.
8. CT scan (axial and coronal views) of the orbits and brain. B-scan ultrasound may be needed to localize the rupture site(s) and to rule out an intraocular or intraorbital foreign body.
9. Arrange for surgical repair to be done as soon as possible.

❖ **Note** *In any severely traumatized eye in which there is no chance of restoring vision, enucleation should be considered initially or within 7–14 days post-trauma.*

3.16 INTRAOCULAR FOREIGN BODY

Symptoms
Eye pain, decreased vision, or may be asymptomatic; often suggestive history (e.g., ocular foreign body after hammering metal).

Critical Signs
May or may not have a clinically detectable corneal or scleral perforation site or an intraocular foreign body. Intraocular foreign bodies are usually seen on CT scan and/or B-scan ultrasound.

Other Signs
Microcystic (epithelial) edema of the peripheral cornea (a clue that a foreign body may be hidden in the anterior-chamber angle in the same sector of the eye), an iris transillumination defect (see Work-up), an irregular pupil, anterior and/or posterior segment inflammation, vitreous hemorrhage, decreased intraocular pressure (IOP).

Types of Foreign Bodies
A. Frequently produce severe inflammatory reactions when left in the eye
   1. Magnetic: Iron and steel.
   2. Nonmagnetic: Copper and vegetable matter.
B. Typically produce mild inflammatory reactions when left in the eye
   1. Magnetic: Nickel.
   2. Nonmagnetic: Aluminum, mercury, and zinc.
C. Inert foreign bodies: Carbon, coal, glass, lead, plaster, platinum, porcelain, rubber, silver, and stone.

❖ **Notes**

1. *Even inert foreign bodies can be toxic to the eye because of a coating or chemical additive.*
2. *Most BBs and gunshot pellets are made of 80–90% lead and 10–20% iron.*

Work-up

1. History: Composition of foreign body, time of last meal, tetanus immunization status.
2. Ocular examination, including visual-acuity assessment and careful evaluation of whether the globe is intact. If there is an obvious perforation site, the remainder of the examination may be deferred until surgery. If there does not appear to be a risk of extrusion of the intraocular contents, the globe is inspected gently to localize the site of perforation and detect the foreign body.
   a. Slit-lamp examination; search the anterior chamber and iris for a foreign body and look for an iris transillumination defect (direct a small beam of light directly through the pupil and look at the iris for a red reflex penetrating through it). Examine the lens for disruption, cataract, or embedded foreign body. Check the IOP.
   b. Consider gonioscopy of the anterior-chamber angle if no wound leak can be detected and the globe appears intact. (This may produce an aqueous leak if the cornea has been perforated.)
   c. Dilated retinal examination using indirect ophthalmoscopy.
3. Obtain a CT scan of the orbit and brain (coronal and axial views). (MRI is contraindicated in the presence of an intraocular foreign body that may be metallic).
4. B-scan ultrasound of the globe and orbit. (Note that intraocular air can mimic a foreign body).
5. Culture the object from which the foreign body arose, if possible. Culture the wound site, if present.
6. Determine whether the foreign body is magnetic (e.g., examine the hammer, nail, or piece of metal from which the foreign body came).

Treatment

1. Hospitalization.
2. No food or drink (NPO).
3. Place a protective shield over the involved eye.
4. Tetanus prophylaxis as needed (see Appendix 10).
5. IV antibiotics (e.g., gentamicin 2.0 mg/kg IV load, then 1 mg/kg q 8 h and cefazolin 1 g IV q 8 h or clindamycin 600 mg IV q 8 h).[3]

---

[3]Dosages may need to be adjusted in the presence of renal dysfunction. Peak and trough levels of gentamicin are obtained one-half hour before and after the fifth dose, and blood urea nitrogen and creatinine levels are evaluated every other day.

6. Cycloplegic (e.g., atropine 1% tid).
7. Surgical removal of the intraocular foreign body may be advisable in the following situations:
   a. The foreign body is composed of iron, steel, copper, or vegetable matter.
   b. A large foreign body (even if inert) in the visual axis.
   c. Any foreign body associated with severe recurrent inflammation.
   d. A foreign body that can be extracted without much difficulty during the surgical repair of an ocular structure.

Follow-up

Observe the patient closely in the hospital for signs of inflammation. Periodic follow-up for years is required; watch for a delayed inflammatory reaction. When an intraocular foreign body is left in place, an electroretinogram (ERG) should be obtained as soon as it can be done safely, and the patient should have serial ERGs performed to look for toxic retinal metallosis. If found, this retinal toxicity often reverses after the foreign body is removed.

3.17 TRAUMATIC OPTIC NEUROPATHY

Symptoms

Decreased vision after a traumatic injury, other trauma symptoms (e.g., pain).

Critical Signs

A new afferent pupillary defect in a traumatized eye that cannot be accounted for by retinal pathology (which would have to be severe) or chiasmal damage.

Other Signs

Relatively poor color vision in the affected eye, a visual field defect, and other signs of trauma. Optic disc acutely appears normal in most cases.

❖ **Note** *Optic disc pallor usually does not appear for weeks following a traumatic optic-nerve injury. If pallor is present immediately after trauma, a preexisting optic neuropathy should be suspected.*

Etiology

Shearing injury from blunt trauma; compression of the nerve by bone, hemorrhage, or perineural edema; laceration of the nerve by bone or an intraorbital foreign body (which may or may not still be present in the orbit).

Differential Diagnosis

(Other causes of a traumatic afferent pupillary defect)

- Severe retinal trauma   (Retinal pathology evident on examination.)
- Traumatic vitreous hemorrhage   (Obscured retinal view on dilated fundus examination. The relative afferent pupillary defect is mild.)
- Intracranial trauma with damage to the optic chiasm.

Work-up

1. Complete ocular examination (if a penetrating injury or ruptured globe is ruled out and it is determined to be safe to fully examine the globe without risking extrusion of the intraocular contents). A pupillary evaluation is essential in order to diagnose a traumatic optic neuropathy.
2. Color vision testing in each eye (color plates).
3. Visual fields by confrontation. (Formal visual-field testing may be deferred.)
4. CT scan of the head and orbit (coronal and axial views) to rule out an intraorbital foreign body and possibly to determine the cause of the optic neuropathy. (Thin cuts through the optic canal should be done.)
5. B-scan ultrasound when a foreign body is suspected but not discovered by CT scan.

Treatment

1. Consider hospitalization in acute cases.
2. Systemic antibiotics in the presence of a sinus wall fracture or penetrating orbital injury (e.g., gentamicin 2.0 mg/kg IV load, then 1 mg/kg IV q 8 h and cefazolin 1 g IV q 8 h or clindamycin 600 mg IV q 8 h).
   - Consider IV steroids (e.g., methylprednisolone 250 mg IV q 6 h for 12 doses) plus a histamine H_2 antagonist (e.g., ranitidine 150 mg po bid— controversial).
   - Surgical intervention is indicated if vision is decreasing.

Follow-up

Daily evaluate vision, pupillary reactions, and color vision. If vision deteriorates after discontinuing steroids, they should be reinstituted as previously described. If visual deterioration occurs despite steroids, surgery is indicated.

4

CORNEA

4.1 SUPERFICIAL PUNCTATE KERATITIS (SPK)

Symptoms
Pain, photophobia, red eye, foreign-body sensation.

Critical Signs
Small pinpoint corneal epithelial defects (stain with fluorescein).

Other Signs
Conjunctival injection, watery or mucoid discharge.

Etiology
SPK is nonspecific, but is most commonly seen with the following disorders:

- Dry eye syndrome   (Poor tear lake or a decreased tear break-up time.)
- Blepharitis   (Erythema, telangiectasias, and crusting of the eyelid margins.)
- Trauma   (Can occur from relatively mild trauma, such as chronic eye rubbing.)
- Exposure keratopathy   (Poor eyelid closure with failure to cover the entire globe.)
- Topical drug toxicity (e.g., neomycin, tobramycin, or any drops with preservatives, including artificial tears)
- Ultraviolet burn/photokeratopathy   (Often in welders or from sun lamps.)

The Wills Eye Manual: Office and Emergency Room Diagnosis and Treatment of Eye Diseases,
Second Edition, edited by R. Douglas Cullom, Jr., M.D., and Benjamin Chang, M.D. © 1994 J. B.
Lippincott Company.

- Mild chemical injury
- Contact lens–related disorder (e.g., chemical toxicity, tight-lens syndrome, contact lens overwear syndrome, giant papillary conjunctivitis)
- Thygeson's SPK (Bilateral, recurrent SPK without conjunctival injection.)
- Foreign body under the upper eyelid (Typically linear SPK, fine scratches arranged vertically.)
- Conjunctivitis (Discharge, eyelids stuck together upon awakening.)
- Trichiasis/distiachiasis [Eyelash(es) rubbing on the cornea.]
- Entropion or ectropion (SPK are superior or inferior.)
- Floppy lid syndrome [Extremely loose lids that pull away from the eye very easily (see Section 6.5).]

Work-up

1. History: Trauma? Contact lens wear? Eyedrops? Discharge or eyelid matting?
2. Evaluate the cornea and tear film. Evert the upper and lower eyelids and look for a foreign body. Check eyelid closure and eyelid laxity and look for inward-growing lashes.
3. Inspect contact lenses for fit (if still in the eye) and for the presence of deposits, sharp edges, and cracks.

❖ **Note** *A soft contact lens should be removed prior to placing fluorescein in the eye.*

Treatment

See the appropriate section to treat the underlying disorder. SPK are often treated nonspecifically as follows:

A. Non–contact lens wearer with a small amount of SPK
   1. Artificial tears, preferably nonpreserved (e.g., Refresh Plus) qid.
   2. Can add a lubricating ointment qhs (e.g., Refresh PM).
B. Non–contact lens wearer with a large amount of SPK
   1. Antibiotic ointment (e.g., erythromycin ointment), cycloplegics (e.g., tropicamide 1% and cyclopentolate 2%), and a pressure patch for 24 hours.
   2. Antibiotic [e.g., erythromycin ointment 2–3 times per day or trimethoprim/polymyxin (e.g., Polytrim) drops qid] for 4 days after the patch is removed.
C. Contact lens wearer with a small amount of SPK
   1. Artificial tears, preferably nonpreserved (e.g., Refresh Plus) qid.
   2. Lenses may or may not be worn, depending on the symptoms and the degree of SPK.
D. Contact lens wearer with a large amount of SPK

1. Discontinue contact lens wear.
2. Tobramycin drops 4–6 times per day and tobramycin ointment qhs.
3. Consider a cycloplegic drop (e.g., scopolamine 0.25%) for pain.

Follow-up
A. Non–contact lens wearers with SPK (especially traumatic SPK) are not seen again solely for the SPK unless the patient is a child or is unreliable. Reliable patients are told to return if their symptoms worsen or do not improve. When underlying ocular pathology is responsible for the SPK, follow-up is in accordance with the guidelines for the underlying problem (see the specific section).
B. Contact lens wearers with a large amount of SPK are seen every day until significant improvement is demonstrated. Contact lenses are not to be worn until the condition clears. The tobramycin may be discontinued when the SPK resolves. The patient's contact lens habits (e.g., wearing time, cleaning routine) are corrected and/or the contact lenses are changed if either is thought to be responsible (see Section 4.17). Contact lens wearers with a small amount of SPK are rechecked in several days to 1 week, depending on their symptoms and degree of SPK.

❖ **Note** *In general, contact lens wearers should not wear their lenses whenever their eyes feel irritated.*

4.2 DRY EYE SYNDROME

Symptoms
Burning or foreign-body sensations, may have *excess* tearing, often exacerbated by smoke, wind, heat, low humidity, or prolonged use of the eye. Usually bilateral and chronic (although patients sometimes present with recent onset in one eye). Often causes more discomfort than the clinical signs would suggest.

Critical Signs
(Either or both may be present.)

• Scanty tear meniscus seen at the inferior eyelid margin. The meniscus should be at least 1 mm in height and have a convex shape.
• Decreased tear break-up time. The time measured from a blink to the appearance of a tear film defect (using fluorescein stain) should be longer than 10 seconds.

Other Signs
Punctate corneal and/or conjunctival fluorescein or rose bengal staining, usually inferiorly or in the interpalpebral area. Excess mucus or debris in the tear
film and filaments on the cornea may be found.

Differential Diagnosis
- Blepharitis   (Eyelid margin crusting, thickening, erythema, and telangiectasias, often seen in combination with dry eyes. See Section 5.10.)
- Eyelid abnormality leading to exposure (exposure keratopathy)   (Often
  secondary to a seventh-nerve palsy, trauma, a chemical or thermal burn,
  a congenital anomaly, senile ectropion, or other causes. See Section 4.4.)
- Nocturnal lagophthalmos   (Eyelids remain partially open while asleep.)

Etiology
- Idiopathic
- Collagen-vascular diseases (e.g., Sjögren's syndrome, rheumatoid arthritis,
  Wegener's granulomatosis, systemic lupus erythematosis)
- Conjunctival scarring (e.g., ocular pemphigoid, Stevens-Johnson syn-
  drome, trachoma, chemical burn)
- Drugs (e.g., oral contraceptives, antihistamines, beta-blockers, phenothi-
  azines, atropine)
- Infiltration of the lacrimal glands (e.g., sarcoidosis, tumor)
- Postradiation fibrosis of the lacrimal glands
- Vitamin A deficiency   (Usually from malnutrition or intestinal malabsorp-
  tion.) (see Section 14.10)

Work-up
1. History and external examination to detect underlying etiology.
2. Slit-lamp examination: Using fluorescein stain and/or rose bengal staining,
   examine the tear meniscus and tear break-up time.
3. Schirmer's test
   Technique: Schirmer filter paper is placed at the junction of the middle
   and lateral one third of the lower eyelid in each eye for 5 minutes, after
   drying the eye of excess tears.
   a. Unanesthetized—Measures basal and reflex tearing.
      Normal = wetting of $\geq$ 15 mm in 5 minutes
   b. Anesthetized—Topical anesthetic (e.g., proparacaine) is applied before
      drying with cotton swab and placing filter paper—Measures basal tearing
      only.
      Normal = wetting of $\geq$ 10 mm in 5 minutes
   We prefer the anesthetized method.

Treatment

MILD

Artificial tears qid (e.g., Tears Plus, Hypo tears, Tears Naturale II)

MODERATE

1. Increase frequency of artificial tear application up to every 1–2 hours—use preservative-free artificial tears (e.g., Refresh Plus, Aquasite, Bion tears, Celluvisc).
2. Can add a lubricating ointment at bedtime (e.g., Hypo tears ointment, Refresh PM, Lacri-lube).

SEVERE

1. Lubricating ointment (e.g., Refresh PM) 2–3 times per day during the daytime with preservative-free artificial tears q 1–2 h.
2. Patch with lubrication at night (may need to patch during the day).
3. If mucus strands or filaments are present, remove with forceps and consider 10% acetylcysteine (e.g., Mucomyst) qid.
4. Consider an artificial-tear insert (e.g., Lacrisert) with tears and ointment.
5. If the above measures are unsuccessful, consider punctal occlusion with collagen or silicone plugs or by electric cautery (after a trial of the former).
6. Consider lateral tarsorrhaphy if all of the previous measures fail. A temporary adhesive-tape tarsorrhaphy (to tape the lateral one third of the eyelid closed) can also be used before a surgical tarsorrhaphy.

❖ **Notes**
1. *In addition to treating the dry eye, treatment for contributing disorders (e.g., blepharitis, exposure keratopathy) should be instituted if these conditions are present.*
2. *Always use preservative-free artificial tears if using them more frequently than every 3 hours to prevent preservative toxicity.*
3. *If the history suggests the presence of a previously undiagnosed collagen-vascular disease (e.g., history of arthritic pain), referral should be made to an internist or rheumatologist for further evaluation.*

Follow-up

In days to weeks, depending upon the severity of the drying changes and the symptoms. Anyone with severe dry eyes caused by an underlying chronic systemic disease (e.g., rheumatoid arthritis, sarcoidosis, ocular pemphigoid) may need to be monitored more closely.

❖ **Note** *Patients with severe dry eyes should be discouraged from contact lens wear. Patients with Sjögren's syndrome have an increased incidence of lymphoma and mucous-membrane problems and may require internal medicine, rheumatological, dental, and gynecological follow-up.*

4.3 FILAMENTARY KERATOPATHY

Symptoms

Moderate-to-severe pain, red eye, foreign-body sensation, photophobia.

Critical Signs

Short strands of epithelial cells and mucus attached to the anterior surface of the cornea at one end of the strand. The strands stain with fluorescein.

Other Signs

Conjunctival injection, poor tear film, superficial punctate keratitis (SPK).

Etiology

- Dry eye syndrome   [Most common cause. Can be associated with an autoimmune collagen-vascular disease such as Sjögren's syndrome (dryness of the mouth and other mucous membranes). See Section 4.2.]
- Superior limbic keratoconjunctivitis   (Superior conjunctival injection and fluorescein staining, superior corneal pannus. See Section 5.5.)
- Recurrent corneal erosions   (Recurrent spontaneous corneal abrasions often occurring upon awakening. See Section 4.6.)
- Patching (e.g., postoperative, following corneal abrasions)
- Neurotrophic keratopathy (see Section 4.5)
- Chronic bullous keratopathy (see Section 4.28)

Work-up

1. History, especially for the above conditions.
2. Slit-lamp examination with fluorescein staining.

Treatment

1. Treat the underlying condition (see the specific sections).
2. Consider debridement of the filaments: After applying topical anesthesia (e.g., proparacaine), gently remove filaments at their base with fine forceps or a cotton-tipped applicator.
3. Lubrication with one of the following regimens:
   a. Artificial tears (e.g., Refresh Plus) 4–8 times per day and artificial-tear ointment (e.g., Refresh PM) qhs.
   b. Sodium chloride 5%: drops qid and ointment qhs.
   c. Acetylcysteine 10% (e.g., Mucomyst) qid.
4. If the symptoms are severe or the above treatment fails, then consider a bandage soft contact lens, unless the patient has severe dry eyes. Extended-wear bandage soft contact lenses may need to be worn for months.

Follow-up

In 1–4 weeks. If the condition is not improved, then consider or repeat the debridement and/or apply a bandage soft contact lens if not yet tried. Lubrication must be maintained chronically if the underlying condition cannot be eliminated.

4.4 EXPOSURE KERATOPATHY

Symptoms

Ocular irritation, burning, foreign-body sensation, and redness of one or both eyes. Usually worse in the morning.

Critical Signs

Inadequate blinking or closure of the eyelids leading to corneal drying. Superficial punctate keratitis (SPK) is found on the lower one third of the cornea or as a horizontal band in the region of the palpebral fissure.

Other Signs

Conjunctival injection, corneal infiltrate or ulcer, eyelid deformity, or abnormal eyelid closure.

Etiology

- Seventh-nerve palsy (orbicularis oculi weakness—e.g., Bell's palsy. See Section 11.8.)
- Eyelid deformity (e.g., ectropion or eyelid scarring from trauma, chemical burn, or herpes zoster ophthalmicus.)
- Nocturnal lagophthalmos (Failure to close the eyes during sleep.)
- Proptosis (e.g., due to an orbital process, such as thyroid eye disease.)
- Following ptosis repair or blepharoplasty procedures.

Differential Diagnosis

See Section 4.1.

Work-up

1. History: Previous Bell's palsy or eyelid surgery? Thyroid disease?
2. Evaluate eyelid closure and corneal exposure. Ask the patient to close his or her eyes gently (as if sleeping). Assess Bell's phenomenon.
3. Slit-lamp examination: Evaluate the tear film and corneal integrity with fluorescein dye. Look for signs of secondary infection (corneal infiltrate, anterior-chamber reaction, severe conjunctival injection).
4. Investigate any underlying disorder (e.g., etiology of seventh-nerve palsy).

Treatment
In the presence of secondary infection, see Section 4.12.

1. Correct any underlying disorder.
2. Artificial tears (e.g., Refresh Plus or Celluvisc drops q 1–6 h).
3. Lubricating ointment (e.g., Refresh PM qhs or qid).
4. Consider eyelid taping or patching at bedtime to maintain the eyelids in the closed position. If severe, consider taping the lateral one third of the eyelids closed (allowing the patient to see) during the day. (Taping is rarely a definitive therapy, but may be tried when the underlying disorder is thought to be temporary.)
5. When maximal medical therapy fails to prevent progressive corneal deterioration, one of the following surgical procedures may be beneficial:
   a. Eyelid reconstruction (e.g., for ectropion).
   b. Tarsorrhaphy.
   c. Orbital decompression (e.g., for proptosis).
   d. Conjunctival flap.

Follow-up
Reevaluate every 1–2 days in the presence of corneal ulceration. Less frequent examinations (e.g, weeks to months) are required for less severe corneal pathology.

4.5 NEUROTROPHIC KERATOPATHY

Symptoms
Red eye, foreign-body sensation, swollen eyelid.

Critical Signs
Loss of corneal sensation, epithelial defects with fluorescein staining.

Other Signs
Early Perilimbal injection progressing to corneal superficial punctate keratitis (SPK).
Late Corneal ulcer with associated iritis. The ulcer often has a gray, heaped-up border, tends to be in the lower one half of the cornea, and is oval.

Etiology
- Status post-infection by varicella-zoster of herpes simplex virus
- Stroke
- Complication of trigeminal nerve surgery
- Complication of irradiation to the eye or an adnexal structure
- Tumor (especially an acoustic neuroma)

Work-up

1. History: Previous episodes of a red and painful eye (herpes)? Previous eye surgery, irradiation, stroke, or hearing problem?
2. Test corneal sensation bilaterally with a sterile cotton wisp (before topical anesthesia).
3. Slit-lamp examination with fluorescein staining.
4. Check the skin for herpetic lesions or scars from a previous herpes zoster infection.
5. Look for signs of a corneal exposure problem (e.g., inability to close an eyelid, seventh-nerve palsy, absent Bell's phenomenon).
6. If suspicious of a CNS lesion, obtain a CT scan (axial and coronal views) of the brain.

Treatment

Mild to moderate punctate epithelial staining   Artificial tears (e.g., Refresh Plus or Celluvisc drops) q 2 h and artificial-tear ointment (e.g., Refresh PM) qhs.

Small corneal epithelial defect   Erythromycin ointment and pressure patch for 24 hours, then erythromycin ointment qid for 4 days or until resolved. Usually requires chronic artificial-tear treatment as above.

Corneal ulcer   See 'Infectious Corneal Infiltrate/Ulcer," Section 4.12, for the work-up and treatment of an infected ulcer. If the ulcer is sterile, then prescribe erythromycin ointment and patch for several days. A tarsorrhaphy, bandage soft contact lens, or conjunctival flap may be required.

❖ **Note** *Patients with neurotrophic keratopathy and a corneal exposure problem often will not respond to treatment unless a tarsorrhaphy is performed (eyelids partly sewn together). A temporary adhesive-tape tarsorrhaphy (the lateral one third of the eyelid is taped closed) may be beneficial.*

Follow-up

Mild to moderate epithelial staining   In 3–7 days.

Corneal epithelial defect   Every 1–2 days until improvement demonstrated, then every 3–5 days until resolved.

Corneal ulcer   Hospitalization is required for severe ulcers (see Section 4.12). Follow daily until significant improvement is demonstrated.

4.6 RECURRENT CORNEAL EROSION

Symptoms

Recurrent attacks of acute ocular pain, photophobia, and tearing often at the time of awakening or during sleep when the eyelids are rubbed or opened; often a history of a prior corneal abrasion in the involved eye.

Critical Signs

Localized roughening of the corneal epithelium (fluorescein dye may lightly outline the area) or a corneal abrasion. Epithelial changes may resolve within hours of the onset of symptoms so that no abnormality is present when the patient is examined.

Other Signs

Corneal epithelial dots or small cysts (microcysts), a fingerprint pattern, or maplike lines may be seen in both eyes if map-dot-fingerprint (MDF) dystrophy is the underlying problem.

Etiology

Damage to the corneal epithelium or epithelial basement membrane from one of the following:

- Anterior corneal dystrophy [e.g., MDF (most common), Meesmann's, and Reis-Bückler dystrophies]
- Previous traumatic corneal abrasion
- Stromal corneal dystrophy (lattice, macular, and granular dystrophies)
- Radial keratotomy or cataract surgery

Work-up

1. History: Recent trauma? Previous corneal abrasion? Family history?
2. Slit-lamp examination with fluorescein staining.

Treatment

1. Acute episodes: A cycloplegic (e.g., cyclopentolate 2% or homatropine 2%), an antibiotic ointment (e.g., erythromycin), and a pressure patch are applied. The patch is left over the eye for 24–48 hours. This treatment may need to be repeated in large or persistent epithelial defects.
2. After epithelial healing is complete: Artificial tears (e.g., Refresh Plus or Celluvisc) 4–8 times per day and artificial-tear ointment (e.g., Refresh PM) qhs for at least 3 months, or 5% sodium chloride drops 4–8 times per day and 5% sodium chloride ointment at bedtime for at least 3 months.
3. If the corneal epithelium is loose and heaped and is not healing, consider debridement of the abnormal epithelium. Apply a topical anesthetic (e.g., proparacaine) and use a sterile cotton-tipped applicator to gently remove the loose epithelium.
4. Erosions not responsive to the above treatment:
   a. Consider an extended wear bandage soft contact lens for several months.

b. Consider anterior stromal puncture (Fig. 4.1). Generally used in extremely symptomatic, refractory cases, with erosions outside the visual axis. It can be performed with or without an intact epithelium. The patient must be very cooperative. This treatment causes small permanent corneal scars.

Technique: Anesthetize the eye with a topical anesthetic (e.g., proparacaine). At the slit lamp, use a 25-gauge needle to perform multiple punctures into the superficial cornea through Bowman's membrane, just into the anterior stroma. Depending on the size of the erosion, between 20 and 100 punctures are placed close together until the entire area of the erosion has been punctured. A cycloplegic drop, antibiotic ointment, and pressure patch as above are placed onto the eye following the procedure, and the patient is reexamined in 24 hours.

5. Excimer laser superficial stromal ablation is showing promising results in the treatment of recalcitrant recurrent erosions from MDF, posttraumatic, and other corneal dystrophies.

Follow-up

Every 1–2 days until the epithelium has healed, then every 1–6 months, depending on the severity and frequency of the episodes.

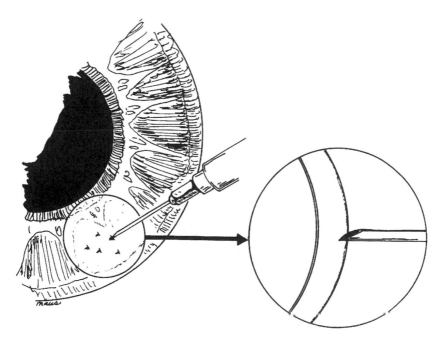

Figure 4.1

Anterior stromal puncture. In the area of the erosion, multiple superficial corneal punctures are made to the depth illustrated.

4.7 THERMAL/ULTRAVIOLET KERATOPATHY

Symptoms

Moderate-to-severe ocular pain, foreign-body sensation, red eye, tearing, photophobia, blurred vision; often a history of welding or using a sunlamp without protective eyewear. The symptoms are typically worse 6–12 hours after the exposure.

Critical Sign

Confluent superficial punctate keratitis (SPK) in an interpalpebral distribution seen with fluorescein staining.

Other Signs

Conjunctival injection, mild-to-moderate eyelid edema, mild-to-no corneal edema, and relatively miotic pupils that react sluggishly.

Differential Diagnosis

- Toxic epithelial keratopathy from exposure to a chemical or drug (e.g., neomycin, tobramycin, antiviral agents)
- Exposure keratopathy   (Poor eyelid closure.)
- Nocturnal lagophthalmos   (Eyelids remain partially open while asleep.)

Work-up

1. History: Welding? Sunlamp use? Topical medications?
2. Slit-lamp examination: Use fluorescein stain. Evert the eyelids to search for a foreign body.

Treatment

1. Cycloplegic (e.g., cyclopentolate 2%).
2. Antibiotic ointment (e.g., erythromycin).
3. Pressure patch for 24 hours. Bilateral patching is desirable, but often impractical in bilateral disease. Generally, the more severely affected eye is patched, and the patient is instructed to place antibiotic ointment in the contralateral eye at home. Sometimes patients are asked to patch the contralateral eye when going to sleep.
4. Oral pain medicine (e.g., acetaminophen with or without codeine) prn.

Follow-up

Patients are instructed to remove the patch after 24 hours.

- If the eye feels much improved, the patient begins topical antibiotics [e.g.,

erythromycin ointment 2–3 times per day or trimethoprim/polymyxin (e.g., Polytrim) drops qid for 3–4 days.]
- If the eye is still significantly symptomatic, the patient should return for reevaluation. If significant SPK is still present, the patient is retreated with a cycloplegic, antibiotic, and pressure patch, as discussed previously.

4.8 THYGESON'S SUPERFICIAL PUNCTATE KERATOPATHY

Symptoms
Foreign-body sensation, photophobia, tearing; no history of recent conjunctivitis. The disease is usually bilateral and has a chronic course with exacerbations and remissions.

Critical Sign
Coarse punctate to stellate shaped gray-white corneal epithelial opacities, often central and slightly elevated with minimal-to-no staining with fluorescein.

Other Signs
No conjunctival injection, corneal edema, anterior-chamber reaction, or eyelid abnormalities.

Differential Diagnosis
See Section 4.1.

Treatment

MILD

1. Artificial tears (e.g., Refresh Plus) 4–8 times per day.
2. Artificial-tear ointment (e.g., Refresh PM) qhs.

MODERATE-TO-SEVERE

1. Mild topical steroid (e.g., fluorometholone 0.1% qid) for 1 week. Then taper very slowly. May need chronic low-dose topical steroid therapy.
2. If no improvement with topical steroids, a therapeutic soft contact lens can be tried.

Follow-up
Every week during an exacerbation, then every 3–12 months. Patients receiving topical steroids require periodic intraocular pressure checks.

4.9 PHLYCTENULOSIS

Symptoms

Tearing, irritation, pain, mild-to-severe photophobia; history of similar episodes. Corneal phlyctenules cause more severe symptoms than conjunctival phlyctenules.

Critical Signs

Conjunctival phlyctenule   A small, white nodule on the bulbar conjunctiva in the center of a hyperemic area. Often occurs at the limbus.

Corneal phlyctenule   A small white nodule, initially at the limbus, with dilated conjunctival blood vessels bordering it. The phlyctenule may migrate toward the center of the cornea, producing wedge-shaped corneal neovascularization and ulceration behind the leading edge of the lesion. Often bilateral.

Other Signs

Conjunctival injection, blepharitis, corneal scarring.

Etiology

Delayed hypersensitivity reaction usually as a result of one of the following:

- Staphylococcus   (Often related to blepharitis. See Section 4.22.)
- Tuberculosis (TB)
- Another infectious agent elsewhere in the body   (Rare.)

Differential Diagnosis

- Inflamed pingueculum   (Located within the palpebral fissure. Connective tissue is often seen to extend from the lesion to the limbus. Usually bilateral.)
- Infectious corneal ulcer   [Corneal phlyctenules which migrate from the limbus toward the center of the cornea may produce a sterile ulcer surrounded by a white infiltrate. When an infectious ulcer is suspected (e.g., increased pain, anterior-chamber reaction), appropriate diagnostic smears and cultures are necessary. See Section 4.12.]
- Ocular rosacea   (Corneal neovascularization with thinning and subepithelial infiltration may develop in an eye with rosacea. Telangiectasias, erythema, and/or pustules are found on the cheeks, nose, forehead, and eyelid margins. See Section 5.8.)
- Herpes simplex keratitis   (May produce corneal neovascularization running into a stromal infiltrate. A history of recurrent herpes is often elicited. Usually unilateral. See Section 4.15.)

Work-up

1. History: TB or recent infection?
2. Slit-lamp examination: Inspect the eyelid margin for signs of blepharitis and rosacea.
3. PPD with anergy panel (tuberculin skin test) in patients who have not had a known positive PPD in the past.

❖ **Note** *The PPD should be read between 48 and 72 hours after placement. A positive reaction is defined as skin induration (not just erythema) of 10 mm or more.*

4. Chest x-ray if the PPD is positive or TB is suspected.

Treatment

Indicated for symptomatic patients.

1. Topical steroid (e.g., prednisolone acetate 1% 4–8 times per day, depending on severity of symptoms).
2. Eyelid hygiene 2–3 times per day (see Section 5.10).
3. Artificial tears (e.g., Refresh Plus drops) 4–6 times per day.
4. Antibiotic ointment at bedtime (e.g., bacitracin or erythromycin ointment).
5. In severe cases of blepharitis, use doxycycline 100 mg po bid or erythromycin 250 mg po qid (see Section 5.10).
6. If the PPD or chest x-ray is positive for TB, then refer the patient to a medical internist to consider antituberculous therapy.
7. Penetrating keratoplasty may benefit patients with central corneal scarring from previous phlyctenules.

Follow-up

Recheck in several days. When the symptoms have significantly improved, start tapering the steroid rapidly. Maintain the antibiotic ointment as long as steroids are being used and for at least 2–3 weeks. Continue eyelid hygiene indefinitely and artificial tears prn.

4.10 PTERYGIUM/PINGUECULUM

Symptoms

Irritation, redness, decreased vision; may be asymptomatic.

Critical Signs

Pterygium   Wing-shaped fold of fibrovascular tissue arising from the interpalpebral conjunctiva and extending onto the cornea.

Pingueculum   Yellow-white flat or slightly raised conjunctival lesion, usually in the interpalpebral fissure adjacent to the limbus, but not involving the cornea.

Other Signs
Either lesion may be highly vascularized and injected or may be associated with superficial punctate keratitis or dellen (thinning of the cornea secondary to drying). An iron line (Stocker's line) may be seen in the cornea adjacent to a pterygium.

Differential Diagnosis
See Section 8.1 for others.

- Conjunctival intraepithelial neoplasia   [Unilateral jellylike, velvety, or leukoplakic (white) mass, often elevated, vascularized, and not in a wing-shaped configuration.]
- Dermoid   [Congenital white lesion, usually at the inferotemporal limbus. Occasionally associated with a deformity of the ear—often preauricular skin tags—and/or vertebral skeletal defects (Goldenhar's syndrome).]
- Pannus   (Blood vessels growing into the cornea, often secondary to contact lens wear, trachoma, phlyectenular keratitis, atopic disease, blepharitis, ocular rosacea, herpes keratitis, and others. It is usually at the level of Bowman's membrane with minimal to no elevation.)

Work-up
Slit-lamp examination to identify the lesion and evaluate the adjacent corneal integrity and thickness.

Treatment
1. Protect the eyes from sun, dust, and wind (e.g., sunglasses or goggles if appropriate) as sunlight and chronic irritation are thought to be factors in pterygium/pingueculum growth.
2. Reduce ocular irritation if present:
    a. Mild: Artificial tears (e.g., Refresh Plus 4–8 times per day) or a mild topical vasoconstrictor (e.g., naphazoline 3–4 times per day).
    b. Moderate-to-severe: Mild topical steroid (e.g., fluorometholone 0.1% 3–4 times per day).
3. If a delle is present, then apply artificial-tear ointment (e.g., Refresh PM) and patch the eye for 24 hours.
4. Surgical removal may be considered when:
    a. The lesion is interfering with contact lens wear.
    b. The patient is experiencing extreme irritation unrelieved by the above treatment.
    c. The pterygium is beginning to involve or involves the visual axis.

❖ **Note** *An aggressive pterygium may recur after surgical excision.*

Follow-up
Asymptomatic patients may be checked every 1–2 years.

- If treating with a topical vasoconstrictor, then the patient should be checked in 2 weeks. The vasoconstrictor drops should be discontinued when the inflammation has subsided.
- If treating with a topical steroid, then check every 1–2 weeks to monitor inflammation and intraocular pressure. Taper and discontinue the steroid drop over several days once the inflammation has abated.

4.11 BAND KERATOPATHY

Symptoms
Decreased vision, foreign-body sensation, white spot on the cornea; may be asymptomatic.

Critical Sign
Anterior corneal plaque of calcium at the level of Bowman's membrane in the palpebral fissure area, separated from the limbus by clear cornea. Holes are often present in the plaque, giving it a Swiss-cheese appearance. The plaque usually begins at the 3- and 9-o'clock positions, adjacent to the limbus, and can extend across the cornea.

Other Signs
May have other signs of chronic eye disease.

Etiology
More common   Chronic uveitis (e.g., juvenile rheumatoid arthritis), interstitial keratitis, corneal edema, phthisis bulbi, long-standing glaucoma.
Less common   Hypercalcemia (may be secondary to hyperparathyroidism, sarcoidosis, Paget's disease, vitamin D intoxication, and others), gout, corneal dystrophy, chronic exposure to irritants (e.g., mercury fumes), renal failure, and others.

Work-up
1. History: Chronic exposure to environmental irritants? Systemic disease? Chronic eye disease?

2. Slit-lamp examination, intraocular pressure measurement, and optic-nerve evaluation.
3. If no signs of chronic anterior segment disease or long-standing glaucoma are present and the band keratopathy cannot be accounted for, then consider the following work-up:
   a. Serum calcium, albumin, magnesium, phosphorus levels, blood urea nitrogen, and creatinine.
   b. Uric acid level if gout is suspected.

Treatment

MILD (i.e., foreign-body sensation)

Artificial tears (e.g, Refresh Plus or Celluvisc) 4–6 times per day and artificial-tear ointment (e.g., Refresh PM) qhs.

SEVERE (e.g., obstruction of vision, irritation unrelieved with lubricants, cosmetic problem):

Remove the calcium at the slit lamp.

1. Dilute a solution of 15% disodium EDTA (e.g., Endrate) by mixing 2 ml of disodium EDTA with 8 ml of normal saline (0.9% NaCl). This gives a 3% mixture.
2. Anesthetize the eye with a topical anesthetic (e.g., cocaine 4% or proparacaine).
3. Debride the corneal epithelium with a sterile scalpel or a sterile cotton-tipped applicator dipped in topical anesthetic.
4. Wipe a cellulose sponge or cotton swab saturated with the 3% disodium EDTA solution over the band keratopathy until the calcium clears (which may take 10–30 minutes).
5. Place an antibiotic ointment (e.g., erythromycin), a cycloplegic drop (e.g., cyclopentolate 1–2%), and a pressure patch on the eye for 24 hours.
6. Consider giving the patient an analgesic (e.g., acetaminophen with or without codeine).

Follow-up
If surgical removal has been performed, then the patient needs to be examined every day with repatching, an antibiotic, and a cycloplegic until the epithelial defect heals. Surgical removal can be repeated if the band keratopathy recurs. Otherwise, the patient may be checked every 3–12 months, depending on the severity of the symptoms.

4.12 INFECTIOUS CORNEAL INFILTRATE/ULCER

Symptoms

Red eye, mild-to-severe ocular pain, photophobia, decreased vision, discharge.

Critical Signs

Focal white opacity in the corneal stroma (infiltrate). An ulcer exists if there is an overlying epithelial defect that stains with fluorescein with stromal loss.

❖ **Note** *An examiner using a slit beam cannot see through an infiltrate/ulcer to the iris, whereas stromal edema and inflammation are more transparent.*

Other Signs

Conjunctival injection, corneal thinning, stromal edema and inflammation surrounding the infiltrate, folds in Descemet's membrane, anterior-chamber reaction, hypopyon, mucopurulent discharge, upper eyelid edema. Posterior synechiae, hyphema, and glaucoma may occur in severe cases.

Etiology

- Bacterial   (Most common infectious etiology. In general, corneal infections are assumed to be bacterial until proven otherwise by laboratory studies or until a therapeutic trial is unsuccessful.)
- Fungal   [Must be considered after a traumatic corneal injury, particularly from vegetable matter (e.g., a tree branch). Infiltrates commonly have feathery borders and may be surrounded by satellite lesions. *Candida* infections tend to occur in diseased eyes. Hyphae or yeast may be evident on Giemsa stain, although they are also seen with Gomori methenamine silver stain. Most fungi grow on Sabouraud's dextrose agar.]
- Acanthamoeba   (An extremely painful stromal infiltrate usually in a soft contact lens wearer who practices poor lens hygiene or has a history of swimming with his contact lenses. In the late stages, the infiltrate assumes the shape of a ring. Acanthamoeba cysts may be seen with periodic acid-Schiff or Giemsa stain, and the organism may be cultured on nonnutrient agar with *Escherichia coli* overlay.)
- Herpes simplex virus   (May have eyelid vesicles or corneal epithelial dendrites. A history of recurrent eye disease or known ocular herpes is common. Patients with chronic herpes simplex keratitis may develop bacterial superinfections.)
- Atypical mycobacteria   (Usually follows penetrating injuries or corneal grafts. Culture plates must be kept for 8 weeks.)

Differential Diagnosis

- Sterile ulcer (not infectious) (Dry eye syndrome, rheumatoid arthritis or other collagen-vascular diseases, vernal keratoconjunctivitis, neurotrophic keratopathy, vitamin A deficiency, others. Cultures are negative, anterior-chamber inflammation is minimal to none, and the eye may be white and comfortable.)
- Staphylococcal hypersensitivity [Peripheral corneal infiltrate(s), sometimes with an overlying epithelial defect, usually multiple, often bilateral, with a clear space between the infiltrate and the limbus. There is minimal-to-no anterior-chamber reaction.]
- Corneal infiltrates from an immune reaction to contact lenses or solutions (Generally, multiple, small subepithelial infiltrates with an intact overlying epithelium and minimal-to-no anterior-chamber reaction. Usually a diagnosis of exclusion after ruling out an infectious process.)
- Residual corneal foreign body or rust ring (May be accompanied by corneal stromal inflammation, edema, and sometimes, a sterile infiltrate. There may be a mild anterior-chamber reaction. The infiltrate and inflammation generally clear after the foreign body is removed.)

Work-up

1. History: Contact lens wear and lens-care regimen? Swim with lenses? Trauma or corneal foreign body? Eye care prior to visit (e.g., antibiotics or topical steroids)? Previous corneal disease? Systemic illness?
2. Slit-lamp examination: Stain with fluorescein to determine if there is epithelial loss overlying the infiltrate; document the size, depth, and location of the corneal infiltrate; assess the anterior-chamber reaction; and measure the intraocular pressure (IOP).
3. Corneal scrapings for smears and cultures are performed as described below for infiltrates considered to be infectious and for all ulcers. Small, nonstaining infiltrates are sometimes treated with regular-strength antibiotics without prior scraping.

Culture Procedure

EQUIPMENT

Slit lamp; sterile Kimura spatula, knife blade, or moistened calcium alginate swab (i.e., with thioglycolate or trypticase soy broth); culture media; microscopy slides; alcohol lamp.

PROCEDURE

- Anesthetize the cornea with topical drops (proparacaine is best, as it appears to be less bacteriocidal than others.)
- At the slit lamp, scrape the base and the leading edge of the infiltrate firmly with the spatula, blade, or swab, and place the specimen on the

culture medium or slide. Sterilize the spatula over the flame of the alcohol lamp between each separate culture or slide. Be certain that the spatula-tip temperature has returned to normal before touching the cornea again.

MEDIA

Routine:

1. Blood agar (most bacteria)
2. Sabouraud's dextrose agar without cyclohexamide; place at room temperature (fungi)
3. Thioglycolate broth (aerobic and anaerobic bacteria)
4. Chocolate agar; place into a CO_2 jar (*Haemophilus* species *Neisseria gonorrhoeae*)

Optional:

- Löwenstein-Jensen medium (mycobacteria, *Nocardia species*)
- Nonnutrient agar with *E. coli* overlay (acanthamoeba)
- Trypticase soy broth

SLIDES

Routine:

1. Gram's stain (bacteria, fungi)
2. Giemsa stain (bacteria, fungi, acanthamoeba)

Optional:

- Gomori methenamine silver stain, periodic acid-Schiff stain (acanthamoeba, fungi)
- Acid-fast stain (mycobacteria, *Nocardia* species)
- Calcofluor white; a fluorescent microscope is needed (acanthamoeba)

❖ **Note** *When a fungal infection is suspected, deep scrapings into the base of the ulcer are essential. Sometimes a corneal biopsy is necessary to obtain diagnostic information.*

In contact lens wearers suspected of having an infectious ulcer, the contact lenses and case are cultured if at all possible. Explain to the patient that the cultured contact lenses can never be worn again.

Treatment

As mentioned above, ulcers and infiltrates are generally treated as bacterial initially unless there is a high index of suspicion of another form of infection (see "Fungal Keratitis," Section 4.13; "Acanthamoeba," Section 4.14; and "Herpes Simplex Virus," Section 4.15).

1. Cycloplegic (e.g., scopolamine 0.25% tid).
2. Topical antibiotics:

    a. Small nonstaining infiltrate with minimal-to-no anterior-chamber reaction and minimal-to-no discharge:

       Non–contact lens wearer Broad-spectrum topical antibiotics (e.g., polymyxin B/bacitracin ointment qid or ciprofloxacin drops q 2–6 h).

       Contact lens wearer Tobramycin or ciprofloxacin drops q 2–6 h; can add tobramycin ointment qhs.

    b. Large or staining infiltrate or moderate-to-severe anterior-chamber reaction or purulent discharge: Fortified tobramycin or gentamicin (15 mg/ml) every hour alternating with fortified cefazolin (50 mg/ml) or vancomycin (25 mg/ml) every hour. This means that the patient will be placing either one drop or the other drop in the eye every one-half hour. See Appendix 9 for directions on making fortified antibiotics. An alternative choice for smaller, peripheral, staining infiltrates is ciprofloxacin 0.3% 2 drops every 15 minutes for 6 hours, then 2 drops every 30 minutes.

3. Consider subconjunctival antibiotics [e.g., gentamicin (20–40 mg) and cefazolin (100 mg) or vancomycin (25 mg)] in very severe cases or when fortified antibiotics cannot be started within a short time period. See Appendix 7 for the injection technique.

4. Eyes with corneal thinning should be protected by a shield without a patch (a patch is never placed over an eye thought to have an infection).

5. No contact lens wear.

6. Oral pain medication as needed (e.g., acetaminophen).

7. Admission to the hospital may be necessary if:
   - There is a sight-threatening infection.
   - The patient is unable to give him or herself the antibiotics at the above frequency without difficulty.
   - There is a likelihood of noncompliance.
   - The patient is unable or unwilling to return daily.
   - Systemic antibiotics are needed (e.g., corneal perforation, scleral extension of the infection, gonococcal or *Haemophilus* infection)

8. For atypical mycobacteria, consider amikacin 10 mg/ml drops 2 q h for one week and then qid for 2 months (kanamycin or cefoxitin may be substituted).

Follow-up
- The patient needs daily evaluation with repeat measurements of the size of the infiltrate and ulcer. The most important criteria in evaluating the response to treatment include the degree of eye pain, the size of the epithelial defect over the infiltrate, the size and depth of the infiltrate, and the anterior-chamber reaction. Less pain, a smaller epithelial defect and infiltrate, and a less-inflamed eye are all favorable responses. The IOP must be checked and glaucoma treated if present (see Section 10.4).

- If the ulcer is improving, the antibiotic regimen is gradually tapered. Otherwise, the antibiotic regimen is adjusted according to the culture and sensitivity results.
- If the infiltrate or ulcer was not cultured originally and is now worsening, cultures, stains, and treatment with fortified antibiotics are needed. Hospitalization is considered.
- Reculture the ulcer (with the addition of optional media and stains) if it does not seem to be responding to the current antibiotic regimen and the original cultures are negative.
- A corneal biopsy may need to be performed if the condition is worsening and infection is still suspected despite negative cultures.
- In an impending or completed corneal perforation, a corneal transplant or patch graft is considered. Cyanoacrylate glue may also work in a treated corneal ulcer.

❖ **Note** *Outpatients are told to return immediately if the pain increases or the vision decreases.*

4.13 FUNGAL KERATITIS

Symptoms
Pain, photophobia, red eye, tearing, discharge, foreign-body sensation; a history of trauma, particularly with vegetable matter (e.g., a tree branch), or chronic eye disease.

Critical Signs
Corneal stromal gray-white opacity (infiltrate) with a feathery border. The epithelium over the infiltrate may be elevated above the remainder of the corneal surface, or there may be an epithelial defect with stromal thinning (ulcer).

Other Signs
Satellite lesions surrounding the primary infiltrate, conjunctival injection, mucopurulent discharge, anterior-chamber reaction, hypopyon.

Etiology
- Nonfilamentous fungi (typically *Candida* species)   (Usually in previously unhealthy eyes.)
- Filamentous fungi (typically *Fusarium* or *Aspergillus* species)   (Usually from trauma with vegetable matter.)

Differential Diagnosis

See Section 4.12.

Work-up

See Section 4.12 for complete work-up and culture procedure.

❖ **Notes**

1. *Be certain to obtain a Giemsa stain when a fungus is suspected (periodic acid-Schiff and Gomori methenamine silver stains can also be used), and scrape deep into the base of the ulcer for material.*
2. *If all cultures are negative, yet an infectious etiology is still suspected, consider a corneal biopsy to obtain further diagnostic information.*
3. *Irrigate the lacrimal sac and culture any reflux [rule out fungal dacryocystitis and consider a dacryocystorhinostomy (DCR) if positive].*

Treatment

In general, corneal infiltrates and ulcers of unknown etiology are treated as bacterial until proven otherwise by laboratory studies (see Section 4.12). If the stains and/or cultures indicate a fungal keratitis institute the following measures:

1. Admission to the hospital is usually necessary, unless the patient is very reliable. It may take weeks to achieve complete healing.
2. Natamycin 5% (50 mg/ml) drops q 1–2 h while awake, q 2 h at night.
3. Cycloplegic (e.g., scopolamine 0.25% tid).
4. Treat glaucoma if present (see Section 10.4).
5. No topical steroids. If the patient is currently taking steroids, they should be tapered rapidly.
6. No eye patch.
7. An eye shield, without a patch, may be advisable when the cornea is thinned.
   - If the infection involves the deep corneal stroma or is worsening despite appropriate treatment, one or more of the following medications may be added:
   a. Amphotericin B 0.15% (1.5 mg/ml) drops q 1 h. (May be especially effective in *Candida* infections.)
   b. Fluconazole 400 mg loading dose, then 200 mg po qd.
   c. Miconazole or clotrimazole 0.1–1.0% (1–10 mg/ml) drops q 1 h. (Clotrimazole may be especially effective in *Aspergillus* infections.)
   A corneal transplant may be necessary for a progressive fungal infection in a patient receiving maximal medical therapy. A corneal transplant or patch graft may also be required in an impending or complete corneal perforation.

❖ **Note** *Natamycin is the only commercially available topical antifungal; all others must be made from IV solutions with proper approval and sterile techniques. Other medications such as itraconazole have been used topically and systemically in recalcitrant fungal infections.*

Follow-up

Daily, as per Section 4.12. The response to treatment is slower than in a bacterial infection. Lack of progression is a favorable sign.

4.14 ACANTHAMOEBA

Corneal infection with acanthamoeba should be considered in any patient with a history of soft contact lens wear, poor contact lens hygiene (e.g., using nonsterile homemade saline solutions to clean lenses, infrequent disinfection), and/or swimming or hot-tub use with the contact lenses in.

Symptoms

Severe ocular pain, redness, and photophobia over a period of several weeks.

Critical Signs

Early   Less corneal and anterior segment inflammation than would be expected for the degree of pain the patient is experiencing, epithelial and subepithelial infiltrates (sometimes along corneal nerves, producing a radial keratitis), pseudodendrites on the epithelium.

Late   A corneal stromal infiltrate in the shape of a ring.

❖ **Note** *Cultures for bacteria are negative, and the condition generally does not improve with antibiotic or antiviral medications.*

Other Signs

Eyelid swelling, conjunctival injection, especially circumcorneal cells and flare in the anterior chamber. Generally little discharge or corneal vascularization. Corneal ulceration may occur later in the course.

Differential Diagnosis

- Herpes simplex keratitis   (The patient often has a history of previous attacks in the same eye; typical branching corneal dendrites are common; the condition is much less painful than acanthamoeba; and multinucleated giant cells may be seen on Giemsa stain. See Section 14.15.)

- Fungal ulcer   (Hyphae may be seen on histologic staining; fungi should grow on Sabouraud's dextrose agar. See Section 14.13.)
- Bacterial (e.g., *Pseudomonas* species) ulcer   (Much more acute course, over hours to days, should grow on bacterial culture and respond to fortified antibiotic drops. See Section 14.12.)

Work-up

See Section 4.12 for a general work-up. The following are obtained when acanthamoeba is suspected:

1. Corneal scrapings for Giemsa periodic acid-Schiff (PAS) and Gram's stains (Giemsa and PAS stains may show typical cysts).
2. Calcofluor white stain if available (requires a fluorescent microscope).
3. Culture on nonnutrient agar with *Escherichia coli* overlay.
4. Consider a corneal biopsy if the stains and cultures are negative and the condition is not improving on the current regimen.
5. Consider cultures and smears of contact lens and case.

Treatment

The treatment of acanthamoeba is controversial and often ineffective. The following are modes of therapy which have been found to be successful in some cases.

One or more of the following are generally used in combination, usually in the hospital:

1. Polymyxin-neomycin-gramicidin (e.g., Neosporin) drops q 0.5–2 h.
2. Propamidine isethionate 0.1% (e.g., Brolene) drops q 0.5–2 h.
3. Clotrimazole 1% drops q 2 h.
4. Ketoconazole 200 mg po bid or itraconazole 200 mg po qd.

Topical polyhexamethylene biguanide has also been used recently with some success. Alternative therapy to clotrimazole includes miconazole 1% drops or paromomycin drops q 2 h. Dibromopropamidine isethionate 0.15% (e.g., Brolene) ointment is also available.

All patients:

5. Discontinue contact lens wear.
6. Cycloplegic (e.g., atropine 1% tid).
7. Nonsteroidal antiinflammatory agent (e.g., sulindac 200 mg po bid) for pain.
   - A corneal transplant may be indicated for medical failures, but this procedure can be complicated by recurrent infection.
8. Oral pain medication as needed, e.g., acetaminophen, codeine or oxycodone.

Follow-up

Every day in the hospital until the condition is consistently improving. Medication may then be tapered judiciously and the patient checked as an outpatient. The required duration of therapy is not established, varying from 6–18 months.

❖ **Note** *Brolene is available in England and may be obtained with FDA approval. Clotrimazole is not currently formulated as an ophthalmic suspension, but it can be formulated in artificial tears from a powder (with FDA approval). This solution must be shaken before each use.*

4.15 HERPES SIMPLEX VIRUS (HSV)

Symptoms

Usually, unilateral red eye, pain, photophobia, tearing, decreased vision, skin (e.g., eyelid) rash; history of previous episodes.

Signs

Any or all of the following may be present.

EYELID/SKIN INVOLVEMENT

Clear vesicles on an erythematous base that progress to crusting.

CONJUNCTIVITIS

Conjunctival injection with follicles and a palpable preauricular node.

CORNEAL EPITHELIAL DISEASE

May present as superficial punctate keratitis (SPK), stellate keratitis, dendritic keratitis (a thin, linear, branching lesion with club-shaped terminal bulbs at the end of each branch), or a geographic ulcer (a large, amoeba-shaped corneal ulcer with a dendritic edge). The edges of herpetic lesions are mildly heaped-up with swollen epithelial cells that stain well with rose bengal; the central ulceration stains well with fluorescein. Corneal sensitivity may be decreased. Scars may develop underneath the epithelial lesions.

NEUROTROPHIC ULCER

A sterile ulcer with smooth margins over an area of interpalpebral stromal disease that persists despite antiviral therapy. May be associated with stromal melting and perforation.

CORNEAL STROMAL DISEASE

    A. Disciform keratitis: Disc-shaped stromal edema with an intact epithelium. A mild iritis with localized granulomatous keratic precipitates is typical, and increased intraocular pressure (IOP) may be present. No necrosis nor corneal neovascularization is present.

    B. Necrotizing interstitial keratitis: Multiple or diffuse whitish gray corneal stromal infiltrates often accompanied by stromal inflammation, thinning, and neovascularization. Concomitant iritis, hypopyon, or glaucoma may be present. Bacterial superinfection must be ruled out.

UVEITIS

An anterior-chamber reaction may develop secondary to severe corneal stromal involvement. Less commonly, anterior-chamber reaction can develop without active corneal disease.

RETINITIS

Rare. In neonates, it is usually associated with a severe systemic HSV infection and is often bilateral.

Differential Diagnosis

(Conditions that produce dendritic-appearing corneal lesions)

- Herpes zoster virus   [Frequently painful skin vesicles along a dermatomal distribution of the face, not crossing the midline, are present. (NOTE   Pain may be present before vesicles develop.) The dendrites in this condition do not have true terminal bulbs and do not stain well with fluorescein. See Section 4.16.]

- Recurrent corneal erosion   (A healing erosion often appears as a pseudo-dendrite. Patients frequently provide a history of a corneal abrasion in the involved eye or have underlying anterior basement membrane dystrophy. Pain frequently develops upon awakening from sleep. See Section 4.6.)

- Contact lens–related pseudodendrites   (No skin involvement. Dendrites do not typically branch, do not have terminal bulbs, and stain minimally. See Section 4.17.)

Work-up

1. History: Previous episodes? History of corneal abrasion; contact lens wear; or previous nasal, oral, or genital sores? Recent topical or systemic steroids? Immune deficiency state?

2. External examination: Note the distribution of skin vesicles if present.

3. Slit-lamp examination with IOP measurement.

4. Check corneal sensation before topical anesthetic.

Most cases of herpes simplex are diagnosed clinically and require no confirmatory laboratory tests. However, if the diagnosis is in doubt, any of the following tests may be supportive of the diagnosis:

5. Scrapings of a corneal or skin lesion (scrape the *edge* of a corneal ulcer or the *base* of a skin lesion) for Giemsa stain, which shows multinucleated giant cells. (A papanicolaou stain will show intranuclear eosinophilic inclusion bodies). ELISA testing is also available.
6. Viral culture: A sterile, cotton-tipped applicator is used to swab the cornea, conjunctiva, or skin after unroofing vesicles with a sterile needle and is then placed into the viral transport medium.

❖ **Note** *Smears and cultures for bacteria should be taken if a corneal ulceration suddenly worsens. See Section 4.12.*

Treatment

EYELID/SKIN INVOLVEMENT

1. Topical acyclovir ointment tid to the skin lesions [expensive and not proven to be effective; some physicians treat with an antibiotic ointment instead (e.g., erythromycin or bacitracin)].
2. Warm soaks to skin lesions tid.
3. If the eyelid margin is involved, add trifluorothymidine 1% drops (e.g., Viroptic) or vidarabine 3% ointment (e.g., Vira-A) 5 times per day to the eye (good for small children).

The above medications are continued for 7–14 days until resolution of the symptoms.

❖ **Note** *Oral acyclovir 400 mg po 5 times per day for 7–14 days is given by some physicians to adults suspected of having primary herpetic disease (e.g., flu-like illness, fever, lymphadenopathy. Contraindicated in pregnancy and renal disease.)*

CONJUNCTIVITIS

Trifluorothymidine 1% drops (e.g., Viroptic) or vidarabine 3% ointment (e.g., Vira-A) 5 times per day. Discontinue the antiviral agent when the conjunctivitis has resolved after 7–14 days.

CORNEAL EPITHELIAL DISEASE

1. Trifluorothymidine 1% drops (e.g., Viroptic) 9 times per day or vidarabine 3% ointment (e.g., Vira-A) 5 times per day.
2. Cycloplegic agent (e.g., scopolamine 0.25% tid) if an anterior-chamber reaction is present.
3. Patients on topical steroids should have them tapered in the presence of corneal epithelial disease.

4. Consider gentle debridement of the infected epithelium as an adjunct to the antiviral agents.
   Technique: After topical anesthesia (e.g., proparacaine), a sterile, cotton-tipped applicator or semisharp instrument is used to carefully peel off the lesions at the slit lamp. Following debridement, antiviral treatment should be instituted as above.

❖ **Note** *Avoid debridement in children, in the presence of deep stromal lesions, or when a lesion has been previously treated with topical steroids.*

In epithelial defects that do not resolve after several weeks, antiviral toxicity and/or a neurotrophic ulcer should be suspected. At that point, the antiviral agent should be discontinued and a nonpreserved artificial-tear ointment (e.g., Refresh PM) or an antibiotic ointment (e.g., erythromycin) should be used 2–4 times per day with or without a pressure patch for several days.

NEUROTROPHIC ULCER

See Section 4.5.

CORNEAL STROMAL DISEASE

A. Disciform keratitis
   Mild   Cycloplegic (e.g., scopolamine 0.25% tid) alone.
   Severe and/or central   (i.e., vision is reduced)
   1. Cycloplegic (e.g., scopolamine 0.25% tid).
   2. Topical steroid (e.g., prednisolone acetate 1% qid).
   3. Antiviral drops for prophylaxis (e.g., trifluorothymidine 1% 3–4 times per day).
      • Consider a corneal transplant if inactive postherpetic scars significantly affect vision.

❖ **Notes**
   1. *Topical steroids are contraindicated in those with corneal epithelial disease.*
   2. *Rarely, a systemic steroid (e.g., prednisone 60–80 mg po once a day tapered rapidly) is given to patients with severe stromal disease accompanied by an epithelial defect.*
   3. *Acyclovir has not been shown to be beneficial in the treatment of stromal disease.*

B. Necrotizing interstitial keratitis: Treated as severe disciform keratitis. A corneal transplant may be required if the cornea perforates.

❖ **Note** *The persistence of an ulcer in the presence of stromal inflammation commonly is due to the underlying inflammation (requiring cautious steroid therapy); however, it may be due to antiviral toxicity. When an ulcer deepens,* *a new infiltrate develops, or the anterior-chamber reaction increases, smears and cultures should be taken for bacteria and fungi. See Section 4.12.*

Follow-up
Patients are reexamined in 2–3 days to evaluate the response to treatment and then every 1–7 days, depending on the clinical findings. The following clinical parameters are evaluated: the size of the epithelial defect and ulcer, the corneal thickness and the depth to which the cornea is involved, the anterior-chamber reaction, and the IOP (see Section 10.4 for glaucoma management). Antiviral medications for corneal dendrites and geographic ulcers should be continued 5–9 times per day for 7–14 days and then tapered over one week. Topical steroids used for corneal stromal disease are tapered slowly (often over months to years). The initial concentration of the steroid (e.g., 1%) is eventually reduced (e.g., 0.125%). Prophylactic antiviral agents are used tid. No antiviral coverage is needed when the steroid is given once a day or less.

❖ **Note** *The topical antivirals can cause a local toxic or allergic reaction (usually a papillary or follicular conjunctivitis). If such a reaction should occur, the antiviral agent should be replaced with another antiviral agent, because cross-reactivity is rare.*

4.16 HERPES ZOSTER VIRUS (HZV)

Symptoms
Skin rash, skin "pain," headache, fever, malaise, blurred vision, eye pain, red eye.

Critical Sign
Acute vesicular skin rash which follows a dermatome of the fifth cranial nerve and can progress to scarring. Characteristically, the rash appears on one side of the forehead, does not cross the midline, and involves the upper eyelid only.

Other Signs
Less commonly, the rash involves the lower eyelid and cheek on one side and rarely, one side of the jaw. Conjunctivitis, corneal involvement [e.g., pseudodendrites on the epithelium (raised mucous plaques), superficial punctate keratitis (SPK), immune stromal keratitis, neurotrophic keratitis], uveitis, iris atrophy, scleritis, retinitis, choroiditis, optic neuritis, cranial-nerve palsy, and glaucoma can occur. Late postherpetic neuralgia also may occur.

❖ **Note** *Corneal disease may follow the acute skin rash by many months to years. Rarely, it can precede the skin rash.*

Differential Diagnosis
- Herpes simplex virus (HSV) (The rash does not follow a dermatome nor obey the midline. Patients are typically young. Corneal dendrites of HSV have true terminal bulbs and stain well with fluorescein; dendrites of HZV generally appear stuck on the epithelium, do not have true terminal bulbs, and stain poorly with fluorescein. See Section 4.15.)

Work-up
1. History: Duration of rash and pain? Immunocompromised or risk factors for AIDS?
2. Complete ocular examination, including a slit-lamp evaluation with fluorescein staining, intraocular pressure (IOP) check, and dilated optic-nerve and retinal examination.
3. Systemic evaluation:
   a. *Patients <40 years of age:* Medical evaluation to determine whether the patient may be immunocompromised.
   b. *Patients 40–60 years of age:* None (unless immunodeficiency is suspected from the history).
   c. *Patients >60 years of age:* If systemic steroid therapy is to be instituted, obtain a steroid work-up as required.
   Immunocompromised patients should *not* receive systemic steroids.

Treatment
See Section 14.1 for the treatment of zoster in immunocompromised patients.

SKIN INVOLVEMENT

A. Adults with an acute moderate to severe skin rash present less than 3–5 days in which active skin lesions are present
   1. Acyclovir[1] 800 mg po 5 times per day or famciclovir 500 mg 3× day for 7–10 days; if the condition is severe or the patient is systemically ill, hospitalize and prescribe acyclovir 5–10 mg/kg IV q 8 h for 5–10 days.
   2. Bacitracin ointment to the skin lesions bid.
   3. Warm compresses to periocular skin tid (to keep it clean).

In patients > 60 years of age who are not immunocompromised and who do not have diabetes nor TB, consider adding the following to minimize postherpetic neuralgia:

---

[1]The dosage of acyclovir must be reduced in patients with renal insufficiency and is contraindicated in pregnancy.

4. Prednisone 60 mg po for 3 days, then 40 mg po for 3 days, then 20 mg po for 4 days, then discontinue, plus:
5. Anti-ulcer therapy (e.g., antacid, H_2-blocker) (Although it is unproved, some physicians believe cimetidine relieves some of the discomfort from the acute skin rash. Therefore, cimetidine 400 mg po bid may serve a dual purpose.)

B. Adults with a skin rash of more than 3–5 days' duration or no active skin lesions
1. Warm compresses to periocular skin tid.
2. Bacitracin ointment to skin lesions bid.

C. Children
Treat as in (B) unless there is evidence of systemic spread. For systemic spread, hospitalize and prescribe acyclovir[2] 500 mg/m²/day in 3 divided doses for 7 days. The hospital pharmacy should have a conversion chart for height, weight, and surface area in square meters. The patient is usually transferred to the pediatric service.

OCULAR INVOLVEMENT

A. Conjunctival involvement: Cool compresses and erythromycin ointment to the eye bid.
B. Corneal pseudodendrites or SPK: A lubrication with preservative-free drops (e.g., Refresh Plus) 6–10 × day and ointment (e.g., Refresh PM) qhs. Topical steroids (e.g., prednisolone acetate 1% qid) are occasionally helpful.
C. Uveitis (with or without immune stromal keratitis): Topical steroid (e.g., prednisolone acetate 1% qid), cycloplegic (e.g., cyclopentolate 1–2% qid), and erythromycin ointment qhs.
D. Neurotrophic keratitis: Treat mild epithelial defects with erythromycin or preservative-free artificial tear ointment qid. If corneal ulceration occurs, obtain appropriate smears and cultures to rule out infection (see Section 4.12). If the ulcer is sterile, consider a tarsorrhaphy or conjunctival flap when there is no response to ointment and patching. See Section 4.5.
E. Scleritis: Treat as any other scleritis (see Section 5.7).
F. Retinitis, choroiditis, optic neuritis, or cranial-nerve palsy: Acyclovir[2] 5–10 mg/kg IV q 8 h for 1 week and prednisone 60 mg po for 3 days, tapering as described above.
G. Glaucoma: May be secondary to the uveitis or steroids. If uveitis is present, increase the frequency of the steroid administration for a few days. If IOP remains elevated, substitute fluorometholone 0.1% (e.g., FML) drops for prednisolone acetate. Timolol 0.5% bid and a carbonic anhydrase inhibitor (e.g., methazolamide 25–50 mg po 2–3 times per day) will additionally help lower IOP.

---

[2]The dosage of acyclovir must be reduced in patients with renal insufficiency, and it is contraindicated in pregnancy.

❖ **Note** *Pain may be severe during the first 2 weeks, and analgesics (e.g., aceta-minophen with or without codeine) may be required. An antidepressant (e.g., amitryptyline 25 mg po tid) may be beneficial, as depression frequently develops during the acute phase of HZV infection. Antidepressants may also help postherpetic neuralgia. Capsaicin 0.025% (e.g., Zostrix) ointment 3–4 times per day may be applied to the* skin *(not around the eyes) for post-herpetic neuralgia after the initial skin lesions heal.*

Follow-up

If ocular involvement is present, examine the patient every 1–7 days, depending on the severity. Patients without ocular involvement can be followed every 1–2 weeks. After the acute episode resolves, check the patient every 3–6 months, because relapses may occur months to years later, particularly as steroids are tapered. Systemic steroid administration requires collaboration with the patient's medical doctor.

❖ **Note** *HZV is contagious for children and adults who have not had chicken pox—it can be spread by inhalation. Pregnant women who have not had chicken pox must be especially careful to avoid contact with a herpes zoster patient.*

4.17 CONTACT LENS–RELATED PROBLEMS

Symptoms

Pain, photophobia, foreign-body sensation, decreased vision, red eye, itching.

Signs

See the distinguishing characteristics of each etiology.

Etiology

- Corneal infiltrate/ulcer (bacterial, fungal, acanthamoeba)   (White corneal lesion that may stain with fluorescein. Must always be ruled out in contact lens patients with eye pain. See "Infectious Corneal Infiltrate/Ulcer," Section 4.12; "Acanthamoeba," Section 4.14; and "Fungal Keratitis," Section 4.13.)
- Hypersensitivity/toxicity reactions to preservatives in solutions   [Conjunctival injection and ocular irritation typically develop shortly after lens cleaning and insertion, but can be present chronically. A recent change from one type or brand of solution to another often is elicited in the history. Commonly occurs in patients using preserved solutions (e.g., thimerosal or chlorhexidine as a component). May be due to inadequate rinsing of

lenses after enzyme use. Signs include superficial punctate keratitis (SPK), conjunctival injection, bulbar conjunctival follicles, and subepithelial or stromal corneal infiltrates.]

- Pseudo–superior limbic keratoconjunctivitis [Hyperemia and fluorescein staining of the superior bulbar conjunctiva, particularly at the limbus. Subepithelial infiltrates, haze, and irregularity may be found on the superior cornea. This may represent a hypersensitivity or toxicity reaction to a solution or contact lens–related product (especially thimerosal). Unlike superior limbic keratoconjunctivitis unassociated with contact lenses, there are no corneal filaments, papillary reaction, nor an association with thyroid disease.]
- Giant papillary conjunctivitis (Itching, mucus discharge, and lens intolerance in a patient with large superior tarsal conjunctival papillae. See Section 4.18.)
- Contact lens deposits (Multiple small deposits on the contact lens, leading to corneal and conjunctival irritation. The contact lens is often old and may not have been cleaned or enzymed properly in the past.)
- Tight-lens syndrome [Symptoms may be severe and often develop within 1 or 2 days of being fit with the responsible contact lens (usually a soft lens). The lens does not move with blinking and appears "sucked-on" to the cornea. An imprint in the conjunctiva is often observed after the lens is removed. Corneal edema, SPK, anterior-chamber reaction, and sometimes a sterile hypopyon may develop.]
- Corneal warpage [Seen predominantly in long-term polymethylmethacrylate (PMMA) hard contact lens wearers. Initially, the vision becomes blurred with glasses but remains good with contact lenses. Gradually, blurred vision and sometimes, discomfort develop with contact lenses. There may or may not be SPK. Keratometry and corneal topography reveal distorted mires.]
- Corneal neovascularization [Patients are often asymptomatic until the visual axis is involved. Superficial corneal neovascularization for 1–2 mm is common and generally unalarming in aphakes, with the exception of corneal transplants (which are at a greater risk for graft rejection). Phakic and corneal transplant patients are generally treated.]
- Corneal epithelial changes (Range from epithelial thickening to pseudo-dendritic changes. Not infectious in origin, but rather a toxic/traumatic reaction to the contact lens.)
- Inadequate/incomplete blinking (Can lead to chronic inflammation and staining at the 3- and 9-o'clock positions.)
- Others [Contact lens inside out, corneal abrasion (see Section 3.2), poor lens fit, change in refractive error, others.]

Work-up

1. History: What is the main complaint (severe pain, mild discomfort, itching)? What kind of contact lens does the patient wear (soft, hard, gas-permeable,

daily-wear, extended-wear, or disposable)? How old are the lenses? For how many hours/days/weeks straight are the lenses worn? How are the lenses cleaned and disinfected? Are enzyme tablets used? Are the products preservative-free? Any recent changes in contact lens habits?

2. In noninfectious conditions, while the contact lens is still in the eye, evaluate its fit and examine its surface for deposits at the slit lamp.

3. Ocular examination, including slit-lamp examination with the contact lens in (if not too uncomfortable) to check fit. Then remove lens and examine with fluorescein. Evert the upper eyelids of both eyes and inspect the superior tarsal conjunctiva for papillae.

4. Smears and cultures are taken when a corneal ulcer is suspected (see "Infectious Corneal Infiltrate/Ulcer," Section 4.12; "Acanthamoeba," Section 4.14; and "Fungal Keratitis," Section 4.13).

5. The contact lenses and lens case are cultured, if possible, when an infectious corneal process is suspected.

Treatment

I. When the diagnosis of infection cannot be ruled out, patients are treated as follows:

A. Possible corneal ulcer (corneal infiltrate, epithelial defect, anterior-chamber reaction, pain): Appropriate smears and cultures are obtained, fortified antibiotics and a cycloplegic are started, and contact lens wear is discontinued (see Section 4.12).

B. Small subepithelial infiltrates, corneal abrasion, or diffuse SPK
   1. Discontinue contact lens wear.
   2. Topical antibiotic (e.g., tobramycin drops 4–8 times per day; can also add tobramycin ointment qhs. Beware of toxicity with long-term use.)
   3. No pressure patch.

II. When a specific contact lens problem is suspected, it may be treated as follows (see "Contact Lens–Induced Giant Papillary Conjunctivitis," Section 4.18, for treatment of this condition):

A. Hypersensitivity/toxicity reaction
   1. Discontinue contact lens wear.
   2. Preservative-free artificial tears (e.g., Refresh Plus drops 4–6 times per day).
   3. New contact lenses and preservative-free solutions are used upon resolution of the condition, and appropriate lens hygiene is explained.[3]

---

[3]The following regimen for contact lens care is one recommended system. We do not recommend extended-wear contact lenses to most patients.

Daily cleaning regimen: Preservative-free daily cleaner (e.g., Miraflow), preservative-free saline (e.g., Unisol), disinfectant—preferably heat or hydrogen peroxide (4 hours).

Weekly: Enzyme tablets.

    4. Patients are taught to rinse their lenses thoroughly after using enzymes.

B. Pseudo–superior limbic keratoconjunctivitis: Treated as described for hypersensitivity/toxicity reactions. When a large subepithelial opacity extends toward the visual axis, topical steroids may be added (e.g., prednisolone acetate 1% q 6 h), but they are often ineffective.

C. Contact lens deposits
    1. Discontinue contact lens wear.
    2. Replace with a new contact lens once the symptoms resolve. Consider changing the brand of contact lens.
    3. Teach proper contact lens care, stressing weekly enzyme treatments.

D. Tight-lens syndrome
    1. Discontinue contact lens wear.
    2. Consider a topical cycloplegic (e.g, scopolamine 0.25% tid or atropine 1% tid) in the presence of anterior-chamber reaction.
    3. Patients should be refit with a flatter contact lens after the symptoms and signs resolve.

❖ **Note** *Patients do not need to be cultured for their hypopyon when this syndrome is highly suspected.*

E. Corneal warpage
    1. Discontinue contact lens wear (it is explained to patients that vision may be poor for the following 2–4 weeks).
    2. A gas-permeable hard contact lens should be fit when the refraction and keratometric readings have returned to normal (obtain the original keratometric readings).

F. Corneal neovascularization
    1. Discontinue contact lens wear.
    2. Consider a topical steroid (e.g., prednisolone acetate 1% qid) for extensive neovascularization.
    3. Consider refitting with a highly oxygen transmissible daily-wear contact lens that moves adequately over the cornea.

G. Corneal epithelial changes
    1. Discontinue contact lens wear.
    2. Consider a new contact lens when the epithelial changes resolve, which may take weeks or months.
    3. Use preservative-free solutions.

H. Inadequate/incomplete blinking: Frequently apply preservative-free artificial tears (e.g., Refresh Plus).

Follow-up
- When a corneal infection cannot be ruled out, patients are reevaluated the following day. Eyes of contact lens patients are not patched. Treatment is maintained until the condition clears.

- In noninfectious conditions, patients are reevaluated in 1–4 weeks, depending on the clinical situation. Contact lens wear is resumed when the condition resolves. Patients using topical steroids should be followed more closely and their intraocular pressure monitored.

4.18 CONTACT LENS–INDUCED GIANT PAPILLARY CONJUNCTIVITIS (GPC)

Symptoms
Itching, mucus discharge, decreased lens-wearing time, increased lens awareness, excessive lens movement.

Critical Sign
Giant papillae on the superior tarsal conjunctiva. (NOTE The upper eyelid must be everted to make the diagnosis.)

Other Signs
Contact lens coatings, high-riding lens, ptosis, mild conjunctival injection.

Work-up
1. History: Details of contact lens use, including age of lenses and cleaning and enzyming regimen.
2. Slit-lamp examination: Evert the upper eyelids and examine for papillae.

Treatment

MILD TO MODERATE

1. Replace the contact lens if it is older than 4–6 months or if it has numerous deposits. Refit with a new brand of soft contact lens or refit with a gas-permeable rigid contact lens.
2. Reduce contact lens wearing time (switch extended-wear contact lens patients to daily wear).
3. Lodoxamide (e.g., Alomide) drops qid.
4. Have the patient clean the lenses more thoroughly—preferably using preservative-free solutions (e.g., Miraflow daily cleaner) and preservative-free saline (e.g., Unisol).
5. Increase enzyme use (use at least every week).

SEVERE

1. Discontinue contact lens wearing.
2. Lodaxamide (e.g., Alomide) 4–6 times per day.
3. Restart with a new contact lens in 1–4 months (when the condition clears).
4. Teach lens hygiene as above.

Follow-up
In 2–4 weeks. Lodaxamide is tapered slowly.

❖ **Note** *GPC can also result secondary to an exposed suture or ocular prosthesis. Exposed sutures are removed. Prostheses should be cleaned and polished. A coating (e.g., Biocoat) can be placed on the prosthesis to reduce GPC. Otherwise, these entities are treated with lodoxamide, as described previously.*

4.19 INTERSTITIAL KERATITIS (IK)

Acute symptomatic IK most commonly occurs within the first or second decade of life. Signs of old IK often persist throughout life.

Acute Phase

Symptoms
Pain, tearing, photophobia, red eye.

Critical Signs
Corneal stromal blood vessels and edema.

Other Signs
Anterior-chamber cells and flare, fine keratic precipitates on the corneal endothelium, conjunctival injection.

Signs of Old Disease

Deep corneal haze or scarring, often, corneal stromal blood vessels containing no blood (ghost vessels), corneal stromal thinning.

Etiology
More common   Congenital syphilis (usually affects both eyes within 1 year of each other).
Less common   Acquired syphilis (unilateral—often sectorial), TB (unilateral—often sectorial), Cogan's syndrome (vertigo, tinnitus, hearing loss, negative FTA-ABS, often associated with systemic vasculitis, typically polyarteritis nodosa), leprosy, herpes simplex virus, and Lyme disease.

Work-up

For active IK and old, previously untreated IK:

1. History: Venereal disease in the mother during pregnancy or in the patient? Difficulty hearing or tinnitus?
2. External examination: Look for saddle-nose deformity, Hutchinson's teeth, frontal bossing, or other signs of congenital syphilis; hypopigmented or anesthetic skin lesions and thickened skin folds, loss of the temporal eyebrow, and loss of eyelashes, as in leprosy.
3. Slit-lamp examination: Note whether the corneal nerves are segmentally thickened like beads on a string and whether iris nodules are present (leprosy); look for patchy hyperemia of the iris with fleshy, pink nodules (syphilis). Check intraocular pressure.
4. Dilated fundus examination: Look for the classic salt-and-pepper chorioretinitis or optic atrophy of syphilis.
5. VDRL or RPR, FTA-ABS or MHA-TP.
6. PPD with anergy panel.
7. Chest x-ray if negative FTA-ABS (or MHA-TP) or positive PPD.
8. Consider ESR, ANA, rheumatoid factor, Lyme titer.

Treatment

A. Acute disease
   1. Topical cycloplegic (e.g., atropine 1% tid).
   2. Topical steroid (e.g., prednisolone acetate 1% q 1–6 h, depending on the degree of inflammation).
   3. Treat any underlying disease.
B. Old inactive disease: Corneal transplant surgery may improve vision when it has been impaired by central corneal scarring and no amblyopia is present.
C. Acute or old, inactive disease
   - If FTA-ABS is positive and
     a. The patient has not been treated for syphilis in the past (or is unsure about treatment)
     b. There are signs of active syphilitic disease (e.g., active chorioretinitis or papillitis)
     c. The VDRL or RPR titer is positive and has not declined the expected amount after treatment (see "Congenital Syphilis," Section 14.3, or "Acquired Syphilis," Section 14.2)
     then treatment for syphilis is indicated (see "Congenital Syphilis," Section 14.3, or "Acquired Syphilis," Section 14.2).
   - If PPD is positive (>10 mm of induration at 48–72 hours) and
     a. Patient <35 years old and has not been treated for TB in the past
     b. There is evidence of active systemic TB (e.g., positive finding on chest x-ray)
     then refer the patient to a medical internist for treatment of TB.

- If Cogan's syndrome is present, then refer the patient to an ear, nose, and throat specialist and consider rheumatologic follow-up.

Follow-up
A. Acute disease   Every 3–7 days initially, then every 2–4 weeks. The frequency of steroid administration is slowly reduced as the inflammation subsides. IOP is monitored closely and lowered with medication when it is thought to be dangerously high (e.g., >30 mm Hg in a patient with a healthy optic nerve). See "Inflammatory Open-Angle Glaucoma," Section 10.4.
B. Old inactive disease   Routine follow-up every year unless treatment is required for underlying etiology.

4.20 PERIPHERAL CORNEAL THINNING

Symptoms
Pain, photophobia; may be asymptomatic.

Critical Sign
Corneal thinning (seen best with a narrow slit of light from the slit lamp), may have a sterile infiltrate or ulcer.

Etiology
- Collagen-vascular disease (e.g., rheumatoid arthritis, relapsing polychondritis, Wegener's granulomatosis, polyarteritis nodosa, systemic lupus erythematosus, others)   (Peripheral, unilateral, or bilateral corneal thinning/ulcers may progress circumferentially to involve the entire peripheral cornea. Perforation may occur. This may be the first manifestation of systemic disease.)
- Terrien's degeneration   [Usually bilateral, slowly progressive thinning of the peripheral cornea typically superiorly, most often in men. The anterior chamber is quiet and the eye is typically not injected. A yellow line (lipid) may appear, with a fine pannus over the thinned areas of involvement. The ulceration may slowly spread circumferentially. Irregular and against-the-rule astigmatism is often present. The epithelium usually remains intact, and perforation is rare.]
- Mooren's ulcer   (Unilateral or bilateral, idiopathic, painful corneal thinning and ulceration with inflammation, initially involving a focal area of peripheral cornea nasally or temporally and without an adjacent perilimbal lucid zone, but later extending circumferentially or centrally. An epithelial

defect, stromal thinning, and a leading undermined edge are present. Limbal blood vessels may grow into the ulcer, and perforation can occur. This diagnosis can only be made after other etiologies are ruled out.)

- Pellucid marginal degeneration   [Painless, bilateral corneal thinning of the inferior peripheral cornea (usually from the 4- to 8-o'clock portions)]. There is no anterior-chamber reaction, conjunctival injection, lipid deposition, nor vascularization. The epithelium is intact. Corneal protrusion may be seen above the area of thinning. The thinning may slowly progress.]
- Furrow degeneration   (Corneal thinning just peripheral to an arcus senilis, typically in the elderly. There is no vascular infiltration nor ocular inflammation, and perforation is rare. Usually nonprogressive and does not require treatment.)
- Dellen   (Oval corneal thinning secondary to corneal drying and stromal dehydration adjacent to an abnormal conjunctival or corneal elevation. The epithelium is usually intact. See Section 4.21.)
- Staphylococcal hypersensitivity (marginal keratitis)   (A peripheral, white corneal infiltrate that is separated from the limbus by a zone of clear cornea, it is often multiple, may stain with fluorescein, may be mildly thinned, and is typically associated with blepharitis. See Section 4.22.)
- Dry eye syndrome   (Peripheral corneal ulcers may result from severe cases of dry eye. Patients may demonstrate a poor tear lake, decreased tear break-up time, SPK inferiorly or centrally, and corneal filaments. See Section 4.2.)
- Exposure/neurotrophic keratopathy   (Typically, a sterile oval ulcer develops inferiorly on the cornea without signs of significant inflammation. An eyelid abnormality, a fifth- or seventh-cranial-nerve defect, or proptosis is common. The ulcer may become superinfected. See Section 4.4 and 4.5.)
- Sclerokeratitis   (Corneal ulceration is associated with severe ocular pain radiating to the temple and/or jaw due to accompanying scleritis. The sclera develops a blue hue, scleral vessels are engorged, and scleral edema with or without nodules is present. An underlying collagen-vascular disease, especially Wegener's granulomatosis, must be ruled out. See Section 5.7.)
- Vernal keratoconjunctivitis   (Superior, shallow shield-shaped sterile corneal ulcer accompanied by giant papillae on the superior tarsal conjunctiva and/or limbal papillae. The conjunctivitis is usually bilateral, often occurs in children, and recurs during the summer months, but it can occur anytime in warm climates. See Section 5.1.)
- Ocular rosacea   (Typically affects the inferior cornea in middle-aged patients. Erythema and telangiectasias of the eyelid margins, nose, forehead, and cheeks are characteristic, and can progress to rhinophyma. See Section 5.8.)

- Others (Cataract surgery, inflammatory bowel disease, and leukemia can rarely cause peripheral corneal thinning/ulceration.)

Differential Diagnosis
- Infectious infiltrate or ulcer (A dense, gray-white stromal infiltrate or ulcer that stains with fluorescein. The conjunctiva is injected, and an anterior-chamber reaction is usually present. Often, lesions are treated as infectious until cultures are noted to be negative. See Section 4.12.)

Work-up
1. History: Contact lens wearer or previous herpes simplex keratitis (infectious)? Known collagen-vascular disease or inflammatory bowel disease? Other systemic symptoms? Seasonal conjunctivitis with itching (vernal)?
2. External examination: Old facial scars of herpes zoster? Eyelid-closure problem causing exposure? Blue tinge to the sclera? Rosacea facies?
3. Slit-lamp examination: Look for infiltrate, corneal ulcer, hypopyon, uveitis, scleritis, old herpetic scarring, poor tear lake, SPK, blepharitis, or giant papillae on the superior tarsal conjunctiva or limbal papillae. Measure intraocular pressure (IOP).
4. Schirmer's test (see Section 4.2).
5. Dilated fundus examination: Look for cotton-wool spots consistent with collagen-vascular disease or evidence of posterior scleritis (e.g., viritis, subretinal fluid, chorioretinal folds, exudative retinal detachment).
6. Corneal scrapings and cultures when infection is suspected (see "Infectious Corneal Infiltrate/Ulcer," Section 4.12).
7. Serum ANA, rheumatoid factor, ESR, and complete blood count with differential to rule out collagen-vascular disease and leukemia, if suspected. Serum anti-neutrophilic cytoplasmic antibody (ANCA) level can be obtained if Wegener's granulomatosis is suspected.
8. Scleritis work-up, when present (see Section 5.7).
9. Refer to an internist (or rheumatologist) when collagen-vascular disease or leukemia is suspected.

Treatment
The treatment of dellen, staphylococcal hypersensitivity, dry eye syndrome, exposure and neurotrophic keratopathies, scleritis, vernal conjunctivitis, and ocular rosacea are discussed elsewhere in this book.

A. Corneal thinning due to collagen-vascular disease: Management is usually coordinated with a rheumatologist or internist.
    1. Antibiotic ointment (e.g., erythromycin ointment) and a pressure patch qhs.

2. Ocular lubricants while awake (e.g., Refresh tears q 1 h or Refresh PM ointment qid).
3. Cycloplegic drops (e.g., atropine 1%) when an anterior-chamber reaction and/or pain are present.
4. Systemic steroids (e.g., prednisone 60–100 mg po once per day; the dosage is adjusted according to the response) and an H_2-blocker (e.g., ranitidine 150 mg po bid) are used for significant and progressive corneal thinning, but not for perforation.
5. An immunosuppressive agent such as cyclophosphamide is usually required, especially for Wegener's granulomatosis. This should be done in cooperation with the patient's medical physician.
6. Excision of adjacent conjunctiva is occasionally helpful when the condition progresses despite treatment.
7. Punctal occlusion if dry eye syndrome is also present.
8. Consider cyanoacrylate tissue adhesive or corneal transplant surgery for an impending or actual corneal perforation. A conjunctival flap can also be used for an impending corneal perforation.
9. Patients with significant corneal thinning should wear their glasses [or protective glasses (e.g., polycarbonate lens)] during the day and an eye shield at night.

❖ **Note** *Topical steroids are generally not used when significant corneal thinning is present because of the risk of perforation. Topical steroids should be gradually tapered if the patient is already taking them. Corneal thinning due to relapsing polychondritis, however, seems to improve with topical steroids (e.g., predniso-lone acetate 1% q 1–2 h).*

B. Terrien's degeneration: Correct astigmatism with glasses or contact lenses if possible. Protective eyewear (e.g., polycarbonate lens) during the day and an eye shield at night should be worn to prevent traumatic perforation if significant thinning is present. Lamellar grafts can be used if thinning is extreme.
C. Mooren's ulcer: Underlying systemic diseases must be ruled out before this diagnosis can be made. A stepwise approach to treatment is taken, using any or all of the following therapeutic modalities. If the epithelial defect over the ulcer is not healing within a few days of initiating treatment, more aggressive therapy is pursued. Some cases are resistant to all forms of treatment.
1. Topical steroid (e.g., prednisolone acetate 1% q 1 h).
2. Systemic steroid (e.g., prednisone 60–100 mg po once per day) and an H_2-blocker (e.g, ranitidine 150 mg po bid).
3. Immunosuppressive agents (e.g., cyclophosphamide, methotrexate) after consultation with a medical physician familiar with these agents.

4. Consider conjunctival excision, a conjunctival flap, or cryotherapy if the ulceration progresses.
5. Consider cyanoacrylate tissue adhesive or corneal surgery to prevent or treat a corneal perforation.

All patients are given the following:

6. Topical antibiotic drops [e.g., trimethoprim/polymyxin (e.g., Polytrim) qid] to prevent secondary bacterial infection.
7. Cycloplegic (e.g., atropine 1% tid).
8. Glasses during the day and an eye shield at night because of the risk of perforation with minor trauma.

D. Pellucid marginal degeneration: See "Keratoconus," Section 4.23.
E. Furrow degeneration: No treatment is required.

❖ **Note** *If systemic steroid therapy is to be instituted, obtain a steroid work-up as indicated.*

Follow-up

Patients with severe disease are examined daily in the hospital or as outpatients if compliant; those with milder conditions are checked less frequently. Watch carefully for signs of superinfection (e.g., increased pain, stromal infiltration, anterior-chamber cells and flare, conjunctival injection), increased IOP, and progressive corneal thinning. Treatment is maintained until the epithelial defect over the ulcer heals and is then gradually tapered. As long as an epithelial defect is present, there is a risk of progressive thinning and perforation.

4.21 DELLEN

Symptoms

Usually asymptomatic; irritation, foreign-body sensation.

Critical Sign

Corneal thinning, usually at the limbus, often in the shape of an ellipse, accompanied by an adjacent focal conjunctival or corneal elevation.

Other Signs

Fluorescein pooling in the area, but minimal staining. No infiltrate, no anterior-chamber reaction, often no hyperemia.

Etiology

Poor spread of the tear film over a focal area of cornea (with resultant stromal dehydration) due to an adjacent surface elevation (e.g., chemosis, conjunctival hemorrhage, filtering bleb from glaucoma surgery, pterygium, tumor, following muscle surgery).

Differential Diagnosis
See "Peripheral Corneal Thinning," Section 4.20.

Work-up
1. History: Previous eye surgery?
2. Slit-lamp examination with fluorescein staining. Look for an adjacent area of elevation.

Treatment
1. Lubricating or antibiotic ointment (e.g., Refresh PM, erythromycin ointment) and a pressure patch for 24 hours.
2. Lubricating ointment qhs following removal of the pressure patch. Maintain the ointment until the adjacent elevation is eliminated.
3. If the cause cannot be removed (e.g., filtering bleb), lubricating ointment should be applied nightly, and artificial-tear drops (e.g., Refresh Plus) used 4–8 times per day, chronically. (Most conjunctival elevations will regress with patching.)

Follow-up
Unless there is severe thinning, reexamination can be performed in 1–7 days, at which time the cornea can be expected to be of normal thickness. If it is not, full-time patching and lubrication should again be instituted.

4.22 STAPHYLOCOCCAL HYPERSENSITIVITY

Symptoms
Acute photophobia, mild pain, red eye, chronic eyelid crusting and itching; history of recurrent acute episodes.

Critical Signs
Usually, multiple peripheral corneal stromal infiltrates with a clear space between the infiltrates and the limbus, and minimal-to-no staining with fluorescein. The anterior chamber is usually quiet, and only a sector of the conjunctiva is typically injected.

Other Signs

Blepharitis, inferior superficial punctate keratitis (SPK), phlyctenule (a wedge-shaped, raised, sterile infiltrate near the limbus), peripheral scarring and corneal neovascularization in the contralateral eye.

Etiology

Staphylococcal blepharitis   (Infiltrates are a noninfectious reaction of the host's antibodies to the staphylococcal antigens.)

❖ **Note** *Patients with ocular rosacea (e.g., telangiectasias of the eyelids, nose, cheeks, and forehead that may progress to rhinophyma) are especially suscepti-ble to this condition.*

Differential Diagnosis

- Infectious corneal infiltrates   (A dense, white-gray stromal infiltrate, often central, painful, and associated with a marked anterior-chamber reaction. Not usually multiple and recurrent. See Section 4.12.)
- See Section 4.20 for other causes of marginal thinning/infiltrates.

Work-up

1. History: Recurrent episodes? Contact lens wearer (a risk of infection)?
2. Slit-lamp examination with fluorescein staining and intraocular pressure (IOP) check.
3. If an infectious infiltrate is suspected, then corneal scrapings for culture and smears should be obtained. See Section 4.12.

Treatment

MILD

Warm compresses, eyelid hygiene, and erythromycin or bacitracin ointment qhs (see "Blepharitis/Meibomianitis," Section 5.10).

MODERATE-TO-SEVERE

Treat as described previously and add a topical steroid (e.g., prednisolone acetate 0.125% qid) or a combination antibiotic/steroid (e.g., dexamethasone/tobramycin qid). Maintain until the symptoms improve, then slowly taper.

If recurrent episodes are not prevented by eyelid hygiene, consider systemic tetracycline 250 mg po qid for 1 month, then bid for 1 month, then once per day until the ocular disease is controlled for several months. Instead, doxycy-cline may be used, 100 mg po bid for 1 month, then once per day for 1 month, then titrated as necessary. Low-dose antibiotics may have to be maintained indefinitely.

❖ **Note** *Tetracycline and doxycycline are contraindicated in children under 8 years of age, pregnant women, and breast-feeding mothers. Erythromycin in the same dose as tetracycline may be substituted.*

Follow-up

In 2–7 days, depending on the clinical picture. IOP is monitored while patients are on topical steroids.

4.23 KERATOCONUS

Symptoms

Progressive decreased vision usually beginning in the adolescence and continuing into middle age. Acute corneal hydrops can cause a sudden decrease in vision, pain, red eye, photophobia, and profuse tearing.

Critical Signs

Slowly progressive irregular astigmatism secondary to paracentral thinning and bulging of the cornea (maximal thinning near the apex of the protrusion), vertical tension lines in the posterior cornea (Vogt's stria), an irregular corneal retinoscopic reflex, and egg-shaped mires on keratometry. Inferior steepening is seen on corneal topographic evaluation. Usually bilateral but often asymmetric.

Other Signs

Fleischer's ring (epithelial iron deposits at the base of the cone), bulging of the lower eyelid when looking downward (Munson's sign), superficial corneal scarring. Corneal hydrops (sudden development of corneal edema) results from a rupture in Descemet's membrane.

Associations

Keratoconus is often seen in Down's syndrome, atopic disease, and others. It may be related to chronic eye rubbing.

Differential Diagnosis

- Pellucid marginal degeneration   (Corneal thinning in the inferior periphery. The cornea protrudes superior to the band of thinning.)
- Keratoglobus   (Rare. Uniform circularly thinned cornea with maximal thinning in the midperiphery of the cornea. The cornea protrudes central to the area of maximal thinning.)

Treatment for these two conditions is the same as for keratoconus, except corneal transplants are not as readily performed, because they are technically more difficult and have a higher failure rate.

Work-up

1. History: Duration and rate of decreased vision? Frequent change in eyeglass prescriptions? History of eye rubbing? Medical problems? Allergies?
2. Slit-lamp examination. (NOTE Fleischer's ring is sometimes best seen with the blue light of the slit lamp.)
3. Retinoscopy and refraction. Look for irregular astigmatism and a waterdrop or scissors red reflex.
4. Computed corneal topography (can show central and inferior steepening) and keratometry (irregular mires and steepening).

Treatment

1. Patients are instructed not to rub their eyes.
2. Correct refractive errors with glasses (for mild cases) or rigid gas permeable contact lenses (successful in most cases).
3. Corneal transplant surgery is usually indicated when contact lenses cannot be tolerated or no longer produce satisfactory vision because of corneal scarring.
4. Thermokeratoplasty, epikeratophakia, and lamellar keratoplasty are occasionally used.

CORNEAL HYDROPS

1. Cycloplegic agent (e.g., scopolamine 0.25%), sodium chloride 5% ointment, and occasionally a pressure patch.
2. Patients are instructed to remove the pressure patch in 24–48 hours and start sodium chloride 5% ointment bid until resolved (usually several weeks).

❖ **Note** *Acute hydrops does not cause corneal perforation and is not an indication for an emergent corneal transplant.*

Follow-up

Every 3–12 months depending on the progression of symptoms. After an episode of hydrops, examine the patient every 1–2 weeks until resolved.

4.24 CORNEAL DYSTROPHIES

Bilateral, inherited, progressive corneal disorders showing no signs of inflammation or corneal vascularization and without associated systemic disease.

Anterior Corneal Dystrophies

Anterior Basement Membrane Dystrophy (Map-Dot-Fingerprint Dystrophy)

Diffuse gray patches (maps), large or tiny cysts (dots), or fine refractile lines (fingerprints) in the corneal epithelium best seen with retroillumination or a broad slit-lamp beam angled from the side; spontaneous corneal epithelial defects (erosions) and associated pain and photophobia may develop, particularly upon opening the eyes after sleep. See Section 4.6 for treatment.

Meesmann's Dystrophy

Rare, autosomal dominant, epithelial dystrophy that presents in the first years of life but is usually asymptomatic until middle age. Retroillumination shows discrete, tiny epithelial vesicles diffusely involving the cornea but concentrated in the palpebral fissure. Although treatment is usually not required, a superficial keratectomy or a lamellar corneal transplant may be beneficial if visual acuity is severely affected.

Reis-Bücklers' Dystrophy

Autosomal dominant, progressive dystrophy that appears early in life. Subepithelial, gray reticular opacities are seen primarily in the central cornea. Painful episodes from recurrent erosions are relatively common and require treatment. Corneal transplant surgery may be necessary to improve vision, but the dystrophy often recurs in the graft. Superficial lamellar keratectomy may be adequate treatment in some cases.

Corneal Stromal Dystrophies

Patients with reduced vision from these conditions usually benefit from a corneal transplant.

Lattice Dystrophy

Refractile branching lines, white subepithelial dots, and scarring of the corneal stroma centrally, best seen with retroillumination. Recurrent erosions arc common (see Section 4.6). The corneal periphery is clear. Autosomal dominant.

Granular Dystrophy

White, anterior stromal deposits in the central cornea, separated by discrete clear intervening spaces. The corneal periphery is typically spared. Appears in the first decade of life but rarely becomes symptomatic before middle age. Erosions uncommon. Autosomal dominant.

Macular Dystrophy

Gray-white stromal opacities with ill-defined edges extending from limbus to limbus with cloudy intervening spaces. Can involve full thickness of the stroma, more superficial centrally and deeper peripherally. Autosomal recessive.

Central Crystalline Dystrophy of Schnyder

Fine, yellow-white anterior stromal crystals located in the central cornea. Can be associated with hyperlipidemia and hypercholesterolemia. Autosomal dominant. Work-up includes fasting serum cholesterol and triglyceride levels.

Corneal Endothelial Dystrophies

Fuchs' Dystrophy

See Section 4.25.

Posterior Polymorphous Dystrophy

Changes at the level of Descemet's membrane, including vesicles arranged in a linear or grouped pattern, gray haze, or broad bands with irregular, scalloped edges. Iris abnormalities, including iridocorneal adhesions and a decentered pupil, may be present and are occasionally associated with corneal edema. Glaucoma may occur. Usually autosomal dominant with marked variability. See "Developmental Anterior Segment Anomalies," Section 9.11, for differential diagnosis.

Congenital Hereditary Endothelial Dystrophy (CHED)

Bilateral corneal edema. Normal corneal diameter, normal IOP, no cornea guttata. See "Congenital Glaucoma," Section 9.10, for differential diagnosis. Some patients may benefit from a corneal transplant.

Types
- Autosomal recessive: Present at birth, nonprogressive, nystagmus present.
- Autosomal dominant: Presents during childhood, slowly progressive, no nystagmus. Pain, tearing, and photophobia are common.

4.25 FUCHS' ENDOTHELIAL DYSTROPHY

Symptoms

Glare and blurred vision, especially upon awakening, that may progress to severe pain. Symptoms rarely develop before 50 years of age. May be autosomal dominant.

Critical Signs

Cornea guttata and corneal stromal edema. Bilateral, but may be asymmetric.

❖ **Note** *Central cornea guttata without stromal edema is called* endothelial dystrophy, *which may progress to Fuchs' dystrophy.*

Other Signs

Fine pigment dusting on the endothelium, central epithelial edema and bullae, folds in Descemet's membrane, subepithelial scar tissue.

Differential Diagnosis

- Aphakic or pseudophakic bullous keratopathy   (History of cataract surgery, unilateral. See Section 4.28.)
- Congenital hereditary endothelial dystrophy   (Bilateral corneal edema at birth. See Section 4.24.)
- Posterior polymorphous dystrophy   (Autosomal dominant, presents early in life. Corneal endothelium shows either grouped vesicles, geographic-shaped gray lesions, or broad bands. Occasionally associated with corneal edema. Iridocorneal adhesions and pupillary abnormalities may be present. See Section 4.21.)

Work-up

1. History: Previous cataract surgery?
2. Slit-lamp examination: Cornea guttata are often best seen with retroillumination. Fluorescein staining may demonstrate ruptured bullae.
3. Measure intraocular pressure (IOP).
4. Consider corneal pachymetry to determine the central corneal thickness.

Treatment

1. Topical sodium chloride 5% drops qid and ointment qhs.
2. May gently blow warm air from a hair dryer at arm's length toward the eyes for 5–10 minutes every morning to dehydrate the cornea.
3. Reduce the IOP with antiglaucoma medications if >20–22 mm Hg (e.g., topical beta-blocker such as timolol or levobunolol 0.25–0.5% bid), if no systemic contraindications.
4. Ruptured corneal bullae are painful and should be treated as a corneal abrasion (see Section 3.2).
5. Corneal transplant surgery is usually indicated when visual acuity decreases or the disease becomes advanced and painful.

Follow-up

Every 3–4 months to check IOP and assess corneal edema. The condition progresses very slowly, and visual acuity typically remains good until epithelial edema develops.

4.26 WILSON'S DISEASE (HEPATOLENTICULAR DEGENERATION)

Symptoms

Typically, no ocular complaints. Patients experience symptoms of cirrhosis, renal disease, or neurologic dysfunction (motor, but not sensory dysfunction). Patient is usually <40 years of age at the onset of clinical manifestations. Autosomal recessive.

Critical Signs

Typically, a greenish brown band (Kayser-Fleischer ring) in the corneal periphery (it may appear red), 1–3 mm in width, at the level of Descemet's membrane (deep in the cornea). It first appears superiorly, but eventually forms a ring that involves the entire corneal periphery. The ring usually extends to the limbus, without interspersed clear cornea. Serum and urine copper levels are elevated, and the serum ceruloplasmin level is low.

Other Ocular Signs

Anterior and posterior subcapsular copper deposition, producing "sunflower" cataract.

Differential Diagnosis

- Other rare causes of a Kayser-Fleischer-like ring   (Primary biliary cirrhosis, chronic active hepatitis, progressive intrahepatic cholestasis, and rarely, multiple myeloma. Normal serum ceruloplasmin levels, no neurologic symptoms.)
- Arcus senilis   (Corneal stromal lipid deposition, first seen inferiorly and superiorly before it extends around the corneal periphery. Appears white, typically with a clear zone of cornea separating the edge of the arcus from the limbus. In patients < 40 years of age, a lipid profile with lipoprotein electrophoresis and serum cholesterol should be obtained to rule out hyperlipidemia, hyperlipoproteinemia, and hypercholesterolemia.)

Work-up

1. Slit-lamp examination: Narrow the beam of light to a thin slit and determine the level at which the deposition is located.
2. Gonioscopy if the Kayser-Fleischer ring is not evident on slit-lamp examination (pigment may be noted in peripheral Descemet's membrane before it is apparent on slit-lamp examination).
3. Serum copper and ceruloplasmin levels.
4. Urine copper level.

5. Serum protein electrophoresis when ceruloplasmin levels are normal.
6. Referral to an internist and a neurologist.

Treatment
Systemic therapy (e.g., penicillamine) is instituted by an internist. The ocular manifestations usually require no treatment.

Follow-up
- In conjunction with an internist and a neurologist who manage systemic therapy and monitor blood cell counts.
- Successful treatment should lead to reabsorption of the corneal copper deposition and clearing of the Kayser-Fleischer ring (although residual corneal changes may remain), and can be used as a guide for monitoring treatment. There are no ocular complications of a Kayser-Fleischer ring.

4.27 CORNEAL GRAFT REJECTION

Symptoms
Decreased vision, mild pain, redness, and photophobia in an eye that has undergone a prior corneal transplant, usually several weeks to years previously.

Critical Signs
Any of the following suggest corneal graft rejection: New keratic precipitates (KP) or a fine line of white blood cells on the corneal endothelium (endothelial rejection line), stromal edema or cellular infiltration, subepithelial infiltrates, epithelial edema, an irregularly elevated epithelial line (epithelial rejection line).

Other Signs
Conjunctival injection (particularly circumcorneal injection), anterior-chamber cells and flare, neovascularization growing up to or extending onto the graft (typically the rejection starts near a blood vessel adjacent to the graft wound). Tearing may occur, but discharge is not present.

Differential Diagnosis
- Suture abscess or corneal infection   [May have a corneal infiltrate, hypopyon, or a purulent discharge. Cultures must be taken, including a culture of the suture (which should be removed). Steroid frequency is usually

reduced slowly rather than increased. Patients are often hospitalized and treated with fortified topical antibiotics. See Section 4.12.]

- Uveitis (May produce anterior-chamber cells and flare with KP. Often, a previous history of uveitis is obtained. It is best to treat uveitis as if it were a graft rejection.)
- Increased intraocular pressure (IOP) (A markedly elevated IOP may produce epithelial corneal edema, but few-to-no other signs of graft rejection are present, and the edema often clears after the IOP is lowered.)
- Other causes of graft failure [Corneal endothelial decompensation in the graft, recurrent disease in the graft (e.g., herpes keratitis, corneal dystrophy)].

Work-up

1. History: Time period since the corneal transplant? Current eye medications? Recent change in topical steroid regimen? Previous ocular disease leading to the corneal transplant?
2. Slit-lamp examination, looking for the critical signs listed above. Look carefully for endothelial rejection line, KP, and subepithelial infiltrates.

Treatment

1. Topical steroids (e.g., prednisolone acetate 1% q 1 h while awake and dexamethasone 0.1% ointment at night) if endothelial rejection is present. If only subepithelial infiltrates, KP, or an epithelial rejection is present, prednisolone acetate 1% qid or twice the current level of topical steroids, whichever is more, should be prescribed.
2. Cycloplegic agent (e.g., scopolamine 0.25% 2–3 times per day).
3. Consider systemic steroids (e.g., prednisone 40–80 mg po once per day) or subconjunctival steroids (e.g., betamethasone 3 mg in 0.5 ml) to be used in addition when the graft rejection does not respond to topical steroids alone or for recurrent rejection.
4. Control IOP if elevated (see "Inflammatory Open-Angle Glaucoma," Section 10.4).
5. For multiple rejection episodes or severe rejection, consider hospitalization and single-pulse dose of methylprednisolone 500 mg IV along with prednisolone acetate 1% q 1 h topically.

Follow-up

Treatment must be instituted immediately to maximize the likelihood of graft survival. Examine the patient every 3–7 days. Once improvement is noted, the steroids are tapered very slowly and may need to be maintained at low doses for months to years. IOP must be checked regularly in patients on topical steroids.

4.28 APHAKIC BULLOUS KERATOPATHY (ABK)/ PSEUDOPHAKIC BULLOUS KERATOPATHY (PBK)

Symptoms
Decreased vision, pain, tearing, photophobia, red eye; history of cataract surgery in the involved eye.

Critical Sign
Corneal edema in an eye in which the natural lens has been removed.

Other Signs
Corneal bullae, corneal neovascularization, preexisting endothelial guttata. Cystoid macular edema may be present.

Etiology
Often results from a combination of the following factors: corneal endothelial damage, intraocular inflammation, vitreous or subluxed intraocular lens touching (or intermittently touching) the cornea.

Work-up
1. Slit-lamp examination: Stain the cornea with fluorescein to check for denuded epithelium, check the position of the intraocular lens if present, determine whether vitreous is touching the corneal endothelium, and evaluate the eye for inflammation. Evaluate the contralateral eye for corneal endothelial dystrophy.
2. Check intraocular pressure (IOP).
3. Dilated fundus examination: Look for cystoid macular edema and vitreous inflammation.
4. Consider a fluorescein angiogram to help detect cystoid macular edema.

Treatment
1. Topical sodium chloride 5% drops qid and ointment qhs if epithelial edema is present.
2. Reduce IOP with antiglaucoma medications if elevated (e.g., >20 mm Hg). Avoid epinephrine derivatives if possible because of the risk of cystoid macular edema. See "Primary Open-Angle Glaucoma," Section 10.1.
3. Ruptured epithelial bullae (producing corneal epithelial defects) may be treated with an antibiotic ointment (e.g., erythromycin), a cycloplegic (e.g., scopolamine 0.25%), and pressure patching for 24–48 hours. A bandage

soft contact lens or anterior stromal puncture can be used for recurrent ruptured epithelial bullae (see Section 4.6).

4. Corneal transplant surgery (possibly including intraocular lens repositioning, replacement, or removal) is indicated when vision fails or the disease becomes advanced and painful.

❖ **Note** *Poor vision may be the result of cystoid macular edema or corneal disease, and the role of each may be difficult to determine.*

Follow-up

In 24–48 hours if the patient is being patched. Otherwise, every 2–6 months, depending on the symptoms.

CONJUNCTIVA/SCLERA/ EXTERNAL DISEASE

5.1 ACUTE CONJUNCTIVITIS

Characterized by a discharge and/or eyelid sticking (worse in the morning), red eye (due to conjunctival injection), and foreign-body sensation of less than 4 weeks' duration. Superficial punctate keratitis (SPK) may be present. Specific signs and symptoms of the individual entities are noted in the following section. A follicular reaction is typically seen with adenoviral, herpes, and prolonged toxic conjunctivitis. See "Red Eye" in Chapter 1 for other diseases that may present similarly.

Hyperacute Onset (within 12 hours)

Gonococcal Conjunctivitis (GC)

Critical Sign
Severe purulent discharge.

Other Signs
Conjunctival papillae, marked chemosis, preauricular adenopathy.

Work-up
Conjunctival scrapings for culture and sensitivities [e.g., blood agar, chocolate agar (37°, 10% CO_2), and Thayer-Martin plate, if available] and immediate Gram's stain.

The Wills Eye Manual: Office and Emergency Room Diagnosis and Treatment of Eye Diseases, Second Edition, edited by R. Douglas Cullom, Jr., M.D., and Benjamin Chang, M.D. © 1994 J. B. Lippincott Company.

Treatment

Initiated if the Gram's stain shows gram-negative intracellular diplococci or there is a high suspicion of GC clinically. Our therapeutic regimen is as follows:

1. Ceftriaxone 1 g IM in single dose. If corneal involvement exists, or the examiner is unable to visualize the cornea because of chemosis and lid swelling, then hospitalize the patient and treat with ceftriaxone 1 g IV q 12–24 h. Care must be taken to look for peripheral corneal ulcers under the swollen lids, which may develop rapidly and perforate. The duration of treatment depends on the clinical response.
2. Topical bacitracin or erythromycin ointment qid or ciprofloxacin drops q 2 h.
3. Eye irrigation with saline qid until the discharge is eliminated.
4. Tetracycline or erythromycin 250–500 mg po qid or doxycycline 100 mg po bid for 2–3 weeks (treatment for chlamydia, which may also be present).

❖ **Note** *If the patient is penicillin/cephalosporin-allergic, an infectious disease consult is obtained.* Neisseria meningitidis *is also a cause of hyperacute conjunctivitis.*

Follow-up

The patient needs to be examined every day until consistent improvement is noted, at which point reexamination is performed every 2–3 days until the condition resolves. The patient and sexual partners need to be evaluated by their medical doctors for other sexually transmitted diseases.

Acute Onset

Viral Conjunctivitis (usually adenoviral)

A recent upper respiratory tract infection or contact with someone with red eye is common. It generally starts in one eye and a few days later involves the contralateral eye.

Critical Sign

Tarsal conjunctival follicles.

Other Signs

Watery mucus discharge, red and edematous eyelids, palpable preauricular node (PAN), pinpoint subconjunctival hemorrhages, membrane/pseudomembrane. Subepithelial infiltrates (SEIs) may develop several weeks after the onset of the conjunctivitis.

Treatment
1. Artificial tears (e.g., Refresh Plus) 4–8 times per day for 1–3 weeks.
2. Cool compresses several times per day for 1–2 weeks.
3. Vasoconstrictor/antihistamine (e.g., naphazoline/pheniramine) qid, if itching is severe.
   - In follow-up, topical steroids (e.g., fluorometholone or prednisolone acetate 0.125% qid) may be used for pseudomembranes or when SEIs reduce vision. The SEIs may recur after stopping the steroid. Therapy is maintained for 1 week and then slowly tapered.
   - If a membrane/pseudomembrane is present, it is gently peeled off and a topical steroid is started as described previously. If a symblepharon is forming, then the membrane/pseudomembrane should be peeled off.

Follow-up
In 1–3 weeks, but sooner if the condition worsens significantly.

❖ **Note** *Viral conjunctivitis typically gets worse for the first 4–7 days after onset and may not resolve for 2–3 weeks.*

Variants (treated the same as above)
- Pharyngoconjunctival fever—As described previously, but associated with pharyngitis and fever.
- Acute hemorrhagic conjunctivitis—As described previously, but associated with a large subconjunctival hemorrhage.

❖ **Note** *Viral conjunctivitis is very contagious, usually for 10–12 days from the day of onset. Patients should avoid touching their eyes, shaking hands with other people, sharing towels, and other similar behaviors. The patient should not attend school or camp as long as the eyes are red and weeping.*

Herpes Simplex Virus Conjunctivitis

Patients may have a known history of ocular herpes simplex.

Critical Signs
Unilateral (sometimes recurrent) follicular conjunctival reaction. Occasionally, concurrent herpetic skin vesicles along the eyelid margin or periocular skin are present. A palpable preauricular node may be found.

Treatment
If the cornea or skin is involved, see "Herpes Simplex Virus," Section 4.15.

1. Antiviral therapy [e.g., trifluorothymidine 1% (e.g., Viroptic) drops 5 times per day or vidarabine 3% ointment (e.g., Vira-A) 5 times per day].
2. Cool compresses several times per day.

Follow-up
Every 2–3 days initially, to monitor for corneal involvement, then every 1–2 weeks until resolved.

Allergic Conjunctivitis (e.g., hayfever)

Itching, watery discharge, and a history of allergies is typical.

Critical Signs
Chemosis, red edematous eyelids, conjunctival papillae, preauricular node not palpable.

Treatment
1. Eliminate the inciting agent.
2. Cool compresses several times per day.
3. Topical drops, depending on the severity.
    a. Mild: Artificial tears (e.g., Refresh Plus) 4–8 times per day.
    b. Moderate: Vasoconstrictor/antihistamine qid (e.g., naphazoline/pheniramine); these should only be used for several days at a time, as rebound vasodilation occurs after prolonged use. Ketorolac 0.5% (e.g., Acular) or levocabastine (e.g., Livostin) 4 times per day may help relieve symptoms as well.
    c. Severe: Mild topical steroid (e.g., fluorometholone qid for 1–2 weeks).
4. Consider an antihistamine (e.g., diphenhydramine 25 mg po 3–4 times per day) in moderate-to-severe cases.

Follow-up
In 1–2 weeks as needed. If topical steroids are being used, patients should be followed weekly.

Vernal/Atopic Conjunctivitis

Itching, thick ropy discharge, seasonal (spring/summer) recurrences, history of atopy. Usually seen in young patients, especially males.

Critical Signs
Large conjunctival papillae under the upper eyelid or along the limbus (limbal vernal). The upper eyelid often must be everted to make the diagnosis.

Other Signs
Superior corneal "shield" ulcer (a well-delineated sterile ulcer), limbal or palpebral raised white dots (Horner-Trantas' dots) of degenerated eosinophils, SPK.

Treatment
- If no shield ulcer is present, treat as for allergic except add topical cromolyn sodium 4% qid.
- If a shield ulcer is present:
  1. Topical steroid (e.g., fluorometholone or prednisolone acetate 1% or dexamethasone 0.1% ointment) 4–6 times per day.
  2. Topical antibiotic [e.g., erythromycin ointment tid or trimethoprim/polymyxin (e.g., Polytrim) drops qid].
  3. Cycloplegic agent (e.g., scopolamine 0.25% tid).
  4. Lodoxamide (e.g., Alomide) qid.
  5. Cool compresses qid.

Follow-up

Every 1–3 days in the presence of a shield ulcer; otherwise, every few weeks. Topical medications are tapered slowly as improvement is noted. Cromolyn sodium is maintained for the duration of the season and often reinitiated a few weeks before the next spring.

Bacterial Conjunctivitis

Critical Sign

Purulent discharge of moderate degree.

Other Signs

Conjunctival papillae, chemosis, typically without preauricular adenopathy, except in hyperacute cases.

Work-up

Conjunctival swab for routine cultures and sensitivities (blood and chocolate agars) and Gram's stain if severe.

Etiology

Common organisms are *Staphylococcus aureus* (often associated with blepharitis, phlyctenules and marginal sterile infiltrates), *Streptococcus pneumoniae,* and *Haemophilus influenzae* (especially children).

❖ **Note** *If suspect GC, then see hyperacute onset as described previously.*

Treatment

Topical antibiotic therapy [e.g., trimethoprim/polymyxin (e.g., Polytrim) qid, ciprofloxacin drops qid, or erythromycin or bacitracin ointment qid] for 5–7 days.
Haemophilus influenzae conjunctivitis should be treated with oral amoxicillin/

clavulanate (20–40 mg/kg/day in 3 divided doses) because of occasional nonocular involvement (i.e., otitis media, pneumonia, and meningitis).

❖ **Note** *Most cases of conjunctivitis are not bacterial but viral or allergic; routine use of antibiotics for the latter is discouraged.*

Follow-up
Every 1–2 days initially, then every 2–5 days until resolved. Antibiotic therapy is adjusted according to culture and sensitivity results if the condition does not respond.

Pediculosis (lice, crabs)

Typically develops from contact with pubic lice (usually sexually transmitted).

Critical Sign
Adult lice, nits, and blood-tinged debris on the eyelids and eyelashes.

Other Signs
Conjunctival follicles.

Treatment
1. Mechanical removal of lice and eggs with jewelers forceps, if feasible.
2. Any bland ophthalmic ointment to the eyelids tid for 10 days to smother the lice and nits. Physostigmine 0.25% (e.g., Eserine) ointment to the eyelids, 2 applications 1 week apart may be used instead, but this therapy has ocular side effects.
3. Anti-lice (e.g., Kwell, Nix, Rid) lotion and shampoo as directed to *non*ocular areas for patient and close contacts.
4. Thoroughly wash all clothes, sheets, and other linens.

Chlamydial Conjunctivitis

See "Chronic Conjunctivitis," Section 5.2.

Toxic Conjunctivitis

See "Chronic Conjunctivitis," Section 5.2.

Molluscum Contagiosum

See "Chronic Conjunctivitis," Section 5.2.

Neonatal Conjunctivitis

See "Ophthalmia Neonatorum," Section 9.8.

Stevens-Johnson Syndrome

See "Stevens-Johnson Syndrome," Section 14.9.

Ocular Pemphigoid

See "Ocular Cicatricial Pemphigoid," Section 5.9.

❖ **Note** *Many systemic diseases can cause a nonspecific conjunctivitis (e.g., measles, mumps, influenza). The underlying disease should be managed appropriately; the eyes are treated with artificial-tear drops 4–8 times per day or artificial-tear ointment 2–3 times per day as needed.*

5.2 CHRONIC CONJUNCTIVITIS

Discharge or eyelid sticking, red eye (due to conjunctival injection), and ocular irritation of longer than 4 weeks' duration. Superficial punctate keratitis (SPK) may be present. A follicular reaction is typically seen with chlamydial diseases, toxicity, and Parinaud's oculoglandular conjunctivitis.

Chlamydial Inclusion Conjunctivitis

Sexually transmitted, typically found in teenagers and young adults. A history of vaginitis, cervicitis, or urethritis may be present.

Signs

Inferior tarsal conjunctival follicles, superior corneal pannus, palpable preauricular node (PAN), and/or tiny, gray-white peripheral subepithelial infiltrates. A stringy, mucous discharge is typical.

Work-up

1. History: (Duration of red eye? Prior treatment? Concomitant vaginitis, cervicitis, or urethritis? Sexual contacts with chlamydia?)
2. Slit-lamp examination.
3. Direct chlamydial immunofluorescence test and/or chlamydial culture of conjunctiva. Topical fluorescein can interfere with immunofluorescence tests.
4. Conjunctival scraping for Giemsa stain: Shows basophilic intracytoplasmic inclusion bodies in epithelial cells, polymorphonuclear leukocytes, and lymphocytes.

Treatment

1. Tetracycline 250–500 mg po qid, doxycycline 100 mg po bid, or erythromycin 250–500 mg po qid for 3 weeks is given to the patient and sexual partners.[1]
2. Erythromycin, tetracycline, or sulfacetamide ointment 2–3 times per day for 2–3 weeks.

Follow-up

In 1–3 weeks, depending on the severity. The patient and sexual partners should be evaluated by their medical doctors for other sexually transmitted diseases.

Trachoma

Principally occurs in underprivileged countries in areas of poor sanitation and crowded conditions (eye-to-eye spread).

Signs

Stage 1   Superior tarsal immature follicles, mild superior superficial punctate keratitis (SPK) and pannus, often preceded by purulent discharge and tender PAN.

Stage 2   Florid superior tarsal follicular reaction (IIa) and/or papillary hypertrophy (IIb) associated with superior corneal subepithelial infiltrates, pannus, and limbal follicles.

Stage 3   Follicles and scarring of superior tarsal conjunctiva.

Stage 4   No follicles, extensive conjunctival scarring.

Late complications   Severe dry eyes, trichiasis, entropion, keratitis, corneal scarring, superficial fibrovascular pannus, Herbert's pits (scarred limbal follicular) corneal bacterial superinfection, and ulceration.

Work-up

1. History of exposure to endemic area (i.e., North Africa, Middle East, India, Southeast Asia, rarely in USA)
2. Exam and diagnostic studies as noted for chlamydial inclusion conjunctivitis, described previously.

Treatment

1. Tetracycline or erythromycin 250–500 mg po qid or doxycycline 100 mg bid for 3–4 weeks.[1]

---

[1]The tetracyclines are contraindicated in children younger than 8 years of age, pregnant women, and breast-feeding mothers.

2. Tetracycline, erythromycin, or sulfacetamide ointment 2–4 times per day for 3–4 weeks.

Follow-up

Every 2–3 weeks initially, then as needed. While the previously described treatment is usually curative, reinfection is common if hygienic conditions do not improve.

Molluscum Contagiosum

Critical Sign

Dome-shaped, usually multiple, umbilicated, shiny nodules on the eyelid or eyelid margin.

Other Signs

Follicular conjunctival response from toxic viral products, corneal pannus.

Treatment

Removal of lesions by simple excision, incision and curettage, or cryosurgery.

Follow-up

Every 2–4 weeks until the conjunctivitis resolves.

Toxic Conjunctivitis (eye drops)

Signs

Inferior papillary reaction, especially with aminoglycosides, antivirals, and preservatives. With long-term use, usually >1 month, a follicular response may be seen with atropine, miotics, epinephrine agents, and antivirals. Inferior SPK and scant discharge is noted.

Treatment

Discontinuing the offending eye drop, if possible, is usually sufficient. Artificial tears without preservatives (e.g., Refresh Plus) 4–8 times per day may help as well.

Follow-up

In 1–2 weeks, as needed.

Silent Dacryocystitis

See "Acute Dacryocystitis," Section 6.8.

Parinaud's Oculoglandular Conjunctivitis

See "Parinaud's Oculoglandular Conjunctivitis," Section 5.3.

5.3 PARINAUD'S OCULOGLANDULAR CONJUNCTIVITIS

Symptoms

Red eye, mucopurulent discharge, foreign-body sensation.

Critical Signs

Granulomatous nodule(s) on the palpebral conjunctiva, visibly swollen preauricular or submandibular lymph node on the same side.

Other Signs

Fever, rash, follicular conjunctivitis.

Etiology

- Cat scratch disease   [Often a history of being scratched or licked by a cat within 2 weeks prior to the onset of symptoms (most common cause).]
- Tularemia   (History of contact with rabbits, other small wild animals, or ticks. Patients have severe headache, fever, and other systemic manifestations.)
- Tuberculosis and other mycobacteria
- Syphilis
- Others   (Leukemia, lymphoma, mumps, mononucleosis, fungi, sarcoidosis, and others.)

Work-up

[Initiated when etiology is not known (e.g., no recent cat scratch)]

1. Conjunctival biopsy with scrapings for Gram's, Giemsa, and acid-fast stains.
2. Blood, Lowenstein-Jensen, Sabouraud's, and thioglycolate cultures.
3. Complete blood count, RPR, FTA-ABS, and, if the patient is febrile, blood cultures.
4. Chest x-ray, PPD, and anergy panel.
5. If tularemia is suspected, serologic titers are necessary.

Treatment

1. Warm compresses for tender lymph nodes.
2. Antipyretics prn.
3. Specifically:

    Cat scratch disease   The disease generally resolves spontaneously in 6 weeks. Consider tetracycline 250 mg qid for 2 weeks plus a topical antibiotic (e.g., bacitracin/polymixin B ointment or gentamicin drops qid) for 2 weeks.

Tularemia Streptomycin 1 g IM bid for 7 days and gentamicin drops q 2 h for 1 week then 5 times per day until resolved. Refer to a medical internist for systemic management.

Tuberculosis Refer to an internist for antituberculous medication (e.g., isoniazid and rifampin).

Syphilis Systemic penicillin (dose depends on the stage of the syphilis) and topical tetracycline ointment. See Section 14.2.

Follow-up
Repeat the ocular examination in 1–2 weeks.

5.4 SUBCONJUNCTIVAL HEMORRHAGE

Symptoms
Red eye, may have mild irritation.

Critical Sign
Blood underneath the conjunctiva, often in a sector of the eye. Following trauma, the entire view of the sclera may be obstructed by blood.

Etiology
- Valsalva (e.g., coughing or straining)
- Traumatic (May be isolated or associated with a retrobular hemorrhage or ruptured globe.)
- Hypertension
- Bleeding disorder
- Idiopathic

Differential Diagnosis
- Kaposi's sarcoma (Red or purple lesion beneath the conjunctiva, usually elevated slightly. These patients should be evaluated for AIDS.)
- Other conjunctival neoplasms (e.g., lymphoma) with secondary hemorrhage.

Work-up
1. History: Bleeding or clotting problems? Medications (e.g., aspirin, Coumadin)? Eye rubbing, trauma, heavy lifting or Valsalva? Recurrent subconjunctival hemorrhage? Acute or chronic cough?

2. Ocular examination: Rule out a conjunctival lesion and check intraocular pressure (IOP). In traumatic cases, rule out a ruptured globe (abnormally deep anterior chamber, significant subconjunctival edema, hyphema, vitreous hemorrhage, and/or limitation of extraocular motility) and a retrobulbar hemorrhage (associated with proptosis, increased IOP, and occasionally, conjunctival swelling).
3. Check blood pressure.
4. If the patient has recurrent subconjunctival hemorrhages or a history of bleeding problems, a bleeding time, prothrombin time, partial thromboplastin time, and complete blood count with platelets should be obtained and a medical consultation considered. In addition, elective use of aspririn products should be discouraged.

Treatment

None required. Artificial-tear drops (e.g., Refresh Plus) qid can be given if mild ocular irritation is present.

Follow-up

This condition usually clears spontaneously within 1–2 weeks. Patients are told to return if the blood does not fully resolve or if they suffer a recurrence. Referral to an internist or family physician should be made as indicated for hypertension or a bleeding diathesis.

5.5 SUPERIOR LIMBIC KERATOCONJUNCTIVITIS (SLK)

Symptoms

Red eye, burning, foreign-body sensation, pain, tearing, mild photophobia. The course may be chronic with exacerbations and remissions.

Critical Sign

Thickening and inflammation of the superior bulbar conjunctiva, especially at the limbus.

Other Signs

Papillae on the superior palpebral conjunctiva; fine punctate fluorescein staining on the superior cornea, limbus, and conjunctiva; superior corneal micropannus and filaments. Usually bilateral.

Work-up

1. History: Recurrent episodes?
2. Slit-lamp examination with fluorescein staining, particularly of the superior cornea and adjacent conjunctiva. The upper eyelid often must be lifted by the examiner to see the superior limbal area, and then should be everted to visualize the tarsus. Sometimes the localized thickening, inflammation, and staining of the superior bulbar conjunctiva is best appreciated by direct inspection without a slit lamp.
3. Thyroid function tests (T3, T4, TSH), because 50% of patients have associated dysthyroid disease.

Treatment

MILD

1. Artificial tears (e.g., Refresh Plus) 4–8 times per day.
2. Artificial-tear ointment (e.g., Refresh PM) qhs.

MODERATE-TO-SEVERE

1. Silver nitrate 0.5-1.0% solution (from wax ampules) applied on a cotton-tipped applicator for 10–20 seconds to the superior tarsal and superior bulbar conjunctiva after topical anesthesia (e.g., proparacaine), then antibiotic ointment (e.g., erythromycin) qhs for 1 week.

❖ **Note** *Do* not *use silver nitrate cautery sticks, which cause severe burns.*

2. If significant amounts of mucus or filaments are present, then acetylcysteine 10% drops (e.g., Mucomyst) 3–5 times per day are usually added.
3. If 3–4 separate silver nitrate solution applications are unsuccessful, then consider mechanical scraping, cryotherapy, cautery, or surgical resection or recession of the superior bulbar conjunctiva.
4. Dry eye syndrome and/or blepharitis must be treated if present (see the appropriate sections).

Follow-up

Every week during an exacerbation. If signs and symptoms persist, a reapplication of silver nitrate solution as described previously may be performed at the weekly follow-up visit.

5.6 EPISCLERITIS

Symptoms

Acute onset of redness and mild pain in one or both eyes, typically in young adults; a history of recurrent episodes is common.

Critical Signs

Sectorial (and less commonly, diffuse) redness of one or both eyes, mostly due to engorgement of the episcleral vessels. These vessels are large, run in a radial direction, and can be seen beneath the conjunctiva.

Other Signs

Tenderness over the area of episcleral injection or a nodule that can be moved slightly over the underlying sclera may be seen. The cornea is rarely affected, and there are no aqueous cells nor flare. Vision is normal.

Etiology

- Idiopathic   (Most common.)
- Collagen-vascular disease (e.g., rheumatoid arthritis, polyarteritis nodosa, systemic lupus erythematosus, Wegener's granulomatosis)
- Gout   (Serum uric acid elevated.)
- Herpes zoster virus   (Scars from an old facial rash may be present.)
- Syphilis (FTA-ABS–positive.)
- Others   (e.g., Lyme disease, hepatitis B, Crohn's disease)

Differential Diagnosis

- Scleritis   [Pain is deep, severe, and often radiates to the ipsilateral side of the head or face. The sclera may have a bluish hue when observed in natural light. Scleral (and deep episcleral) vessels, as well as conjunctival and superficial episcleral vessels, are injected. The scleral vessels do not blanch on application of topical phenylephrine 2.5%. Corneal involvement may be present.]
- Iritis   (Cells and flare are present in the anterior chamber. May be present with scleritis. See Section 5.7.)
- Conjunctivitis   (Characterized by a discharge, eyelids sticking together in the morning, and inferior tarsal conjunctival follicles or papillae. See Sections 5.1 and 5.2.)

Work-up

1. History: Rash? Arthritis? Venereal disease? Recent viral illness? Medical problems?
2. External examination in natural light: Look for the bluish hue of scleritis.
3. Slit-lamp examination: Anesthetize (e.g., topical proparacaine) and move the conjunctiva with a cotton-tipped applicator to determine the depth of the injected blood vessels. Determine whether there is any corneal or anterior-chamber involvement. Check intraocular pressure (IOP).
4. Place a drop of phenylephrine 2.5% in the affected eye and reexamine the vascular pattern 10–15 minutes later. Episcleral vessels should blanch.
5. If the history suggests an underlying etiology, the appropriate laboratory tests should be obtained (e.g., ANA, rheumatoid factor, ESR, serum uric acid level, RPR, FTA-ABS).

Treatment
- If mild, treat with artificial tears (e.g., Refresh Plus) qid or a topical vasoconstrictor/antihistamine (e.g., naphazoline/pheniramine) qid.
- If moderate to severe, a topical steroid (e.g., fluorometholone) qid often relieves the discomfort. Rarely, more frequent topical steroid application is necessary.
- In the very rare cases where topical steroids do not provide relief, oral nonsteroidal antiinflammatory drugs may help (e.g., ibruprofen 200–600 mg po 3–4 times per day or aspirin 325–1000 mg po 3–4 times per day, with food and/or antacids).

Follow-up
Patients placed on topical steroids are checked weekly (including an IOP check) until their symptoms have resolved. The frequency of steroid administration is then tapered. Patients treated with artificial tears or a topical vasoconstrictor/antihistamine need not be seen for several weeks for their episcleritis unless it worsens or discomfort continues. Patients are informed that episcleritis may recur in the same or contralateral eye.

5.7 SCLERITIS

Symptoms
Severe and boring eye pain (most prominent feature) which may radiate to the forehead, brow, or jaw and may awaken the patient at night. Onset is gradual in most cases. Red eye, tearing photophobia, insidious decrease in vision. Recurrent episodes are common. No discharge.

Critical Signs
Inflammation of scleral, episcleral, and conjunctival vessels (scleral vessels are deep, large vessels which cannot be moved with a cotton swab and which do not blanch with topical phenylephrine)—can be sectorial or diffuse. The sclera has a characteristic bluish hue (best seen in natural light by gross inspection) and may be thin or edematous.

Other Signs
Scleral nodules, corneal changes (peripheral keratitis, limbal guttering, and/or keratolysis), glaucoma, subretinal granuloma, uveitis, exudative retinal detachment (RD), cataract, proptosis (posterior scleritis), or rapid onset hyperopia (posterior scleritis).

❖ **Note** *The patient should be examined in all directions of gaze in daylight or with adequate room illumination without a slit lamp.*

Classification
Diffuse anterior scleritis:

* Widespread inflammation of the anterior segment.

Nodular anterior scleritis:

* Immovable inflamed nodule(s).

Necrotizing anterior scleritis with inflammation:

* Extreme pain.
* The sclera becomes transparent (choroidal pigment visible) secondary to the inflammation.
* High mortality rate due to a systemic inflammatory disease.

Necrotizing anterior scleritis without inflammation (scleromalacia perforans):

* Almost complete lack of symptoms.
* Mainly seen in patients with long-standing rheumatoid arthritis (RA).

Posterior scleritis:

* May start posteriorly or be an extension of anterior scleritis.
* May simulate an amelanotic choroidal mass.
* Exudative RD, disc swelling, retinal hemorrhage, choroidal folds, choroidal detachment.
* Restricted extraocular movements.
* Proptosis, pain, tenderness.
* Usually unrelated to systemic disease.

Etiology
Fifty percent of patients with scleritis have an associated systemic disease.

More common   Connective tissue disease (e.g., RA, ankylosing spondylitis, systemic lupus erythematosus, polyarteritis nodosa, Wegener's granulomatosis), post–herpes zoster ophthalmicus, syphilis, gout.

Less common   Tuberculosis (TB), other bacteria (*Pseudomonas* species), Lyme disease, sarcoidosis, hypertension, foreign body, status postsurgery parasite.

Differential Diagnosis
* Episcleritis   (Sclera not involved. Blood vessels blanch with topical phenylephrine. More acute onset than scleritis.)

Work-up

1. History: Previous episodes? Medical problems?
2. Examine the sclera in natural light or adequate room light.
3. Slit-lamp examination with a red-free filter (green light) to determine whether avascular areas of the sclera exist.
4. Dilated fundus examination to rule out posterior involvement.
5. Complete physical examination (especially joints, skin, cardiovascular and respiratory systems, often performed by an internist or rheumatologist).
6. Complete blood count, ESR, uric acid, RPR, FTA-ABS, rheumatoid factor, ANA, fasting blood sugar.
7. Serum anti-neutrophilic cytoplasmic antibody (ANCA) can be obtained if Wegener's granulomatosis is suspected.
8. Other tests if clinical suspicion warrants additional work-up: PPD with anergy panel, chest x-ray, x-ray of sacroiliac joints, B-scan ultrasonography to detect posterior scleritis, MRI or CT scan if indicated.

Treatment

1. Symptomatic scleritis: One or more of the following may be required. [An antacid or H$_2$-blocker (e.g., ranitidine 150 mg po bid) is often used in conjunction.]
   a. Nonsteroidal antiinflammatory drug (NSAID; e.g., ibuprofen 400–600 mg po qid or indomethacin 25 mg po tid for at least 1 week).
   b. Systemic steroids: Highly recommended in the presence of severe or necrotizing scleritis, pronounced uveitis, or areas of vascular closure diagnosed by slit-lamp examination or fluorescein angiogram or after no response to the NSAID (e.g., prednisone 60–100 mg po once per day for several days, then taper slowly. The addition of a NSAID often facilitates the tapering of the steroid.)
   c. Immunosuppressive therapy (e.g., cyclophosphamide): Particularly useful in patients with systemic vasculitis, polyarteritis nodosa, and Wegener's granulomatosis. It can be used as an adjunct when high-dose steroids alone cannot improve the disease. Use in collaboration with an internist or rheumatologist.
   d. Surgery: Only when persistence of scleritis is thought to be caused by production of local antibodies following a local ocular problem (e.g., foreign body, parasite, caterpillar hair).
2. Scleromalacia perforans: No ocular treatment is available. Patients are referred to a rheumatologist for systemic treatment and consideration of immunosuppression, as the associated systemic disease is often severe

❖ **Note** *Glasses or an eye shield should be worn at all times if there is significant corneal thinning and a risk of perforation with minor trauma.*

Follow-up
Depends on the severity of the symptoms and the degree of corneal thinning.

❖ **Notes**
   1. Decreased pain is a sign of response to treatment, even if inflammation appears unchanged.
   2. Topical steroids are rarely indicated in scleritis and are not effective. (A trial of topical steroids can be given to distinguish between episcleritis and scleritis since the former will often respond.)
   3. Subconjunctival steroids are contraindicated *in scleritis and may lead to scleral thinning and perforation at the injection sites.*

5.8 OCULAR ROSACEA

Symptoms
Bilateral chronic ocular irritation, redness, burning, and foreign-body sensation. Patients are typically middle-aged adults.

Critical Signs
Telangiectasias, pustules, papules, and/or erythema of the cheeks, forehead, and nose. The findings may be subtle and are often best seen in natural light. Superficial or deep corneal vascularization, particularly in the inferior cornea, is sometimes seen, and it may extend into a stromal infiltrate.

Other Signs
Rhinophyma of the nose occurs in the late stages of the disease. Blepharitis (telangiectasias of the eyelid margin with inflammation) and chalazia are common. Conjunctival injection, superficial punctate keratitis (SPK), phlyctenules, perilimbal infiltrates of staphylococcal hypersensitivity, iritis, or even corneal perforation may occur.

Differential Diagnosis
   • Herpes simplex keratitis (Usually unilateral. The keratitis is often dendritic, but may appear similar. The typical facial lesions of rosacea are absent.)
   • See "Superficial Punctate Keratitis," Section 4.1, for additional differential diagnoses.

Work-up
   1. External examination: Look at the face for the characteristic skin findings and inspect the eyelids for chalazia.

2. Slit-lamp examination: Look for telangiectasias of the eyelid margins, conjunctival injection, and corneal vascularization, in particular, inferiorly.
3. Perform Schirmer's test (see Section 4.2).

Treatment

1. Tetracycline 250 mg po qid or doxycycline 100 mg po bid for 3–6 weeks; taper the dose slowly once relief of symptoms is obtained. Some patients are maintained on low-dose tetracycline (e.g., 250 mg q day) indefinitely if active disease recurs when the patient is off medication. Erythromycin, in the same dose as tetracycline, may be substituted if tetracycline or doxycycline cannot be used (e.g., in a pregnant woman or a nursing mother.)

❖ **Note** *Patients diagnosed with ocular rosacea who are asymptomatic and who do not demonstrate progressively worsening eye disease need not be treated with oral antibiotics.*

2. Warm compresses and eyelid hygiene for blepharitis or meibomianitis (see Section 5.10). Treat dry eyes if present (see Section 4.2).
3. Treat chalazia as needed (see Section 6.1).
4. Corneal perforations may be treated with cyanoacrylate adhesive if small, whereas larger perforations may require surgical correction. (Tetracycline is usually administered in the preoperative and postoperative periods.)
5. If infiltrates stain with fluorescein, smears, cultures, and antibiotic treatment may be necessary (see Section 4.12).

Follow-up

Variable; depends on the severity of disease. Patients without corneal involvement are seen weeks to months later. Those with corneal disease are examined more often.

❖ **Note** *Tetracycline and doxycycline should not be given to pregnant women, nursing women, or children <8 years of age. Patients should be told to take the tetracycline on an empty stomach and be warned of susceptibility to sunburn while on tetracycline and doxycycline.*

5.9 OCULAR CICATRICIAL PEMPHIGOID

Symptoms

Insidious onset of redness, foreign-body sensation, tearing, and photophobia. Bilateral involvement. The course is characterized by remissions and exacerbations. Usually occurs in patients >55 years of age.

Critical Signs

Inferior symblepharon (linear folds of conjunctiva connecting the palpebral conjunctiva of the lower eyelid to the inferior bulbar conjunctiva), foreshortening and tightness of the lower fornix.

Other Signs

Superficial punctate keratitis (SPK), secondary bacterial conjunctivitis, corneal ulcer. Later, poor tear film resulting in severe dry eye syndrome, entropion, trichiasis, corneal opacification with pannus and keratinization, obliteration of the fornices with eventual limitation of ocular motility, and ankyloblepharon can occur. Open-angle glaucoma may be present also.

Systemic Signs

Mucous membrane (nose, oral cavity, pharynx, larynx, esophagus, anus, vagina, urethra) vesicles, scarring and/or strictures; ruptured or formed bullae; denuded epithelium. In the mouth, a desquamative gingivitis is common. Vesicles and bullae may also be noted on the skin, sometimes with erythematous plaques or scars near affected mucous membranes.

Differential Diagnosis

- Stevens-Johnson syndrome (erythema multiforme major)   [Acute onset, usually with fever and malaise. Similar ocular involvement as ocular pemphigoid. The lips are typically swollen and crusted and target lesions of the skin (red centers surrounded by a pale zone) are often found. Often precipitated by drugs (e.g., sulfa, other antibiotics, dilantin) or infections (e.g., herpes and mycoplasma).]
- Membranous conjunctivitis with scarring   (Usually adenovirus or beta-hemolytic streptococcus. Symblepharon can follow any severe membranous/pseudomembranous conjunctivitis.)
- Severe chemical burn.
- Chronic topical medicine (e.g., epinephrine, pilocarpine, antiviral agents).
- Others   (Atopic keratoconjunctivitis, radiation treatment, squamous cell carcinoma).

Work-up

1. History: Chronic topical medications? Acute onset of severe systemic illness in the past?
2. Skin and mucous membrane (especially the mouth) examination.
3. Slit-lamp examination: especially examine for inferior symblepharon. (Pull down the lower eyelid and have the patient look up.) Check intraocular pressure (IOP).
4. Gram's stain and culture of the conjunctiva if secondary bacterial infection is suspected.

5. Consider a conjunctival biopsy for immunofluorescence studies.
6. Dermatology; ear, nose, and throat; gastrointestinal; and pulmonary consults if needed.

Treatment

(Often needs to be coordinated with an internist and/or dermatologist.)

1. Artificial tears (e.g., Refresh Plus drops) 4–10 times per day. Can add an artificial-tear ointment (e.g., Refresh PM) 2–4 times per day and qhs.
2. Treat blepharitis vigorously with eyelid hygiene, warm compresses, and antibiotic ointment (e.g., bacitracin tid). Oral tetracycline can be used if eyelid disease is severe. See "Blepharitis/Meibomianitis," Section 5.10.
3. Goggles or glasses with sides to provide a moist environment for the eyes.
4. Punctal occlusion if puncta are not closed already by scarring.
5. Topical steroids (e.g., prednisolone acetate 1% qid) may rarely help in suppressing acute exacerbations, but be cautious of corneal melting.
6. Systemic steroids (e.g., prednisone 60 mg po once per day) may additionally help in suppressing acute exacerbations.
7. Dapsone is often used for progressive disease. Starting dose is 25 mg po for 3 days, increase by 25 mg every 4–5 days until the desired result is achieved (usually 100–150 mg po qid).

❖ **Note** *Dapsone can cause a dose-related hemolysis; therefore, complete blood count and G6PD must be checked before administration. Dapsone should be avoided in patients with G6PD deficiency. A complete blood count is made weekly as the dose is increased, every 3–4 weeks until blood counts are stable, and then every few months.*

8. Immunosuppressive agents (e.g., cyclophosphamide) are occasionally used for progressive disease.
9. Consider surgical correction of entropion and cryotherapy or electrolysis of trichiasis. (May be necessary, but carries a risk of further scarring and of provoking an acute exacerbation.)
10. Mucous membrane grafts (e.g., buccal) can be used to reconstruct the fornices if needed.
11. Consider a keratoprosthesis in an end-stage eye with apparently good macular function.

Follow-up

Every 1–2 weeks during acute exacerbations, every 1–3 months during remissions.

5.10 BLEPHARITIS/MEIBOMIANITIS

Symptoms
Itching, burning, mild pain, foreign-body sensation, tearing, crusting around the eyes on awakening.

Critical Sign
Crusty, red, thickened eyelid margins with prominent blood vessels (blepharitis) and/or inspissated oil glands at the eyelid margins (meibomianitis).

Other Signs
Conjunctival injection, swollen eyelids, mild mucus discharge, superficial punctate keratitis (SPK); acne rosacea may be present.

Treatment
See Section 5.8 in the presence of acne rosacea.

1. Scrub the eyelid margins with mild shampoo (e.g., Johnson's baby shampoo) 2 times per day on a cotton-tipped applicator or a wash cloth.
2. Warm compresses for 15 minutes qid.
3. If associated with dry eyes, then use artificial tears (e.g., Refresh) 4–8 times per day.
4. If moderately severe, then add erythromycin or bacitracin ointment to the eyelid qhs.
5. Recurrent meibomianitis can be treated with tetracycline 250 mg po qid or doxycycline 100 mg po bid for 6 weeks, then taper slowly.

❖ **Note** *Tetracycline and doxycycline should not be used in pregnant women, nursing mothers, or children <8 years of age. Erythromycin 250 mg po qid can be used instead.*

Follow-up
Follow-up in 3–4 weeks as needed. Eyelid cleaning and warm compresses may be reduced to once per day as the condition improves. They often need to be maintained indefinitely.

❖ **Note** *Rarely, intractable, unilateral or asymmetric blepharitis is the only manifestation of sebaceous-gland carcinoma.*

5.11 CONTACT DERMATITIS

Symptoms

Sudden onset of a periorbital rash or eyelid swelling, mild watery discharge.

Critical Signs

Periorbital edema, erythema, vesicles, lichenification of the skin.

Other Signs

Conjunctivitis, watery discharge; crusting of the skin may develop when secondary infection arises.

Etiology

Most commonly, eye drops and cosmetics, including nail polish.

Treatment

1. Avoid the offending agent(s).
2. Cool compresses 4–6 times per day.
3. Consider a mild steroid cream (e.g., dexamethasone cream 0.05%) applied to the periocular area 2–3 times per day for 4–5 days.
4. Consider an oral antihistamine [e.g., diphenhydramine (e.g., Benadryl) 25–50 mg po 3–4 times per day] for several days.

Follow-up

Reexamine within 1 week.

EYELID

6.1 CHALAZION/HORDEOLUM

Symptoms

Eyelid lump. swelling, pain, tenderness, erythema.

Critical Signs

Visible or palpable, well-defined subcutaneous nodule within the eyelid (in some cases, a nodule cannot be identified).

Other Signs

Blocked meibomian orifice, eyelid swelling and erythema, localized eyelid tenderness, palpable preauricular node. There may be associated blepharitis or acne rosacea.

Differential Diagnosis

- Preseptal cellulitis   (Eyelid erythema, edema, and warmth. Often, there is a periorbital skin abrasion, laceration, or site of infection. Patients may be febrile.)
- Sebaceous cell carcinoma   (Should be suspected in recurrent chalazion, thickening of both the upper of lower eyelids, and a chalazion associated with loss of the eyelashes. It usually develops in older patients. A biopsy with frozen sections can establish the diagnosis. A special request must be made for lipid stains on frozen sections.)
- Pyogenic granuloma   [Deep red, pedunculated lesion that may be associ-

The Wills Eye Manual: Office and Emergency Room Diagnosis and Treatment of Eye Diseases, Second Edition, edited by R. Douglas Cullom, Jr., M.D., and Benjamin Chang, M.D. © 1994 J. B. Lippincott Company.

ated with a chalazion/hordeolum or may develop after trauma or surgery to the conjunctiva or skin. If associated with a chalazion/hordeolum, it may be excised or treated with a topical antibiotic-steroid combination (e.g., gentamicin/prednisolone acetate qid for 1–2 weeks). Intraocular pressure must be followed if topical steroids are used.]

Work-up
1. History: Previous chalazion excision?
2. Palpate the involved eyelid, feeling for a nodule.
3. Slit-lamp examination: Evaluate the meibomian glands and evert the involved eyelid (this may allow better visualization of the nodule).

Treatment
1. Warm compresses for 15–20 minutes qid.
2. Consider a topical antibiotic (e.g., bacitracin or erythromycin ointment bid).
3. Light massage over the lesion several times a day may help.

If the chalazion does not disappear after 3–4 weeks of appropriate medical therapy and the patient wishes to have it removed, incision and curettage are performed. Rarely, an injection of steroids into the lesion is performed instead of minor surgery, especially if the chalazion is near the lacrimal apparatus (e.g., 0.2–1.0 ml of triamcinolone 40 mg/ml is injected into and around the chalazion; the total dosage depends on the size of the lesion).

❖ **Note** *A steroid injection can lead to permanent depigmentation of the skin at the injection site.*

Follow-up
Patients are not seen after instituting medical therapy unless the lesion persists beyond 3–4 weeks. Patients who have incision and curettage are reexamined in 1 week.

6.2 ECTROPION

Symptoms
Tearing, eye or eyelid irritation; may be asymptomatic.

Critical Sign
Outward turning of the eyelid margin.

Other Signs
Superficial punctate keratitis (SPK); may result from exposure keratopathy), conjunctival injection and, eventually, keratinization (may result from conjunctival drying).

Etiology
- Congenital
- Paralytic (Seventh-nerve palsy.)
- Involutional (Aging.)
- Cicatricial (Due to chemical burn, surgery, eyelid laceration scar, and others.)
- Mechanical (Due to herniated orbital fat, eyelid tumor, and others.)
- Allergic (Contact dermatitis.)

Work-up
1. History: Previous surgery, trauma, chemical burn, or seventh-nerve palsy?
2. External examination: Check orbicularis oculi function, look for an eyelid tumor, eyelid scarring, herniated orbital fat, and other causes.
3. Slit-lamp examination: Check for SPK due to exposure and evaluate conjunctival integrity.

Treatment
1. Treat exposure keratopathy with lubricating agents (see Section 4.4).
2. Treat an inflamed, exposed eyelid margin with warm compresses and antibiotic ointment (e.g., bacitracin or erythromycin tid).
3. Taping the eyelids into position with adhesive tape may be a temporizing measure.
4. Definitive treatment usually requires surgery. Surgery is delayed for 3–6 months in patients with a seventh-nerve palsy, as the ectropion may resolve spontaneously (see Section 11.8).

Follow-up
Patients with signs of corneal or conjunctival drying are reevaluated in 1–2 weeks to evaluate the efficacy of therapy. Otherwise, follow-up is not urgent.

6.3 ENTROPION

Symptoms
Ocular irritation, foreign-body sensation, tearing, red eye.

Critical Sign
Inward turning of the eyelid margin.

Other Signs
Superficial punctate keratitis (SPK) (from eyelashes contacting the globe), conjunctival injection.

Etiology
- Involutional   (Aging.)
- Cicatricial   (Due to conjunctival scarring in ocular pemphigoid, Stevens-Johnson syndrome, chemical burns, trauma, trachoma, and others.)
- Spastic   (Due to surgical trauma, ocular irritation, or blepharospasm.)
- Congenital

Work-up
1. History: Previous surgery, trauma, chemical burn, severe eye disease?
2. Slit-lamp examination: Check for SPK, conjunctival and eyelid scarring.

Treatment
See Section 6.6 if blepharospasm is present.

1. Antibiotic ointment (e.g., erythromycin or bacitracin tid) for SPK.
2. Everting the eyelid margin away from the globe and taping it in place with adhesive tape may be a temporizing measure.
3. Surgery is often required for permanent correction (spastic entropion may respond to the above measures and not require surgery).

Follow-up
If the cornea is relatively healthy, the condition does not require urgent attention. If the cornea is significantly damaged, aggressive treatment is indicated (see "Superficial Punctate Keratitis," Section 4.1).

6.4 TRICHIASIS

Symptoms
Ocular irritation, foreign-body sensation, tearing, red eye.

Critical Sign
Misdirected eyelashes rubbing against the globe.

Other Signs
SPK, conjunctival injection.

Etiology
- Chronic blepharitis   (Thickened crusty, erythematous, inflamed eyelid margin with mild discharge and telangiectatic blood vessels.)
- Entropion   (Inward turning of the eyelid margin. May be due to Stevens-

Johnson syndrome, ocular pemphigoid, chemical burns, trachoma, or others.)
- Idiopathic

Work-up
1. History: Recurrent episodes? Severe systemic illness in the past?
2. Slit-lamp examination with fluorescein staining: Evert the eyelids and inspect the palpebral conjunctiva.

Treatment
See Sections 6.3 and 5.10 for treatment of entropion and blepharitis.

1. Remove the misdirected lashes.
   a. A few misdirected lashes: Remove them at the slit lamp with fine forceps (recurrence is common).
   b. Diffuse, severe, or recurrent trichiasis: Can attempt to remove the misdirected lashes as above; however, definitive therapy generally requires electrolysis, cryotherapy, or surgery.
2. Treat SPK with antibiotic ointment (e.g., erythromycin or bacitracin tid) for several days.

Follow-up
As needed.

6.5 FLOPPY EYELID SYNDROME

Symptoms
Chronically red, irritated eye, often worst on awakening from sleep, and a mild mucus discharge. Patients are typically obese.

Critical Signs
Upper eyelid is easily everted, without an accessory finger or cotton-tipped applicator exerting counterpressure.

Other Signs
Soft and rubbery superior tarsal plate, superior tarsal papillary conjunctivitis, superficial punctate keratitis (SPK).

❖ **Note** *The symptoms are thought to result from spontaneous eversion of the upper eyelid during sleep, allowing the superior palpebral conjunctiva to rub against a pillow or mattress.*

Differential Diagnosis

All of the following may produce superior tarsal papillary conjunctivitis, but in none of them are the eyelids easily everted as described previously.

- Vernal conjunctivitis (Seasonal, itching, ropy discharge, large papillary reaction.)
- Giant papillary conjunctivitis (Often related to contact lens wear or an exposed suture.)
- Superior limbic keratoconjunctivitis (Hyperemia and thickening of the superior bulbar conjunctiva, often with filaments and corneal pannus.)
- Toxic keratoconjunctivitis (Papillae and/or follicles are usually more abundant on the inferior tarsal conjunctiva in a patient using eyedrops.)

Work-up

1. Pull the skin of the upper eyelid toward the patient's forehead and watch to see if the eyelid spontaneously everts or is abnormally lax.
2. Slit-lamp examination of the cornea and conjunctiva with fluorescein staining.

Treatment

1. Topical antibiotics or lubricants for any mild corneal or conjunctival abnormality [e.g., erythromycin ointment 2–3 times per day for SPK, then artificial-tear ointment (e.g., Refresh PM) qhs when corneal pathology resolves].
2. The eyelids are taped closed during sleep and/or an eye shield is worn to protect the eyelid from rubbing against the pillow or bed. Sometimes, an eyelid-tightening surgical procedure is performed.
3. Patients are asked to refrain from sleeping face down on their pillow or mattress.

Follow-up

Every 2–7 days initially, then every few weeks to months as the condition stabilizes.

6.6 BLEPHAROSPASM

Symptoms

Uncontrolled blinking, twitching, or closure of the eyelids; decreased vision; always bilateral.

Critical Signs

Episodic involuntary contractions of the orbicularis oculi muscles.

Other Signs

Disappears during sleep, may have uncontrollable orofacial, head, and neck movements.

Differential Diagnosis

- Hemifacial spasm   [Unilateral, contractures involve the entire side of the face, does not disappear during sleep; damage to the seventh nerve at the level of the brainstem is the most common etiology. MRI of the cerebellopontine angle should be obtained to rule out tumor. Treatment options include observation, botulism toxin injections or neurosurgical decompression of the seventh cranial nerve (Janetta procedure).]
- Ocular irritation (e.g., corneal or conjunctival foreign body, trichiasis, blepharitis, dry eye)
- Tourette's syndrome   (Multiple compulsive muscle spasms associated with utterances of bizarre sounds or vile words.)
- Tic douloureux (trigeminal neuralgia)   (Acute episodes of pain in the distribution of the fifth cranial nerve, often causing a wince or tic.)
- Tardive dyskinesia   (Orofacial dyskinesia, often with restlessness and dystonic movements of the trunk and limbs, typically from long-term use of antipsychotic medications.)
- Eyelid myokymia   (Eyelid twitches, often brought on by stress and caffeine.)

Work-up

1. History: Unilateral or bilateral? Are the eyelids alone involved, or are the facial and limb muscles also involved? Medication?
2. Slit-lamp examination: Search for a local ocular disorder.
3. Neuro-ophthalmic examination to rule out other accompanying abnormalities.
4. CT scan (axial and coronal views) and/or MRI of the posterior fossa in atypical cases.

Treatment

1. Treat any underlying eye disorder (e.g., treat dry eye/blepharitis with eyelid hygiene and artificial tears 4–6 times per day).
2. Consider botulinum toxin injections into the orbicularis muscles around the eyelids if the blepharospasm is severe (usually lasts 3–4 months).
3. If the spasm is not relieved with botulinum toxin injections, consider surgical excision of the orbicularis muscle from the upper eyelids and brow.

Follow-up
Not an urgent condition, but with severe blepharospasm, patients can be functionally blind.

6.7 CANALICULITIS

Symptoms
Tearing or discharge, red eye, mild tenderness over the nasal aspect of the lower or upper eyelid.

Critical Signs
Erythmatous pouting punctum, erythema of the skin surrounding the punctum. Mucopurulent discharge or concretions may be expressed from the punctum when pressure is applied over the nasal corner of the lower eyelid (the lacrimal sac).

Other Signs
Recurrent conjunctivitis confined to the nasal aspect of the eye, gritty sensation on probing of the canaliculus.

Etiology
- Actinomyces israelii (streptothrix)   (Most common; Gram positive rod with fine, branching filaments seen on Gram's stain.)
- Fungal (e.g., *Candida, Fusarium,* and *Aspergillus* species)
- Viral (e.g., herpes simplex and varicella-zoster)
- Other bacteria (e.g., *Fusobacterium* and *Nocardia* species)

Differential Diagnosis
- Dacryocystitis   (Much more swelling, tenderness, and pain than canaliculitis. Swelling of the skin is more prominent than pouting of the punctum.)
- Nasolacrimal duct obstruction   (Tearing, minimal-to-no erythema nor tenderness around the punctum.)
- Conjunctivitis   (Conjunctival follicles and/or papillae, discharge. No pouting punctum nor punctal discharge.)

Work-up
1. Apply gentle pressure over the lacrimal sac with a cotton-tipped swab and roll it toward the punctum; observe for a punctal discharge.
2. Smears and cultures of the material expressed from the punctum: Gram's stain, Giemsa stain, and a KOH smear if available (1 drop of KOH 10–20%

is placed on a slide, the discharge is added to the drop with a spatula, and a cover-slip is placed over the mixture before microscopic examination); consider thioglycolate and Sabouraud's cultures.

Treatment
1. Remove obstructing concretions. Can try expressing the concretions through the punctum at the slit lamp, but a surgical canaliculotomy (with marsupialization of the canaliculus) is usually required to remove them all.
2. After removing the concretions, irrigate the canaliculus with penicillin G solution 100,000 units/ml or iodine 1% solution. The patient is irrigated while in the upright position so the solution drains out of the nose and not into the nasopharynx.

   If a fungus is found on smears and cultures, nystatin 1:20,000 drops tid and nystatin 1:20,000 solution irrigation several times per week may be effective.

   If a herpes virus is found on smears, treat with trifluorothymidine 1% drops (e.g., Viroptic) 5 times per day for several weeks. Silicone intubation is sometimes required in viral cases, along with appropriate antiviral therapy.

3. Warm compresses to the punctal area qid.
4. More extensive surgical treatment is occasionally required.

Follow-up
This is generally not an urgent condition.

6.8 DACRYOCYSTITIS
INFLAMMATION OF THE LACRIMAL SAC

Symptoms
Pain, redness, and swelling over the innermost aspect of the lower eyelid (over the lacrimal sac); tearing; discharge; fever; may be recurrent.

Critical Signs
Erythematous, tender swelling centered over the nasal aspect of the lower eyelid and extending around the periorbital area nasally. A mucoid or purulent discharge can be expressed from the punctum when pressure is applied over the lacrimal sac.

Other Signs

Fistula formation (often emerging from the skin beneath the medial canthal tendon), a lacrimal sac cyst, or a mucocele can occur in chronic cases. Rarely, orbital or facial cellulitis may develop as a complication.

Etiology

Nasolacrimal duct obstruction, diverticulum of the lacrimal sac, dacryolith, nasal or sinus surgery, trauma.

Differential Diagnosis

All of the following may produce inflammation of the periorbital area nasally.

- Facial cellulitis involving the medial canthus   (Discharge cannot be expressed from the punctum by placing pressure over the lacrimal sac. The lacrimal drainage system is patent on irrigation and special lacrimal drainage system radiographic studies.)
- Acute ethmoid sinusitis   (Pain, tenderness, and erythema over the nasal bone, just medial to the inner canthus. Frontal headache and nasal obstruction are common. Patients are often febrile.)
- Acute frontal sinusitis   (Inflammation predominantly involves the upper eyelid. The forehead is tender on palpation.)

Work-up

1. History: Previous episodes? Concomitant ear, nose, or throat infection?
2. External examination, including gentle compression of the lacrimal sac (nasal corner of the lower eyelid) with a cotton-tipped swab in an attempt to express discharge from the punctum. This should be performed bilaterally to uncover a subtle contralateral dacryocystitis.
3. Ocular examination: Specifically check extraocular motility and look for proptosis (Hertel exophthalmometry).
4. Obtain a Gram's stain and blood agar culture (and chocolate agar culture in children) of any discharge expressed from the punctum.
5. Consider a CT scan (axial and coronal views) of the orbit and paranasal sinuses in atypical or severe cases or those which do not respond to, or worsen on, appropriate antibiotics.

❖ **Note** *Do not attempt to probe the lacrimal system during the acute stage of the infection.*

Treatment

1. Systemic antibiotic
   Children:
   a. Afebrile, systemically well, mild case, reliable parent: Amoxicillin/clavulanate (e.g., Augmentin) 20–40 mg/kg/day po in 3 divided doses.

Alternative treatment: Cefaclor (e.g., Ceclor) 20–40 mg/kg/day po in 3 divided doses.
  b. Febrile, acutely ill, moderate-severe case, unreliable parent: Hospitalize and treat with cefuroxime 50–100 mg/kg/day IV in 3 divided doses.
  Adults:
  a. Afebrile, systemically well, mild case, reliable patient: cephalexin (e.g., Keflex) 500 mg po q 6 h.
  Alternative treatment: Amoxicillin/clavulanate (e.g., Augmentin) 500 mg po q 8 h.
  b. Febrile, acutely ill: Hospitalize and treat with cefazolin (e.g., Ancef) 1 g IV q 8 h.
  Alternative treatment: See "Orbital Cellulitis," Section 7.4.
  The antibiotic regimen is adjusted according to the clinical response and the culture and sensitivity results. The IV antibiotics can be changed to comparable oral antibiotics depending on the rate of improvement, but systemic antibiotic therapy should be continued for a full 10- to 14-day course.
2. Topical antibiotic drops [e.g., trimethoprim/polymyxin (e.g., Polytrim) qid].
3. Warm compresses and gentle massage to the inner canthal region qid.
4. Pain medication (e.g., acetaminophen with or without codeine) prn.
5. Consider incision and drainage of a pointing abscess.
6. Consider surgical correction (e.g., dacryocystorhinostomy [DCR] with silicone intubation) once the acute episode has resolved, particularly with chronic dacryocystitis.

Follow-up
  Daily. If the condition of an outpatient worsens, hospitalization and IV antibiotics are recommended.

6.9 ACUTE INFECTIOUS DACRYOADENITIS
INFECTION OF THE LACRIMAL GLAND

Symptoms
  Unilateral pain, redness, and swelling over the outer one third of the upper eyelid, often with tearing or discharge. Typically occurs in children and young adults.

Critical Signs
  Erythema, swelling, and tenderness over the outer one third of the upper eyelid; may be associated with hyperemia of the palpebral lobe of the lacrimal gland.

Other Signs

Ipsilateral preauricular lymphadenopathy, ipsilateral conjunctival chemosis temporally, fever, elevated white blood cell count (WBC).

Etiology

- Bacterial (e.g., *Staphylococcus aureus, Neisseria gonorrhea,* streptococci)
- Viral (e.g., mumps, infectious mononucleosis, influenza, herpes zoster)

Differential Diagnosis

- Chalazion   (A palpable subcutaneous nodule or a blocked meibomian orifice may be present, afebrile, normal WBC.)
- Adenovirus conjunctivitis   (May produce eyelid swelling and erythema with preauricular lymphadenopathy and a discharge. Typically produces inferior tarsal conjunctival follicles, often bilateral.)
- Preseptal cellulitis   [Erythema, edema, and warmth of the eyelid(s) and surrounding soft tissue. May have a periorbital skin laceration or site of infection.]
- Orbital cellulitis   (Proptosis and limitation of ocular motility often accompany eyelid erythema and swelling.)
- Inflammatory dacryoadenitis from orbital pseudotumor   (No preauricular lymphadenopathy. May have concomitant proptosis, downward displacement of the globe, or limitation of ocular motility. Typically afebrile with a normal WBC. Does not respond to antibiotics, but improves dramatically with systemic steroids.)
- Malignant lacrimal gland tumor   (Commonly produces displacement of the globe or proptosis, often palpable, evident on CT scan.)

Work-up

The following is performed when an acute infectious etiology is suspected. When the disease does not respond to medical therapy or another etiology is being considered, see "Lacrimal Gland Mass," Section 7.7.

1. History: Acute or chronic? Fever? Discharge? Systemic infection or viral syndrome?
2. Palpate the eyelid and along the orbital rim for a mass.
3. Evaluate the resistance of each globe to retropulsion.
4. Look for proptosis (Hertel exophthalmometry).
5. Complete ocular examination, particularly extraocular motility assessment.
6. Smears and bacterial cultures of any discharge.
7. Examine the parotid glands (often, but not always, enlarged in mumps, sarcoidosis, tuberculosis, lymphoma, and syphilis.)
8. If the patient is febrile, a complete blood count with differential and, sometimes, blood cultures are obtained.

9. CT scan of the orbit and brain (axial and coronal views) when proptosis or a motility restriction is present or a mass is suspected.

Treatment
  A. Bacterial or infectious (but unidentified) etiology
    If mild-to-moderate: Amoxicillin/clavulanate (e.g., Augmentin)
        Adults: 250–500 mg po q 8 h.
        Children: 20–40 mg/kg/day po in 3 divided doses.
      Alternative treatment: Cephalexin (e.g., Keflex)
        Adults: 250–500 mg po q 6 h.
        Children: 25–50 mg/kg/day po in 4 divided doses.
    If moderate-to-severe: hospitalize and treat with ticaricillin/clavulanate (e.g., Timentin)
        Adults: 3.2 g IV q 4–6 h.
        Children: 200 mg/kg/day IV in 4 divided doses.
      Alternative treatment: Cefazolin (e.g., Ancef)
        Adults: 500–1000 mg IV q 6–8 h.
        Children: 50–100 mg/kg/day IV in 3–4 divided doses.
    The antibiotic regimen should be adjusted according to the clinical response and culture and sensitivity test results. IV antibiotics can be changed to comparable oral antibiotics depending on the rate of improvement, but systemic antibiotics should be continued for a full 7- to 14-day course.

    If an abscess develops, incision and drainage are necessary.

  B. Viral (e.g., mumps, infectious mononucleosis)
    1. Cool compresses to the area of swelling and tenderness.
    2. Analgesic prn (e.g., acetaminophen 650 mg po q 4 h).

❖ **Note** *Do not give aspirin to children with a viral syndrome because of the risk of Reye's syndrome.*

Follow-up
  Daily. Watch for signs or orbital involvement (decreased motility or proptosis). Outpatients are admitted to the hospital for IV antibiotic therapy and an orbital CT scan if the condition worsens. Patients who fail to respond to medical therapy are managed as those with chronic dacryoadenitis (see "Lacrimal Gland Mass," Section 7.7).

6.10 PRESEPTAL CELLULITIS

Symptoms

Tenderness and redness of the eyelid, mild fever, irritability.

Critical Signs

Eyelid erythema, edema, warmth, tenderness. No proptosis, no restriction of extraocular motility, no pain with eye movement (unlike orbital cellulitis). The patient may not be able to open the eye because of the eyelid edema.

Other Signs

Conjunctival chemosis, tightness of the eyelid skin, fluctuant lymphedema of the eyelids.

❖ **Note** *Preseptal cellulitis due to* Haemophilus influenzae *generally occurs in children <5 years of age and is characterized by the presence of an excessive amount of upper- and lower-eyelid edema, which may extend into the cheeks. Classically, there is a distinctive red-purple discoloration of the involved area. The child may have malaise, ipsilateral otitis media, sinusitis, leukocytosis, or a bacteremia.*

Etiology

Puncture wound, laceration, retained foreign body from trauma, vascular extension, or extension from sinuses or another infectious site (e.g., dacryocystitis in children, chalazion). May be primarily infectious or inflammatory with secondary infectious potential.

Organisms

S. aureus and streptococci most common, but *H. influenzae* should be considered in children. Suspect anaerobes if a foul-smelling discharge or necrosis is present or there is a history of an animal or human bite. Consider a viral cause if preseptal cellulitis is associated with a skin rash (e.g., herpes simplex or herpes zoster).

Differential Diagnosis

- Orbital cellulitis   (Proptosis, pain with eye movement, restricted motility, decreased sensation along the first division of the trigeminal nerve, decreased vision, fever, or chemosis.)
- Other orbital disorders   (Proptosis, globe displacement, or restricted ocular motility. See Section 7.1.)
- Chalazion   (Focal eyelid inflammation, palpable mass, pointing meibomian gland.)

- Allergic eyelid swelling (Sudden onset, bright-red eyelid discoloration, prominent itching, absence of tenderness, history of allergies, or new eye or skin medication.)
- Viral conjunctivitis with eyelid swelling (Conjunctival follicles, palpable preauricular lymph node, itching, tearing, eyelid sticking, or watery discharge.)
- Cavernous sinus thrombosis (Proptosis; paresis of the third, fourth, and sixth cranial nerves out of proportion with the eyelid swelling; decreased sensation of the first and second division of the trigeminal nerve; typically bilateral.)
- Erysipelas (Rapidly advancing streptococcal cellulitis, often with a clear demarcation line, high fever, and chills.)
- Others (Insect bite, angioedema, trauma, maxillary osteomyelitis, and others.)

Work-up
1. History: Pain with eye movements? Prior trauma or cancer?
2. Complete ocular examination: Look carefully for restriction of ocular motility or proptosis. An eyelid speculum or Desmarres eyelid retractor may facilitate the ocular examination if the eyelids are excessively swollen.
3. Check facial sensation in the distribution of first and second division of the trigeminal nerve.
4. Palpate the periorbital area and the head and neck lymph nodes for a mass.
5. Check vital signs.
6. Gram's stain and culture of any open wound or drainage.
7. CT scan of the brain and orbits (axial and coronal views) if there is a history of significant trauma or a concern about the possibility of an orbital or intraocular foreign body, orbital cellulitis, a subperiosteal abscess, cavernous sinus thrombosis, or cancer.
8. Consider obtaining a complete blood count with differential and blood cultures in severe cases or when a fever is present.

Treatment
1. Antibiotic therapy
    A. Mild preseptal cellulitis and age >5 years:
        Amoxicillin/clavulanate (e.g., Augmentin)
            Children: 20–40 mg/kg/day po in 3 divided doses.
            Adults: 250–500 mg po q 8 h.
        or cefaclor (e.g., Ceclor)
            Children: 20–40 mg/kg/day po in 3 divided doses; maximum dose 1 g/day.
            Adults: 250–500 mg po q 8 h.
        If the patient is allergic to penicillin, then:
            Trimethoprim/sulfamethoxazole (e.g., Bactrim)

Children: 8 mg/kg/day trimethoprim and 40 mg/kg/day sulfameth-
oxazole po in 2 divided doses.
Adults: 160 mg trimethoprim and 800 mg sulfamethoxazole po
bid.
If the patient is allergic to penicillin and sulfa drugs, then:
Erythromycin
Children: 30–50 mg/kg/day po in 3–4 divided doses.
Adults: 250–500 mg po q 6 h.

❖ **Note** *Oral antibiotics are maintained for 10 days.*

B. Moderate-to-severe preseptal cellulitis or any one of the following:
- Patient appears toxic.
- Patient may be noncompliant with outpatient treatment and follow-
up.
- Child ≤5 years of age.
- Suspect *H. influenzae.*
- No noticeable improvement or worsening after a few days of oral
antibiotics.

Admit to the hospital for IV antibiotics as follows:
Ceftriaxone
Children: 100 mg/kg/day IV in 2 divided doses.
Adults: 1–2 g IV q 12 h.
and Vancomycin
Children: 40 mg/kg/day IV in 2–3 divided doses.
Adults: 0.5–1 g IV q 12 h.

❖ **Note** *IV antibiotics can be changed to comparable oral antibiotics after significant improvement is observed. Systemic antibiotics are maintained for a
complete 10- to 14-day course. See "Orbital Cellulitis," Section 7.4, for alternative treatment.*

2. Warm compresses to the inflamed area tid prn.
3. Polymyxin B/bacitracin ointment (e.g., Polysporin) to the eye qid if secondary conjunctivitis is present.
4. Tetanus toxoid if needed (see Appendix 10).
5. Exploration and debridement of the lesion if a fluctuant mass or abscess
is present. Incise over the mass or reopen a healing laceration with a scalpel,
fully explore the wound, and Gram's stain and culture any drainage. Avoid
the orbital septum if possible. A drain may need to be placed.

Follow-up

Daily until clear and consistent improvement is demonstrated, then every 2–7 days until the condition has totally resolved. If a preseptal cellulitis progresses despite antibiotic therapy, the patient is admitted to the hospital and a repeat (or initial) orbital CT scan is obtained. For patients on oral antibiotics, IV antibiotic treatment is started (see "Orbital Cellulitis," Section 7.4).

6.11 MALIGNANT TUMORS OF THE EYELID

Symptoms

Asymptomatic or mildly irritating eyelid lump.

Signs

Skin ulceration and inflammation and distortion of the normal eyelid anatomy are common findings in malignant lesions.

Etiology

- Basal cell carcinoma (most common malignant eyelid tumor)   (Middle-aged or elderly patients.) There are two clinical presentations:
  1. Nodular: Indurated, firm mass, commonly with telangiectasia over the tumor margins. Sometimes, the center of the lesion is ulcerated.
  2. Morpheaform: Firm, flat, subcutaneous lesion with indistinct borders.

❖ **Note** *Basal cell carcinoma does not metastasize, but it may be highly locally invasive, particularly when it is present in the medial canthal region.*

- Squamous cell carcinoma   (Variable presentation, often appearing similar to a basal cell carcinoma. Metastasis may occur but is uncommon. A premalignant lesion, actinic keratosis, may appear as a scaly erythematous flat lesion or as a cutaneous horn.)
- Sebaceous gland carcinoma   (Usually occurs in middle-aged or elderly patients. Most arise from the meibomian glands. Must be considered in the presence of a recurrent "chalazion" or intractable "blepharitis," as it may simulate each of these condition. Loss of eyelashes and destruction of the meibomian gland orifices in the region of the tumor may occur. The tumor may be multifocal, involving both the upper and lower eyelids. Metastasis or orbital extension can occur.)
- Others   (Malignant melanoma; lymphoma; sweat gland carcinoma; metastasis, usually breast or lung; and others.)

Differential Diagnosis
(Benign eyelid masses)

- Seborrheic keratosis   (Middle-aged or elderly patients. Brown-black well-circumscribed, crustlike lesion, usually elevated slightly and uninflamed. May be removed by shave biopsy if desired.)
- Hordeolum (stye)   (Acute, erythmetous, tender, well-circumscribed lesion, often associated with blepharitis. See Section 6.1 for treatment.)
- Chalazion   (A chronically obstructed meibomian gland. See Section 6.1 for treatment.)
- Keratoacanthoma   [Appears similar to basal and squamous cell carcinomas, as it is elevated and possesses a central ulcer crater. These tumors, however, grow rapidly to a large size (1–2 cm) and then slowly shrink, often resolving spontaneously. Lesions that involve the eyelid or eyelash margin can be destructive and are surgically excised.]
- Cysts (e.g., epidermal inclusion, sudoriforous, sebaceous)   (Well-circumscribed white or yellow lesions on the eyelid margin or underneath the skin. Ultrasound may help differentiate a cyst from a solid lesion. May be surgically excised.)
- Molluscum contagiosum   (Frequently multiple small papules with umbilicated centers. Viral in origin. May produce a chronic follicular conjunctivitis. We usually surgically excise these lesions, but cryotherapy or other methods may be used.)
- Nevus   (Light-to-dark-brown, well-circumscribed lesion, sometimes with hair arising from the surface. It does not grow in size.)
- Xanthelasma   (Multiple, often bilateral, yellow plaques in the upper, and sometimes the lower, eyelids. Patients should have a serum cholesterol and lipid profile evaluation to rule out a cholesterol or lipid disorder. Diabetes may also be present. Cosmetic surgery can be performed as desired.)
- Others [Verrucae (viral warts), papilloma, benign tumors of hair follicles or sweat glands, inverted follicular keratosis, neurofibroma, neurilemoma, capillary hemangioma, cavernous hemangioma, pseudoepitheliomatis hyperplasia, necrobiotic xanthogranuloma nodules of multiple myeloma (yellow plaques or nodules often mistaken for xanthelasma).]

Work-up
1. History: How long has the lesion been present? Rapid or slow growth? Previous malignant skin lesion?
2. External examination: Check the skin for additional lesions, palpate the preauricular and submaxillary nodes for metastasis.
3. Slit-lamp examination: Look for telangiectasias on nodular tumors, evaluate for loss of eyelashes in the region of the tumor, and inspect the meibomian orifices to determine whether they have been destroyed.

4. Photograph and/or draw the lesion and its location for documentation.
5. Biopsy the lesion: An incisional biopsy is most commonly performed when a malignancy is suspected, although an excisional biopsy with wide margins on all sides is preferable to detect malignant melanoma. Margins of potential malignant melanoma are sent for permanent section.
6. When a sebaceous cell carcinoma is suspected, the pathologist should be alerted, and frozen or nonfixed tissue (for oil red O stain for fat) must be obtained. Patients confirmed to have this tumor are referred to a medical internist for a metastatic work-up (typically metastatic to the lymph nodes, lung, brain, liver, and bone).

Treatment

- Basal cell carcinoma: Surgical excision with histologic evaluation of the tumor margins. Cryotherapy and radiation are used rarely. Patients are informed about the etiologic role of the sun and are advised to avoid sunlight when possible and to use protective sunscreens.
- Squamous cell carcinoma: Same as for basal cell carcinoma. Radiation therapy is the second-best treatment after surgical excision. Patients are informed about the etiologic role of the sun.
- Sebaceous gland carcinoma: Surgical excision, taking wide margins of normal tissue on all sides. Frozen section evaluation of the margins is recommended.

Follow-up

After the initial follow-up period (every 1–4 weeks to ensure proper healing of the surgical site), patients are reevaluated every 6–12 months. Patients who have had one skin malignancy are at greater risk for additional malignancies.

ORBIT

7.1 ORBITAL DISEASE

This first section aids in distinguishing a variety of orbital diseases. Specific work-ups and treatments are covered in sections on the individual disease entities.

Symptoms

Eyelid swelling, bulging eye(s), and double vision are common. Pain and decreased vision can occur.

Critical Signs

Proptosis and restriction of ocular motility, which can be confirmed by forced duction testing (see Appendix 6). There is often resistance on attempted retropulsion of the globe.

Other Signs

See the individual entities.

Etiology

One or more of the critical signs are usually present, but it is the specific characteristics listed below that help to distinguish the individual entities.

- Thyroid eye disease   (Eyelid retraction and eyelid lag. Painless unless exposure keratopathy develops. Often bilateral. *CT scan:* Thickening of the extraocular muscles without involvement of the associated tendons.)
- Orbital inflammatory pseudotumor   (Often painful. The patient is usually afebrile with a normal white blood cell count [WBC]. *CT scan:* Extraocular muscles are commonly thickened, with involvement of the associated tendons. The sclera, orbital fat, or lacrimal gland may be involved. Acute disease usually responds dramatically to systemic steroids.)

The Wills Eye Manual: Office and Emergency Room Diagnosis and Treatment of Eye Diseases, Second Edition, edited by R. Douglas Cullom, Jr., M.D., and Benjamin Chang, M.D. © 1994 J. B. Lippincott Company.

- Orbital cellulitis   (Patients are usually febrile and often have an elevated WBC. *CT scan:* Sinusitis, especially ethmoid sinusitis, is usually present.)
- Orbital tumors   (A palpable mass may be present. The globe may be displaced away from the location of the tumor. *CT scan:* A mass lesion is evident.)
- Lacrimal gland tumors   (Tumor is located in the outer one third of the upper eyelid. The globe is usually is displaced inferiorly and medially with ptosis of the involved eyelid. *CT scan:* A mass lesion is present in the lacrimal gland.)
- Trauma (e.g., intraorbital foreign body, retrobulbar hemorrhage)   (An intraorbital foreign body may not produce orbital signs for a long period of time. Retrobulbar hemorrhage can result in optic-nerve compression. CT scan with or without orbital ultrasound is diagnostic.)
- Orbital vasculitis (e.g., Wegener's granulomatosis, polyarteritis nodosa)   - [Systemic signs and symptoms (especially sinus, renal, pulmonary, and skin disease), fever, markedly elevated ESR.)
- Mucormycosis   (Orbital, nasal, and sinus disease in a diabetic, immunocompromised, or debilitated patient. Life-threatening. See "Cavernous Sinus/Superior Orbital Fissure Syndrome," Section 11.8.)
- Varix   [A large dilated vein within the orbit that produces proptosis when it fills and dilates (e.g., during a Valsalva maneuver or while placing the head in the dependent position). When the vein is not engorged, the proptosis is not present. *CT scan:* Demonstrates the dilated vein if an enhanced scan is performed during a Valsalva maneuver. MRI with gadolinium may be done if CT scan is negative.]

Differential Diagnosis
- Arteriovenous fistula (e.g., carotid-cavernous fistula)   (May mimic orbital disease. It follows trauma or can occur spontaneously. A bruit is often heard by the patient and may be heard if ocular auscultation is performed. Arterialized conjunctival vessels and chemosis may be present. *CT scan:* Enlarged superior ophthalmic vein, sometimes accompanied by enlarged extraocular muscles.)
- Cavernous sinus thrombosis   (Orbital cellulitis signs, plus decreased sensation of the fifth cranial nerve, dilated and sluggish pupil, paresis of the third, fourth, and sixth cranial nerves out of proportion to the degree of orbital edema, decreasing level of consciousness, nausea, and vomiting. Usually bilateral with rapid progression.)
- Cranial-nerve palsy   (May produce mild proptosis with limitation of eye movement in specific directions. No resistance to retropulsion or on forced duction testing. Orbital CT scan is normal.)
- Enlarged globe (e.g., myopia)   (May produce pseudoproptosis. Large, myopic eyes frequently have tilted discs and peripapillary crescents, and ultrasound reveals a long axial length.)

- Enophthalmos of the fellow eye (e.g., after an orbital floor fracture)   (May produce pseudoproptosis.)

Work-up
1. History: Rapid or slow onset? Pain? Ocular bruit? Fever, chills, systemic symptoms? History of cancer, diabetes, pulmonary disease, or renal disease? Skin rash? Trauma?
2. External examination:
   a. Look from over the patient's forehead to examine for proptosis. Measure the amount with a Hertel exophthalmometer.[1]
   b. Look for displacement of the globe. Measure from the bridge of the nose with a ruler.
   c. Test for resistance to retropulsion. Have the patient close his or her eyes while gently pushing each globe back into the orbit with your thumb. Assess the resistance of each eye.)
   d. Feel along the orbital rim for a mass.
   e. Measure any ocular misalignment with prisms (see Appendix 2).
3. Ocular examination: Specifically check the pupils, visual fields, color vision (using color plates), intraocular pressure (IOP), optic nerve, and peripheral retina.
4. Orbital CT scan (axial and coronal views).
5. Occasionally, an MRI or orbital ultrasound is obtained in addition when the diagnosis is uncertain or the extent of the lesion must be better defined.
6. Vital signs, particularly temperature.
7. Laboratory tests when appropriate: T3, T4, TSH, complete blood count (CBC), ESR, ANA, blood urea nitrogen (BUN), creatinine, fasting blood sugar, blood cultures, others.
8. Consider a forced duction test (see Appendix 3 for technique.)
9. Consider an excisional, incisional, or fine-needle biopsy as dictated by the working diagnosis.

Additional work-up, treatment, and follow-up vary according to the suspected diagnosis. See individual sections.

7.2 THYROID EYE DISEASE (GRAVES' OPHTHALMOPATHY)

Ocular Symptoms
Prominent eyes, eyelid swelling, double vision, foreign-body sensation, pain, photophobia, decreased vision in one or both eyes.

---

[1]Normal upper limits for proptosis are approximately 22 mm in Caucasians and 24 mm in blacks. There should be no more than a 2-mm difference between the two eyes.

Critical Ocular Signs

Retraction of the eyelids, eyelid lag on downward gaze, and often, unilateral or bilateral proptosis. When extraocular muscles are involved, elevation and outward movement are commonly restricted. There is resistance on forced duction testing. Orbital CT scan shows thickening of the involved extraocular muscles with sparing of the tendon.

❖ **Note** *Optic-nerve compression secondary to thickened extraocular muscles at the orbital apex can produce an afferent pupillary defect, reduced color vision, and visual field and visual acuity loss. The optic disc may be swollen. Optic-nerve compression can develop in the presence of minimal exophthalmos. Involvement of more than one muscle with restriction of both elevation and horizontal eye movements is an indication that the patient is at risk for this complication.*

Other Ocular Signs

Reduced frequency of blinking (stare), injection of the blood vessels over the insertion sites of involved extraocular muscles, resistance to retropulsion, eyelid edema, superficial punctate keratitis or ulceration from exposure keratopathy.

Systemic Signs

Hyperthyroidism common [rapid pulse, hot and dry skin, diffusely enlarged thyroid gland (goiter), weight loss, muscle wasting with proximal muscle weakness, hand tremor, pretibial dermopathy or myxedema, and sometimes, cardiac arrhythmias]. Some patients are euthyroid. Myasthenia gravis with fluctuating double vision and ptosis is often present.

Differential Diagnosis

See "Orbital Disease," Section 7.1, for conditions that produce proptosis. Two rare conditions that may produce eyelid retraction or eyelid lag are:

- Third-nerve palsy with aberrant regeneration   (The upper eyelid may elevate with downward gaze, simulating eyelid lag. Ocular motility may be limited, but forced duction testing and orbital CT scan are normal.)
- Parinaud's syndrome   (Eyelid retraction and limitation of upward gaze may accompany mildly dilated pupils that react poorly to light, but react normally to convergence.)

Work-up

See "Orbital Disease," Section 7.1, for a general work-up of proptosis of unknown etiology.

1. History: Duration of symptoms? Pain? Known thyroid disease or cancer?
2. Complete ocular examination to establish the diagnosis and to determine

whether the patient is developing exposure keratopathy (slit-lamp examination with fluorescein staining) or optic-nerve compression (pupillary assessment and evaluation of color vision using color plates). Limitation of motility is measured with prisms (see Appendix 2) and proptosis is measured with a Hertel exophthalmometer. Check intraocular pressure (IOP).

3. CT scan of the orbit (axial and coronal views) is performed when the diagnosis is uncertain (e.g., proptosis is present without other signs of thyroid disease) or surgery is planned.
4. Forced duction testing as needed to establish the diagnosis (see Appendix 5).
5. Formal visual field examination when signs or symptoms of optic-nerve compression are present (e.g., Humphrey, Octopus, or Goldmann).
6. Thyroid function tests (T3, T4, TSH).
7. Edrophonium chloride (e.g., Tensilon) test for suspected myasthenia gravis (see Section 11.9).

Treatment
1. Refer the patient to a medical internist or endocrinologist for management of systemic thyroid disease, if present.
2. Treat exposure keratopathy with artificial tears and lubricating ointment (e.g., Refresh Plus drops q 1–6 h and/or Refresh PM ointment qhs–tid) or by taping eyelids closed at night (see Section 4.4).
3. Elevate the head of the bed at night if the patient is developing eyelid edema.
4. Orbital disease may need to be treated more aggressively when exposure keratopathy is worsening despite treatment (or is already severe), bothersome diplopia is present (particularly when looking straight ahead or reading), or optic-nerve compression is developing.
   The following recommendations are somewhat controversial:
   a. Proptosis and corneal ulceration: Prednisone 100 mg po once per day for 1–2 days followed by orbital decompression surgery.
   b. Acute disturbing double vision with an inflamed eye: Prednisone 60–100 mg po once per day, which may be tapered slowly as the condition improves. If no improvement occurs within 10 days, then taper the patient off of the steroids quickly. When thyroid disease is no longer active, extraocular muscle surgery may be performed as needed.
   c. Visual loss from optic neuropathy: Treat immediately. Options include prednisone 100 mg po once per day, radiation therapy, and posterior orbital decompression surgery. Often, prednisone is started immediately in preparation for radiation or surgical therapy. If the vision does not improve or continues to deteriorate after 2–7 days of systemic steroids, one of the other modalities is employed. We prefer posterior orbital decompression surgery if it can be performed by a surgeon very familiar with the technique.

❖ **Note** *See the Drug Glossary for systemic steroid work-up.*

Follow-up

Optic-nerve compression is the most urgent ocular complication of thyroid eye disease; it requires immediate attention. Patients with advanced exposure keratopathy and severe proptosis also require prompt attention. Patients with minimal-to-no exposure problems and mild-to-moderate proptosis are reevaluated every 3–6 months. Patients who develop fluctuating diplopia and/or ptosis should be considered for an edrophonium chloride (e.g., Tensilon) test to rule out myasthenia gravis.

7.3 ORBITAL INFLAMMATORY PSEUDOTUMOR
NONSPECIFIC ORBITAL INFLAMMATORY DISEASE

Symptoms

May be acute, recurrent, or chronic. Pain, prominent red eye, double vision, or decreased vision are common in acute disease. Children may have concomitant constitutional symptoms (including fever), which are not typical in adults. Asymptomatic proptosis may develop in chronic disease.

Critical Signs

Proptosis and/or restriction of ocular motility, usually unilateral. Orbital CT scan shows a thickened posterior sclera (or a ring of scleral thickening 360 degrees around the globe), orbital fat or lacrimal gland involvement, or thickening of extraocular muscles (including the tendons). Bone destruction is very rare.

Other Signs

Eyelid erythema and edema, lacrimal gland enlargement or a palpable orbital mass, decreased vision, uveitis, elevated intraocular pressure (IOP), hyperopic shift, optic-nerve swelling or atrophy, decreased sensitivity of the first division of the trigeminal nerve, conjunctival chemosis and injection.

❖ **Note** *Bilateral pseudotumor in adults can occur, but should prompt a careful evaluation to rule out a systemic vasculitis (e.g., Wegener's granulomatosis, polyarteritis nodosa) and lymphoma. Bilateral pseudotumor is more common in children than in adults.*

Etiology

Idiopathic.

Differential Diagnosis

See "Orbital Disease, " Section 7.1.

Work-up

See Section 7.1, for general orbital work-up.

1. History: Previous episodes? Any other systemic symptoms or diseases? History of cancer?
2. Complete ocular examination, including ocular motility, exophthalmometry, IOP, and optic-nerve evaluation.
3. Vital signs, particularly temperature.
4. Orbital CT scan (axial and coronal views).
5. Blood tests as needed (e.g., bilateral or atypical cases): ESR, CBC with differential, ANA, BUN, creatinine (to rule out vasculitis), and fasting blood sugar (to rule out mucormycosis in diabetics and immunocompromised hosts). Consider antineutrophilic cytoplasmic antibody (ANCA) if Wegener's granulomatosis is suspected.
6. Orbital biopsy (fine-needle aspiration or incisional biopsy) when the diagnosis is uncertain, the case is atypical, the patient has a history of cancer, or a patient with an acute case does not respond to systemic steroids within a few days.

Treatment

Prednisone 80–100 mg po once per day and an antiulcer medication (e.g., ranitidine 150 mg po bid). Low-dose radiation therapy may be used when the patient does not respond to systemic steroids, when disease recurs as steroids are tapered, or when steroids pose a significant risk to the patient (see Appendix 5).

Follow-up

Reevaluate in 3–5 days. Patients who respond to the systemic steroids are maintained at the initial dose for 1–2 weeks and then tapered off of them slowly, usually over several months. Patients who do not respond to the steroids usually undergo biopsy (unless the diagnosis is known for certain, in which case radiation therapy is attempted). The IOP must be followed closely in patients being treated with steroids.

7.4 ORBITAL CELLULITIS

Symptoms

Red eye, pain, blurred vision, fever, headache, double vision.

Critical Signs

Eyelid edema, erythema, warmth, tenderness. Conjunctival chemosis and injection, proptosis, and restricted ocular motility with pain on attempted eye movement are usually present.

Other Signs

Decreased vision, retinal venous congestion, optic-disc edema, purulent discharge, decreased periorbital sensation, fever. CT scan usually shows a sinusitis (typically an ethmoid sinusitis).

Etiology

- Direct extension from a sinus infection (especially ethmoiditis), focal orbital infection (e.g., dacryoadenitis, dacryocystitis, panophthalmitis), orbital fracture, or dental infection.
- Status following orbital trauma. (NOTE   When a foreign body is retained, the cellulitis may develop months after injury.)
- Status following eye surgery (especially orbital surgery).
- Vascular extension (from a bacteremia).

Organisms

Staphylococcus species, *Streptococcus* species, *Haemophilus influenzae* (especially in children), bacteroides, gram-negative rods (especially after trauma).

Differential Diagnosis

See "Orbital Disease," Section 7.1.

Work-up

See Section 7.1 for a nonspecific orbital work-up.
1. History: Trauma? Ear, nose, throat, or systemic infection? Stiff neck or mental status changes? Diabetes or an immunosuppressive illness?
2. Complete ophthalmic examination: Look for an afferent pupillary defect, limitation of or pain with eye movements, proptosis, decreased skin sensation, or an optic-nerve or fundus abnormality.
3. Check vital signs, mental status, and neck flexibility.
4. CT scan of the orbits and sinuses (axial and coronal views, with and without contrast, if possible) to confirm the diagnosis and to rule out a foreign body, orbital or subperiosteal abscess, and sinus disease.
5. CBC with differential.
6. Blood cultures.
7. Explore and debride wound, if present, and obtain a Gram's stain and culture of any drainage (e.g., blood and chocolate agars, Sabouraud's dextrose agar, thioglycolate broth.)
8. Obtain a lumbar puncture for suspected meningitis. Consider a neurology consult.

❖ **Note** *Mucormycosis, a life-threatening disease, must be considered in all diabetics and immunocompromised patients with orbital cellulitis. Immediate action may need to be taken. See "Cavernous Sinus/Superior Orbital Fissure Syndrome," Section 11.8.*

Treatment
1. Admit the patient to the hospital.
2. Broad-spectrum IV antibiotics to cover gram-positive, gram-negative, and anaerobic organisms are required for at least 1 week or until the condition improves significantly. The specific recommendations frequently change. We presently prefer the following (or equivalent) drugs:

CHILDREN

vancomycin	40 mg/kg/day IV in 2–3 divided doses
or nafcillin	150 mg/kg/day IV in 6 divided doses
plus ceftriaxone	100 mg/kg/day IV in 2 divided doses

ADULTS

ceftriaxone	1–2 g IV q 12 h
plus vancomycin	1 g IV q 12 h
or nafcillin	1–2 g IV q 4

Consider adding metronidazole 15 mg/kg IV load, then 7.5 mg/kg IV q 6 h for adults with chronic orbital cellulitis or when an anaerobic infection is suspected.

If the patient is allergic to penicillin/cephalosporin:

vancomycin	1 g IV q 12 h
or clindamycin	300 mg IV q 6 h
plus gentamicin	2.0 mg/kg IV loading dose, then 1 mg/kg IV q 8 h.

❖ **Note** *Antibiotic dosages may need to be reduced in the presence of renal insufficiency or failure. Peak and trough levels of vancomycin and gentamicin are usually drawn one-half hour before and after the fifth dose, and dosages are adjusted as needed. BUN and creatinine levels are followed closely.*

3. Ear, nose, and throat consult for surgical drainage of the sinuses as needed, usually after the initial episode is treated.
4. Nasal decongestant spray (e.g., Afrin bid) as needed.
5. Erythromycin ointment qid for corneal exposure if there is severe proptosis.

Follow-up
Reevaluate every day in the hospital; may take 24–36 hours to show improvement.

1. Progress may be monitored by:
   a. Temperature and WBC.
   b. Visual acuity.
   c. Ocular motility.
   d. Degree of proptosis and any displacement of the globe (significant displacement may indicate an abscess).

   If any of the above are worsening, then a CT scan of the orbit and brain should be repeated to look for an abscess. If an abscess is found, then surgical drainage may be required. Other conditions that must be considered when the patient is not improving are cavernous sinus thrombosis and meningitis.

2. Evaluate the cornea for signs of exposure.
3. Check intraocular pressure.
4. Examine the retina and optic nerve for signs of posterior compression (e.g., choroidal folds), inflammation, or exudative retinal detachment.

When orbital cellulitis is clearly and consistently improving, then the regimen can be changed to oral antibiotics (depending on the culture and sensitivity results) to complete a total 14–day course. We often use:

amoxicillin/clavulanate (e.g., Augmentin) 20–40 mg/kg/day in 3 divided doses in children; 250–500 mg tid in adults
or
cefaclor (e.g., Ceclor) 20–40 mg/kg/day in 3 divided doses in children; 250–500 mg tid in adults

The patient is examined every few days as an outpatient until the condition resolves.

7.5 ORBITAL TUMORS IN CHILDREN

Presentation
Proptosis and/or globe displacement. See the specific etiologies below for additional presenting signs.

Etiology
- Dermoid and epidermoid cysts   [Present from birth to young adulthood and progress slowly, unless the cyst ruptures. May develop in the orbit superiorly (especially superotemporally) or outside of the orbit in the temporal upper eyelid or brow. When external to the orbit, the cyst is usually a smooth, round, nontender mass. *CT scan:* Well-defined lesion

that may mold the bone of the orbital walls. *Ultrasound (B-scan):* Cystic lesion with good transmission of echoes.]

- Capillary hemangioma [Presents from birth to early infancy, slow progression, usually in the superonasal orbit. May be observed through the eyelid as a bluish mass or be accompanied by a red hemangioma of the skin (strawberry nevus), which blanches with pressure. Proptosis may be exacerbated by crying. It can enlarge over the first year but spontaneously regresses over the following several years. *CT scan:* Irregular, contrast-enhancing, usually extraconal lesion.]

- Rhabdomyosarcoma (Usually presents around 7 years of age, but may occur from infancy to adulthood. Malignant and may metastasize. Rapid onset and progression. May have edema of the eyelids, a palpable superonasal eyelid or subconjunctival mass, or a history of nosebleeds. Must be managed by urgent biopsy. *CT scan:* Bone destruction is typical. The mass may be well circumscribed and is commonly in the superior orbit, especially nasally.)

- Lymphangioma [Usually presents in the first decade of life with a slowly progressive course, but may abruptly worsen if the tumor bleeds. Proptosis may be intermittent and exacerbated by upper respiratory infections. Concomitant conjunctival, eyelid, or oropharyngeal lymphangiomas may be noted (a conjunctival lesion appears as a multicystic mass). *CT scan:* Nonencapsulated, irregular mass. *Ultrasound [B-scan]:* Cystic spaces are often seen.]

- Optic-nerve glioma (juvenile pilocytic astrocytoma) [Usually presents at 2–6 years of age and is slowly progressive. Decreased visual acuity and a relative afferent pupillary defect usually develop. Optic atrophy or optic-nerve swelling may be present. May be associated with neurofibromatosis (in which case it may be bilateral). *CT scan:* Fusiform enlargement of the optic nerve. The optic canal or chiasm may be involved.]

- Leukemia (granulocytic sarcoma) [Presents in the first decade of life with rapidly evolving unilateral or bilateral proptosis and occasionally, swelling of the temporal fossa area due to a mass. Typically, these lesions precede blood or bone marrow signs of leukemia, usually acute myelogenous leukemia, by several months. *CT scan:* Irregular mass, sometimes with bony erosion. There may also be extension of the mass into the temporal fossa. (NOTE Acute lymphoblastic leukemia can also produce unilateral or bilateral proptosis.)]

- Metastatic neuroblastoma (Presents in the first few years of life. Abrupt presentation with unilateral or bilateral proptosis, eyelid ecchymosis, and globe displacement. The child is usually systemically ill. The vast majority of patients have already been diagnosed with abdominal cancer. *CT scan:* Poorly defined mass with bony destruction, especially of the lateral orbital wall.)

- Plexiform neurofibroma (Presents in the first decade of life and is pathognomonic of neurofibromatosis. Ptosis, eyelid hypertrophy, S-shaped deformity of the upper eyelid, or pulsating proptosis may be present. Facial asymmetry and a palpable anterior orbital mass may also be evident. *CT scan:* Diffuse, irregular soft tissue mass. A defect in the orbital roof may be seen. See Section 14.11.)

- Teratoma   (Presents at birth with severe unilateral proptosis that may progress. Vision is often lost from increased intraocular pressure (IOP), optic-nerve atrophy, and corneal exposure. The mass transilluminates. *CT scan:* Multiloculated soft tissue mass and enlarged orbit; intracranial extension is possible.)

Differential Diagnosis
See Section 7.1.

Work-up
1. History: Determine the age of onset and the rate of progression. Does the proptosis vary in degree (e.g., with crying)? Nosebleeds? Systemic illness?
2. External examination: Look for an anterior orbital mass, a skin hemangioma, or a temporal fossa lesion. Measure any proptosis (Hertel exophthalmometer) or globe displacement (measure from the bridge of the nose with a ruler). Abdominal examination is needed.
3. Complete ocular examination, including visual acuity, pupillary assessment, color vision, IOP, refraction, and optic-nerve evaluation.
4. CT scan (axial and coronal views) of the orbit and brain.
5. Orbital ultrasound or MRI of the orbit as needed to further define the lesion.
6. In cases of acute onset and rapid progression, an emergent incisional biopsy for frozen, permanent, and electron microscopic evaluation may be advisable to rule out an aggressive malignancy (e.g., rhabdomyosarcoma).
7. Other tests as determined by the working diagnosis (usually performed by a pediatric oncologist):

    Rhabdomyosarcoma   Physical examination (look especially for enlarged lymph nodes), chest and bone x-rays, bone marrow aspiration, lumbar puncture, liver function studies.
    Leukemia   CBC with differential, bone marrow studies, others.
    Neuroblastoma   Abdominal CT scan, urine for vanilyllmandelic acid (VMA).

Treatment
- Dermoid and epidermoid cysts: Complete surgical excision with the capsule intact. If the cyst ruptures, the contents can incite an acute inflammatory response.
- Capillary hemangioma: Observe if mild. A local steroid injection (e.g., betamethasone 6 mg and triamcinolone 40 mg) may be given to shrink

the lesion if necessary. Treatment is often indicated if strabismus, anisometropia, or amblyopia develop (see "Amblyopia," Section 9.6).

- Rhabdomyosarcoma (managed by a pediatric oncologist in most cases): Local radiation therapy and systemic chemotherapy are given once the diagnosis is confirmed by biopsy.
- Lymphangioma: Surgical excision is performed for a significant cosmetic deformity, ocular dysfunction (e.g., strabismus and amblyopia), or compressive optic neuropathy from acute orbital hemorrhage. May recur after surgical excision.
- Optic-nerve glioma: Controversial. Observation, surgery, or radiation is used.
- Leukemia (managed by a pediatric oncologist in most cases): Systemic chemotherapy for the leukemia. Some physicians administer orbital radiation therapy alone when systemic leukemia cannot be confirmed on bone marrow studies.
- Metastatic neuroblastoma (managed by a pediatric oncologist in most cases): Local radiation and systemic chemotherapy.
- Plexiform neurofibroma: Surgical excision is reserved for patients with significant symptoms or disfigurement.
- Teratoma: Surgical excision (sometimes with the help of a neurosurgeon). Aspiration of the cyst may facilitate complete removal of large lesions. Preservation of ocular function may be possible.

Follow-up

Tumors with rapid onset and progression require urgent attention to rule out malignancy. Tumors that present more slowly may be managed less urgently.

7.6 ORBITAL TUMORS IN ADULTS

Symptoms

Prominent eye, double vision, pain, decreased vision; may be asymptomatic.

Critical signs

Proptosis, displacement of the globe away from the location of the tumor, orbital mass on CT scan.

Other Signs

A palpable mass, limitation of ocular motility, optic disc edema, or choroidal folds may be present. See the individual tumors below for more specific findings.

Etiology

- Metastatic [Usually occurs in middle-aged to elderly people with a rapid onset of orbital signs. Common primary sources include the breast (most common), lung, genitourinary tract (especially prostate), and gastrointestinal tract. Enophthalmos (not proptosis) may be seen with scirrhous breast carcinoma. *CT scan:* Poorly defined, diffuse tumor which may conform to the shape of the adjacent orbital structures. Bone destruction may be seen.]

- Cavernous hemangioma [Typically occurs in young adulthood to middle age, with a slow onset of orbital signs. *CT scan:* Well-defined mass, usually within the muscle cone. *Ultrasound (A-scan):* High-amplitude internal echoes.]

- Mucocele (Often, a frontal headache and a history of chronic sinusitis. Usually nasally or superonasally located. *CT scan:* A frontal or ethmoid sinus cyst usually seen extending through eroded bone into the orbit. Affected sinuses may be opacified.)

- Lymphoid tumors (Usually occurs in middle-aged adults. Slow onset and progression. Typically develop superiorly in the anterior aspect of the orbit. May be accompanied by a subconjunctival, salmon-colored lesion. *CT scan:* Irregular mass conforming to the shape of the orbital bones or globe. No bony erosion. Less responsive to systemic steroids than orbital pseudotumor. Can occur without evidence of systemic lymphoma.)

- Optic-nerve-sheath meningioma [Typically occurs in middle-aged women with painless, slowly progressive visual loss, often with mild proptosis. An afferent pupillary defect develops with visual loss. Ophthalmoscopy can reveal optic-nerve swelling, optic atrophy, or abnormal collateral vessels around the disc (optociliary shunt vessels). Meningiomas arising intracranially can produce a temporal-fossa mass. *CT scan:* Tubular enlargement of the optic nerve, sometimes with a "railroad-track" appearance (a linear shadow is seen within the lesion).]

- Localized neurofibroma [Occurs in young to middle-aged adults with slow development of orbital signs. Some have neurofibromatosis, but most do not. *CT scan:* Well-defined mass in the superior orbit (rarely inferiorly)].

- Neurilemoma (benign schwannoma) (Progressive painless proptosis. Rarely associated with neurofibromatosis. *CT scan:* Well-circumscribed fusiform or ovoid mass, usually located in the superior orbit.)

- Fibrous histiocytoma (Occurs at any age. *CT scan:* Well-circumscribed mass anywhere in the orbit. Cannot be distinguished from a hemangiopericytoma before biopsy. See the following.)

- Hemangiopericytoma [Occurs at any age. Relatively slow development of signs. Usually superiorly located. *CT scan:* May appear well defined and indistinguishable from a cavernous hemangioma or fibrous histiocytoma. Sometimes extends through the orbital bones into the temporal fossa and cranial cavity. *Ultrasound (A-scan):* Low-to-medium internal reflectivity.]

- Others   (Dermoid cyst, osteoma, hematocele, lymphangioma, extension of an ocular or periocular tumor, others.)

Differential Diagnosis
See Sections 7.1 and 7.7.

Work-up
1. History: Determine the age of onset and rate of progression. Headache or chronic sinusitis? History of cancer? Trauma (e.g., hematocele, orbital foreign body, ruptured dermoid)?
2. Complete ocular examination, particularly visual acuity, pupillary response, ocular motility, color vision and visual field of each eye, measurement of globe displacement (from the bridge of the nose with a ruler) and proptosis (Hertel exophthalmometer), intraocular pressure (IOP), and optic-nerve evaluation.
3. CT scan (axial and coronal views) of the orbit and brain.
4. Orbital ultrasound or MRI as needed to further define the lesion.
5. When a metastasis is suspected and primary tumor is unknown, the following should be performed:
    a. Fine-needle aspiration biopsy or incisional biopsy to confirm the diagnosis, with estrogen-receptor assay if breast carcinoma is suspected.
    b. Breast examination and palpation of axillary lymph nodes.
    c. Medical work-up as directed by the biopsy result (e.g., chest x-ray, mammogram).
6. When a lymphoma is suspected, a medical consult is obtained and a systemic work-up is instituted (e.g., CBC with differential, serum protein electrophoresis, bone marrow biopsy, CT scan of the abdomen and brain). If the work-up is negative, an incisional biopsy is performed (often need nonfixed tissue). If the work-up is positive, the systemic lymphoma is treated and the orbital lesion is observed for its response to treatment. Occasionally, a fine-needle biopsy is performed to confirm the orbital diagnosis.

Treatment

METASTATIC DISEASE

Systemic chemotherapy as required for the primary malignancy. Radiotherapy is often used for the orbital mass. Carcinoid tumors are occasionally resected.

CAVERNOUS HEMANGIOMA

Complete surgical excision is performed when there is compromised visual function or for cosmetic purposes. If the patient is asymptomatic, he or she can be followed every 6–12 months.

MUCOCELE

1. Systemic antibiotics (e.g., vancomycin 1 g IV q 12 h and ceftazidime 1 g IV q 8 h) preoperatively and postoperatively.

2. Surgical drainage of the mucocele and exenteration of the involved sinus.

LYMPHOID TUMORS

Lymphoid hyperplasia and orbital lymphoma without systemic involvement are treated with local radiation therapy. Systemic lymphoma is treated with chemotherapy.

OPTIC-NERVE-SHEATH MENINGIOMA

Surgery is usually indicated when the tumor is growing and producing visual loss. Otherwise, the patient may be followed every 3–6 months with serial clinical examinations and imaging studies (CT scan or MRI) as needed.

LOCALIZED NEUROFIBROMA

Surgical removal is performed for enlarging tumors that are producing symptoms.

NEURILEMOMA

Same as for cavernous hemangioma (see previous).

FIBROUS HISTIOCYTOMA

Complete surgical removal. Recurrences are generally more aggressive and more malignant, sometimes necessitating orbital exenteration.

HEMANGIOPERICYTOMA

Complete surgical excision (because there is a potential for malignant transformation and metastasis).

Follow-up
Variable. Referral for treatment is not emergent, except when optic-nerve compromise is present. Metastatic disease requires work-up without much delay.

❖ **Note** *Also see "Lacrimal Gland Mass," Section 7.7, especially if the mass is in the outer one third of the upper eyelid, and "Orbital Tumors in Children," Section 7.5.*

7.7 LACRIMAL GLAND MASS/ CHRONIC DACRYOADENITIS

Symptoms
Persistent or progressive swelling of the outer one third of the upper eyelid. Pain and/or double vision may or may not be present.

Critical Signs

Chronic eyelid swelling and erythema, predominantly in the outer one third of the upper eyelid, with or without proptosis and displacement of the globe inferiorly and medially.

Other Signs

A palpable mass may be present in the outer one third of the upper eyelid. Extraocular motility may be restricted.

Etiology

- Sarcoidosis   [May have concomitant lung, skin, or ocular disease. Lymphadenopathy, parotid gland enlargement, or seventh-nerve palsy may be present. More common in blacks. Angiotensin-converting enzyme (ACE) level may be elevated.]
- Orbital inflammatory pseudotumor   (Commonly, pain and swelling develop acutely, with or without limitation of ocular motility, displacement of the globe, or proptosis. A rapid response to systemic steroids is typical in acute cases.)
- Benign mixed epithelial tumor (pleomorphic adenoma)   (Slowly progressive, painless proptosis or displacement of the globe in middle-aged adults. CT scan may show a well-circumscribed mass with pressure-induced remodeling and enlargement of the lacrimal gland fossa. No bony erosion occurs.)
- Dermoid   (Typically, a painless, subcutaneous mass that enlarges slowly and is found in a child. Well-defined, extraconal mass noted on CT scan.)
- Lymphoid tumor   (Slowly progressive proptosis and globe displacement in a middle-aged patient. May have a pink-white salmon-patch subconjunctival extension. CT scan shows an irregularly shaped lesion that conforms to the globe and lacrimal fossa. Bony erosion is not usually found.)
- Adenoid cystic carcinoma   (Acute onset of pain and proptosis, which progress rapidly. Globe displacement, ptosis, and a motility disturbance are common. CT scan often shows an irregular mass, often with bony erosion.)
- Malignant mixed epithelial tumor (pleomorphic adenocarcinoma)   (Occurs primarily in elderly patients, acutely producing pain and progressing rapidly. Usually develops within a long-standing benign mixed epithelial tumor, or secondarily, as a recurrence of a previously resected benign mixed tumor. CT scan findings are similar to those for adenoid cystic carcinoma.)
- Lacrimal gland cyst (dacryops)   (Usually an asymptomatic mass that may fluctuate in size. Typically occurs in a young adult or middle-aged patient.)
- Others (Tuberculosis, syphilis, leukemia, mumps, mucoepidermoid carcinoma, plasmacytoma, others.)

❖ **Note** *Primary neoplasms (except lymphoma) are almost always unilateral; inflammatory disease may be bilateral. Lymphoma is more commonly unilateral, but may be bilateral.*

Work-up

1. History: Determine the duration of the abnormality and rate of progression. Associated pain, tenderness, double vision? Weakness, weight loss, fever, or other signs of systemic malignancy? Breathing difficulty, skin rash, or prior history of uveitis (sarcoidosis)? Any known medical problems? Prior lacrimal gland biopsy or surgery?
2. Complete ocular examination: Specifically look for keratic precipitates, iris nodules, posterior synechiae, and old retinal periphlebitis from sarcoidosis.
3. Orbital CT scan (axial and coronal views). MRI is rarely required.
4. Consider a chest x-ray (may diagnose sarcoidosis and rarely, tuberculosis).
5. Consider CBC with differential, ACE, RPR, FTA-ABS, and PPD with anergy panel.
6. Systemic work-up by an internist or hematologist/oncologist when a lymphoma is suspected (e.g., abdominal and head CT scan, bone marrow biopsy).
7. Lacrimal gland biopsy is indicated when:
   a. A malignant tumor is suspected. (This may be unnecessary when a lymphoma is suspected clinically and is found on systemic work-up.)
      or
   b. The diagnosis is uncertain, but a malignancy or inflammatory etiology is suspected.

❖ **Note** *Do not biopsy lesions thought to be benign mixed tumors or dermoids. Incomplete excision of a benign mixed tumor may lead to a recurrence with or without malignant transformation. Rupture of a dermoid cyst may lead to a severe inflammatory reaction. These two lesions must be completely excised without rupturing the capsule or pseudocapsule.*

Treatment
- Sarcoidosis: Systemic steroids (see Section 13.4).
- Orbital inflammatory pseudotumor: Systemic steroids (see Section 7.3).
- Benign mixed epithelial tumor: Complete surgical removal.
- Dermoid cyst: Complete surgical removal.
- Lymphoid tumor:
   a. Confined to the orbit: Orbital irradiation.
   b. Systemic involvement: Chemotherapy (orbital irradiation is usually withheld until the response of the orbital lesion to chemotherapy can be evaluated).
- Adenoid cystic carcinoma: Consider orbital exenteration with irradiation. (Rarely, chemotherapy is used.)
- Malignant mixed epithelial tumor: Same as for adenoid cystic carcinoma.
- Lacrimal gland cyst: Excise if symptomatic.

Follow-up
Depends on the specific cause.

OCULAR TUMORS

8.1 CONJUNCTIVAL TUMORS

The following are the most common and important conjunctival tumors. Phlyctenulosis and pterygium/pingueculum are discussed in Sections 4.9 and 4.10, respectively.

Amelanotic Lesions

Limbal Dermoid

Congenital benign tumor, usually located in the inferotemporal quadrant of the limbus; it may involve the cornea. Lesions are white, solid, fairly well circumscribed, elevated, and may have hair arising from their surface. They may enlarge, particularly at puberty. They may be associated with eyelid colobomas, preauricular skin tags, and vertebral abnormalities (Goldenhar's syndrome). Surgical removal may be performed for cosmetic purposes or if they are affecting the visual axis, although a white corneal scar may persist postoperatively.

❖ **Note** *The cornea or sclera underlying a dermoid may be very thin or even absent, and penetration of the eye can occur with surgical resection.*

Dermolipoma

Congenital benign tumor, usually occurring under the bulbar conjunctiva in the temporal-most aspect of the eye. It appears as a yellow-white solid tumor, and may have hair arising from its surface. Surgical removal is usually avoided if

The Wills Eye Manual: Office and Emergency Room Diagnosis and Treatment of Eye Diseases, Second Edition, edited by R. Douglas Cullom, Jr., M.D., and Benjamin Chang, M.D. © 1994 J.B. Lippincott Company.

possible because of the frequent extension of this tumor into the orbit, involving some of the orbital structures. Partial resection of the anterior portion usually can be done without difficulty if necessary.

Pyogenic Granuloma

Benign, deep-red, pedunculated mass. It typically develops at a site of prior surgery, trauma, or chalazion. It may respond to topical steroids—we usually give a topical steroid–antibiotic combination (e.g., prednisolone acetate-gentamicin qid for 1–2 weeks) because infection may be present, but the tumor often must be excised if it persists.)

Lymphangioma

Probably congenital, but often not detected until years after birth. The lesion is benign yet slowly progressive and appears as a diffuse, multiloculated, cystic mass. This lesion presents most commonly between birth and young adulthood, often before 6 years of age. Hemorrhage into the cystic spaces may produce a "chocolate cyst". Lymphangiomas may enlarge, sometimes due to an upper respiratory tract infection. Concomitant eyelid, orbital, facial, nasal, or oropharyngeal lymphangiomas may be present. Surgical excision may be performed for cosmetic or functional purposes (it often needs to be repeated, because it is difficult to remove the entire tumor with one surgical procedure). Lesions often stabilize in early adulthood. These lesions do not regress like the capillary hemangiomas.

Granuloma

May occur at any age, predominantly on the tarsal conjunctiva. No distinct clinical appearance, but patients may have an associated embedded foreign body, sarcoidosis, tuberculosis, or another granulomatous disease. Management often includes an incisional or excisional biopsy.

Papilloma

Two types:

A. Viral [Frequently multiple pedunculated or sessile lesions in children and young adults. These lesions can occur on palpebral or bulbar conjunctiva. They are benign and are generally left untreated because of their high recurrence rate (which is often multiple) and their tendency for spontaneous resolution.]

B. Nonviral [Typically, a single sessile or pedunculated lesion found in older patients. These are located more commonly near the limbus and may represent precancerous lesions with malignant potential. Complete excisional biopsy flush with the surface is the preferred treatment. Supplemental cryotherapy may be applied.

❖ **Note** *In dark-skinned individuals, papillomas may appear pigmented and may be mistaken for malignant melanoma.*

Kaposi's Sarcoma

Malignant, subconjunctival nodule, usually red or purple. Patients should be evaluated for AIDS (see Section 14.1).

Conjunctival Intraepithelial Neoplasia (Dysplasia and Carcinoma-in-Situ)

Typically occurs in middle-aged to elderly people. The lesion is a leukoplakic or gray-white gelatinous lesion that usually begins at the limbus. Occasionally, a papillomatous, cauliflowerlike appearance develops. The lesions are usually unilateral and unifocal and may evolve into invasive squamous cell carcinoma if not treated early and successfully. They can spread over the cornea or, less commonly, invade the eye or metastasize. A complete excisional biopsy followed by supplemental cryotherapy to the remaining adjacent conjunctiva is the preferred treatment. (Excision may require lamellar dissection into the corneal stroma and sclera.) Periodic follow-up examinations are required to detect recurrences.

Lymphoid Tumors (Range from Benign Reactive Lymphoid Hyperplasia to Lymphoma)

Occurs in young to middle-aged adults. Usually appears as a light pink, salmon-colored lesion. It may appear in the bulbar conjunctiva, where it is typically oval, or in the fornix, where it is usually horizontal, conforming to the contour of the fornix. Excisional or incisional biopsy is performed for immunohistochemical studies (may require nonfixed tissue). Symptomatic benign reactive lymphoid hyperplasia may be treated by excisional biopsy, low-dose radiation, or topical steroid drops. Lymphomas should be completely excised. Patients with the latter tumor are referred to an internist for systemic evaluation. Systemic lymphoma may or may not develop if it is not already present.

Epibulbar Osseous Choristoma

Congenital, benign, hard, bony mass, usually on the superotemporal bulbar conjunctiva. Surgical removal may be performed for cosmetic purposes.

Amyloid

Smooth, waxy, yellow masses seen especially in the lower fornix when the conjunctiva is involved. Often there are associated small hemorrhages; this clinical picture is characteristic of the lesion. Definitive diagnosis is made with biopsy. Consider work-up for systemic amyloidosis.

Amelanotic Melanoma

Pigmentation of conjunctival melanoma is variable. Look for bulbar or limbal lesions with significant vascularity to help make this difficult diagnosis.

Sebaceous Cell Carcinoma

Though usually involving the palpebral conjunctiva, this tumor can involve the bulbar conjunctiva as well when there is pagetoid invasion of the conjunctiva. This diagnosis should always be considered in patients with refractory blepharo-conjunctivitis.

Melanotic Lesions

Ocular or Oculodermal Melanocytosis

Congenital. Not a conjunctival lesion, but an episcleral lesion, as demonstrated (after topical anesthesia) by moving the conjunctiva back and forth over the area of pigmentation with a sterile, cotton-tipped swab. (Conjunctival pigmentation will move with the conjunctiva.) Typically, the lesion is unilateral, blue-gray, and is often accompanied by a darker ipsilateral iris and choroid. In oculodermal disease, also called nevus of Ota, the periocular skin is also pigmented. These lesions may become pigmented at puberty. Both conditions predispose to malignant melanoma of the uveal tract, orbit, and brain (most commonly in Caucasians).

Primary Acquired Melanosis

Appears in middle-aged adults as flat, brown patches of pigmentation without small cysts within the conjunctiva. These tumors usually arise during or after middle age and almost always occur in Caucasians. (Overall, approximately one fifth of these lesions will develop into malignant melanoma of the conjunctiva.) Malignant transformation should be suspected when an elevation or increase in vascularity in one of these areas develops. Management options include careful observation with photographic comparison for any change and incisional or excisional biopsy followed by cryotherapy for suspicious lesions.

Nevus

Commonly develops during puberty, most often within the palpebral fissure on the bulbar conjunctiva. It is usually well demarcated and may or may not be pigmented (the degree of pigmentation may also change with time). A key sign in the diagnosis is the presence of small cysts within the lesion. Benign nevi may enlarge; however, malignant melanoma may occasionally develop from a nevus, and enlargement may be an early sign of malignant transformation. Nevi of the palpebral conjunctiva are rare; primary acquired melanosis and malignant melanoma must be considered in such lesions. A baseline photograph of the nevus should be taken, and the patient should be observed every 6–12 months. Surgical excision is elective.

Malignant Melanoma

Typically occurs in middle-aged to elderly patients. The lesion is a nodular brown mass. The tumor is well vascularized, and a large conjunctival vessel can often be seen to be feeding the tumor. It may develop from a nevus or primary acquired melanosis, but it may also develop de novo. Check for an underlying ciliary body melanoma (dilated fondus examination, transillumination, and B-scan ultrasound). Intraocular and orbital extension may occur. Excisional biopsy (often with supplemental cryotherapy) is performed unless intraocular or orbital involvement is present (in which case an incisional biopsy may be performed if the diagnosis is uncertain, followed by enucleation or exenteration).

Other Less Common Causes of Increased Pigmentation

Ochronosis with alkaptonuria: Autosomal recessive enzyme deficiency. Occurs in young adults with arthritis and dark urine. Pigment is at level of the sclera.

Argyrosis: Silver deposition causes black discoloration. Patients have a history of chronic use of silver nitrate drops.

Hemochromatosis (bronze diabetes):   This can cause increased conjunctival pigmentation.

Ciliary staphyloma: Scleral thinning with uveal show.

Adrenochrome deposits: Chronic epinephrine or dipivifren (e.g., Propine) use.

8.2 MALIGNANT MELANOMA OF THE IRIS

Malignant melonoma (MM) of the iris may occur as a localized or diffuse pigmented (melanotic) or nonpigmented (amelanotic) lesion.

Critical Signs

Unilateral brown or translucent iris mass lesion exhibiting slow growth. It is more common in the inferior one half of the iris and in light-skinned individuals. Rare in blacks.

Other Signs

A *localized* MM is generally >3 mm in diameter at the base and >1 mm in depth and often has prominent feeder vessels that ramify throughout the mass. It may produce secondary glaucoma. Although nonspecific, it may cause a sector cortical cataract, ectropion iridis, spontaneous hyphema, seeding of tumor cells into the anterior chamber, or direct invasion of tumor into the trabecular meshwork.

A *diffuse* MM causes progressive darkening of the involved iris, loss of iris crypts, and increased intraocular pressure (IOP). Focal iris nodules may be present.

Differential Diagnosis

A. Melanotic masses
  • Nevi   [Typically become clinically apparent at puberty, usually flat or minimally elevated (i.e. <1 mm) and uncommonly exceed 3 mm in diameter. Can cause ectropion iridis, sector cortical cataract, or secondary glaucoma. Generally *not* vascular. More common in the inferior one half of the iris. *Nevi do not usually grow.*]
  • Tumors of the iris pigment epithelium   (Usually black, in contrast to melanomas, which are often dark brown or amelanotic.)

B. Amelanotic masses
  • Metastasis   (Grows rapidly. More likely to be multiple or bilateral than is MM. Frequently liberates cells and produces a pseudohypopyon. Involves the superior and inferior halves of the iris equally.)
  • Leiomyoma   (Transparent and vascular. May be difficult to distinguish from a melanoma.)
  • Iris cyst   (Unlike MM, most transmit light with transillumination.)
  • Inflammatory granuloma (e.g., sarcoidosis or tuberculosis)   (Often have other signs of inflammation such as keratic precipitates, synechiae, and posterior subcapsular cataracts. A history of iritis or a systemic inflammatory disease may be elicited.)

C. Diffuse lesions
  • Congenital iris heterochromia   (The darker iris is present at birth or in early childhood. It is nonprogressive and usually is not associated with glaucoma. The iris has a smooth appearance.)
  • Fuchs' heterochromic iridocyclitis   (Asymmetry of iris color, mild iritis in the eye with the lighter-colored iris, usually unilateral. Often associated with a cataract and/or glaucoma.)
  • Iris nevus syndrome   (Corneal edema, peripheral anterior synechiae,

iris atrophy, or an irregular pupil may be present along with multiple iris nodules and glaucoma.)

- Pigment dispersion   [Usually bilateral. The iris is rarely heavily pigmented (although the trabecular meshwork may be), and iris transillumination defects are often present.]
- Hemosiderosis   (A dark iris may result after iron-breakdown products from an old blood deposit on the iris surface. Patients have a history of a traumatic hyphema or vitreous hemorrhage.)

Work-up

1. History: Previous cancer, ocular surgery or trauma? Weight loss? Anorexia?
2. Slit-lamp examination: Carefully evaluate the irides. Check IOP.
3. Gonioscopy of the anterior-chamber angle.
4. Dilated fundus examination using indirect ophthalmoscopy.
5. Transillumination (used to differentiate between epithelial cysts that transmit light and pigmented lesions that do not).
6. Photograph the lesion and accurately draw it in the chart, including dimensions.

Treatment/Follow-up

1. Observe the patient through periodic examinations and photographs every 3–12 months, depending on suspicion of malignancy.
2. Surgical resection is indicated if growth is documented, the tumor interferes with vision, or it produces intractable glaucoma.
3. Diffuse iris MM with secondary glaucoma may require enucleation.
4. Avoid filtering surgery for glaucoma associated with possible malignant melanoma because of the risk of dissemination.

8.3 MALIGNANT MELANOMA OF THE CHOROID

Symptoms

Decreased vision, a visual field defect, floaters, light flashes, pain; may be asymptomatic.

Critical Signs

Gray-green or brown (melanotic) or yellow (amelanotic) choroidal mass that exhibits one or more of the following:

1. Growth.
2. A large amount of subretinal fluid (i.e., retinal detachment).
3. Height >2 mm, especially with an abrupt elevation from the choroid.

4. Ill-defined, large areas of orange pigment over the lesion.
5. A mushroom shape with congested blood vessels in the dome of the tumor.

❖ **Note** *A diffuse choroidal malignant melanoma (MM) can appear as a thickened choroid without a distinct mass.*

Other Signs

Overlying cystoid retinal degeneration, vitreous hemorrhage or vitreous pigment cells, drusen on the tumor surface, a choroidal neovascular membrane, proptosis (from orbital invasion). Choroidal MM rarely occurs in blacks and more commonly occurs in light-skinned individuals.

Differential Diagnosis

A. Pigmented lesions
- Nevi   (Melanotic or amelanotic choroidal lesions that rarely exhibit significant growth, are not mushroom-shaped, are generally <2 mm thick and show gradual elevation from the choroid. They may have an associated shallow retinal detachment or well-defined small areas of orange pigment on their surface, but surface drusen are more typical.)
- Congenital hypertrophy of the retinal pigment epithelium (RPE) (Flat lesions which are often black in color, but may appear gray-green. The margins are often well delineated with a surrounding depigmented halo. Depigmented areas frequently appear on the surface of the lesion.)
- Reactive hyperplasia of the RPE   (Related to previous trauma or inflammation. Lesions are black, flat, have irregular margins, and may have associated white gliosis. Often multifocal.)
- Age-related disciform macular degeneration   [Subretinal blood can simulate a melanoma. This disease is typically bilateral in the posterior pole and associated with extensive exudate. Fluorescein angiography (FA) will allow easy differentiation.]
- Peripheral disciform degeneration   (Peripheral, elevated, yellow-to-red mass with extensive exudation and hemorrhage. It may extend into the vitreous. The contralateral eye often shows peripheral RPE changes.)
- Melanocytoma of the optic nerve   (A black optic-nerve lesion with fibrillated margins. It may grow slowly. FA may allow differentiation.)
- Choroidal detachment   [Follows ocular surgery, trauma, or hypotony of another etiology. Dark peripheral multilobular fundus mass. (The ora serrata is often visible without scleral depression.) Localized suprachoroidal hemorrhage can be very difficult to differentiate from MM based on appearance alone because of their brown-black color. Transillumination will allow differentiation between serous choroidal detachment and MM but is not helpful when there is a hemorrhagic component.

In these situations, FA is the study of choice, usually allowing differentiation between the two entities.

B. Nonpigmented lesions
- Choroidal hemangioma (Red-orange, may be elevated, never mushroom-shaped.)
- Metastatic carcinoma [Cream or light brown, flat or slightly elevated, extensive subretinal fluid, may be multifocal or bilateral. Patient may have a history of cancer (especially breast or lung cancer)].
- Choroidal osteoma (Yellow-orange in color, generally close to the optic disc, pseudopodium-like projections of the margin, often bilateral, typically occurs in young women in their teens or twenties. Ultrasound may show a calcified mass.)
- Posterior scleritis (Patients may have choroidal folds, pain, proptosis, uveitis, or anterior scleritis associated with an amelanotic mass. Look for the T-sign on ultrasound.)

Work-up
1. History: Ocular surgery or trauma, cancer, anorexia, weight loss, or systemic illness?
2. Dilated fundus examination using indirect ophthalmoscopy.
3. FA.
4. Ultrasound A and B scans: Documents thickness and confirms clinical impression. With choroidal melanoma, the ultrasound usually shows low-to-moderate reflectivity with choroidal excavation.
5. Consider a phosphorus 32 test, CT scan or MRI of the orbit and brain, or fine-needle aspiration biopsy in selected cases.
6. If MM is confirmed:
   a. Blood work: LDH, gamma glutamyl transferase (GGT), SGOT, SGPT, and alkaline phosphatase. If liver enzymes are elevated, consider a liver scan to rule out a liver metastasis.
   b. Chest x-ray.
   c. Complete physical examination by a medical internist.
7. Consider a carcinoembryonic antigen (CEA) if a choroidal metastasis is suspected.

Treatment
Depending on the results of the metastatic work-up, the tumor characteristics, the status of the contralateral eye, and the age and general health of the patient, MM of the choroid may be managed by observation, photocoagulation, radiotherapy, local resection, or enucleation.

PEDIATRICS

9.1 LEUKOCORIA

Definition

A white pupillary reflex

Etiology

- Retinoblastoma   [A malignant tumor of the retina that appears as a white, nodular mass extending into the vitreous (endophytic), as a mass lesion underlying a retinal detachment (exophytic), or as a diffusely spreading lesion simulating uveitis (diffuse infiltrating). Iris neovascularization is common. Pseudohypopyon and vitreous seeding may occur. Cataract is uncommon and the eye is normal in size. May be bilateral, unilateral, or multifocal. Diagnosis is usually made between 12 and 24 months of age. A positive family history may be elicited.]
- Toxocariasis   (A nematode infection that may appear as a localized, white, elevated granuloma in the posterior pole or peripheral retina. Signs of inflammation are usually absent but may occur. Vitreous traction bands associated with macular dragging and traction retinal detachment may occur. Toxocariasis can appear as a diffuse endophthalmitis with an acutely inflamed globe. It is rarely bilateral, and is usually diagnosed between 3 and 10 years of age. Paracentesis of the anterior chamber may reveal eosinophils, and a serum ELISA test for *Toxocara* organisms will be positive. The patient may have a history of contact with puppies.)
- Coats' disease   (A retinal vascular abnormality resulting in small multifocal outpouchings of the retinal vessels, associated with yellow intraretinal

The Wills Eye Manual: Office and Emergency Room Diagnosis and Treatment of Eye Diseases, Second Edition, edited by R. Douglas Cullom, Jr., M.D., and Benjamin Chang, M.D. © 1994 J. B. Lippincott Company.

and subretinal exudate. An exudative retinal detachment may acount for the leukocoria. It usually develops in males during the first two decades of life; more severe cases occur in the first decade of life. Coats' disease is rarely bilateral, and a negative family history is elicited.)

- Persistent hyperplastic primary vitreous (PHPV)   (A developmental ocular abnormality consisting of a varied degree of fibroglial and vascular proliferation in the vitreous cavity. It is usually associated with a slightly small eye. Other findings can include cataract, a fibrovascular membrane behind the lens that places traction on the ciliary processes, glaucoma, and retinal detachment. The condition is present at birth but may not be detected until later in childhood. It is rarely bilateral, and a negative family history is elicited.)

- Congenital cataract   (Opacity of the lens present at birth, may be unilateral or bilateral. There may be a positive family history or an associated systemic disorder.)

- Retinal astrocytoma   (A sessile to slightly elevated yellow-white retinal mass that may be calcified and is often associated with tuberous sclerosis, and rarely neurofibromatosis. May be associated with giant drusen of the optic nerve in patients with tuberous sclerosis.)

- Retinopathy of prematurity   (Predominantly occurs in premature children, who may have received supplemental oxygen therapy. Leukocoria is usually the result of a retinal detachment. See "Retinopathy of Prematurity," Section 9.2.)

- Others   (Retinochoroidal coloboma, retinal detachment, familial exudative vitreoretinopathy, myelinated nerve fibers, uveitis, etc.)

Work-up

1. History: Age at onset? Family history of one of the conditions mentioned above? Prematurity or supplemental oxygen therapy? Contact with puppies or habit of eating dirt?

2. Complete ocular examination, including a measurement of corneal diameters (look for a small eye), an examination of the iris (look for neovascularization), and an inspection of the lens (look for a cataract). A hand-held slit lamp is often most helpful. A dilated fundus examination and anterior vitreous examination are essential.

3. Any or all of the following may be helpful in diagnosis and planning treatment:
   a. B-scan ultrasound (retinoblastoma, PHPV, cataract).
   b. IV fluorescein angiogram (Coats' disease, retinopathy of prematurity, retinoblastoma).
   c. CT scan or MRI of the orbit and brain (retinoblastoma), particularly for bilateral cases or those with a positive family history.
   d. Serum ELISA test for toxocara (positive at 1:8 in the vast majority of infected patients.)

e. Systemic examination (retinal astrocytoma, retinoblastoma).

f. Anterior chamber paracentesis (toxocariasis).

❖ **Note** *Paracentesis in a patient with a retinoblastoma can lead to tumor cell dissemination.*

4. Consider examination under anesthesia (EUA) in young or uncooperative children, particularly when retinoblastoma, toxocariasis, Coats' disease, or retinopathy of prematurity is being considered as a diagnosis.

See "Congenital Cataract," Section 9.7, for a more specific cataract work-up.

Treatment
- Retinoblastoma: Enucleation, irradiation, photocoagulation, cryotherapy, or occasionally other therapeutic modalities. Systemic chemotherapy is used in metastatic disease.
- Toxocariasis:
  1. Steroids   (The route and dosage depend on the degree of inflammation and physician preference. In moderate-to-severe cases, a periocular depot steroid may be given during EUA, and topical steroids may be given in the presence of anterior segment inflammation. Systemic steroids may also be used.)
  2. Consider a surgical vitrectomy when vitreoretinal traction bands form or when the condition does not improve or worsens with medical therapy.
- Coats' disease: Laser photocoagulation and/or cryotherapy to leaking vessels; surgery may be required for a retinal detachment.
- PHPV
  1. Cataract extraction.
  2. Possible vitreal membrane excision.
  3. Treat any amblyopia.
- Congenital cataract: See Section 9.7.
- Retinal astrocytoma: Observation.
- Retinopathy of prematurity: See Section 9.2.

Follow-up
Variable, depending on the diagnosis.

9.2 RETINOPATHY OF PREMATURITY (ROP)

Risk Factors
- Prematurity (especially <36 weeks of gestation).
- Birthweight <1500 g (3 lb 5 oz), especially <1250 g (2 lb 12 oz).

- Supplemental oxygen therapy.
- Premature twin.

Critical Signs
An avascular peripheral retina.

Other Signs
Dilation of retinal veins and tortuosity of retinal arteries in the posterior pole (i.e., "plus" disease). Poor pupillary dilation despite mydriatic drops with engorgement of iris vessels. It is usually bilateral and is associated with extraretinal fibrovascular proliferation, vitreous hemorrhage, retinal detachment, and leukocoria. In older children and adults, decreased visual acuity, myopia, strabismus, retinal dragging, lattice-like vitreoretinal degeneration, or retinal detachment may occur.

Differential Diagnosis
- Familial exudative vitreoretinopathy (FEV)   (Appears similar to ROP, except FEV is autosomal dominant, although family members may be asymptomatic; there usually is no history of prematurity or oxygen therapy.)
- Incontinentia pigmenti in females.
- See "Leukocoria," Section 9.1, for additional differential diagnoses.

Work-up
A. *Infants < 1250 g*   Dilated retinal examination with scleral depression at age 4 to 6 weeks, ideally prior to discharge from the hospital, with accurate staging of the disease. Can dilate with phenylephrine 2.5%, tropicamide 0.5–1% and homatropine 2%.
B. *Other premature or low-birth-weight infants*   Examination at age 6 to 10 weeks or prior to discharge from the hospital, as above.

Classification

LOCATION

Zone 1   Posterior pole: 2 times the disc-fovea distance, centered around the disc. (Poorest prognosis.)
Zone 2   From zone 1 to the nasal periphery, temporally equidistant from the disc.
Zone 3   The remaining temporal periphery.

EXTENT

Number of clock hours (30 degree sectors) involved.

SEVERITY

Stage 1   Flat demarcation line separating the vascular posterior retina from the avascular peripheral retina.

Stage 2   Ridged demarcation line.

Stage 3   Ridged demarcation line with orange extraretinal fibrovascular proliferation.

Stage 4A   Extrafoveal retinal detachment.

Stage 4B   Subtotal retinal detachment involving zone 1 (the macula).

Stage 5   Total retinal detachment.

"PLUS" DISEASE

Engorged veins and tortuous arteries in the posterior pole is a critical prognostic sign.

Treatment (Based on Severity)

Stage 1 and Stage 2   No treatment necessary.

Stage 3   Cryotherapy or laser photocoagulaion are employed if zones 1[1] or 2 are involved with at least five contiguous or eight accumulated clock hours of extraretinal fibrovascular proliferation in assocciation with "plus" disease ("threshold disease"). Treatment should be instituted within 72 hours once this degree of involvement is reached. The entire avascular zone is treated.

Stage 4 and Stage 5   Surgical repair of retinal detachment by scleral buckling, vitrectomy surgery, or both.

Follow-up

A. *Infants <1250 g*   Prethreshold disease: Repeat examination every 2 weeks until age 14 weeks, then follow every 1–2 months at first, and later every 6–12 months. These children have a higher incidence of myopia, strabismus, amblyopia, dragged macula, cataracts, glaucoma, and retinal detachment. If any stage of ROP is found in zone 1, if a ridge with "plus" disease is found in zone 2, or if any degree of extraretinal fibrovascular proliferation is found in zone 2, then repeat examinations need to be performed at least weekly, depending on the tempo of the disease.

B. *Other premature or low-birth-weight infants*   If signs of ROP are found on initial examination, follow as outlined for infants <1250 g. If no signs of ROP are present initially, a repeat examination at 12–14 weeks of age may be considered, although the likelihood of ROP is minimal.

---

[1]Treat zone 1 with laser therapy rather than with cryotherapy.

References

Committee for the Classification of Retinopathy of Prematurity. The international classification of retinopathy of prematurity. Arch Ophthalmol 102:1130, 1984.

Cryotherapy for Retinopathy of Prematurity Cooperative Group. Multicenter trial of cryotherapy for retinopathy of prematurity: One-year outcome—structure and function. *Arch Ophthalmol* 108:1408, 1990.

McNamara JA, Tasman W, Brown GC, et al. Laser photocoagulation for stage 3+ retinopathy of prematurity. *Ophthalmology* 98:576, 1991.

9.3 ESODEVIATIONS IN CHILDREN

Critical Signs

Either eye is turned inward (i.e., "cross-eyed"). The nonfixating eye turns outward to refixate straight ahead when the fixating eye is covered during the cover-uncover test (see Appendix 2).

Other Signs

Amblyopia, overaction of the inferior oblique muscles.

Types

A. Comitant esotropic deviations   [A manifest convergent misalignment of the eye (or eyes) in which the measured angle of esodeviation is nearly constant in all fields of gaze at distance fixation.]

- Congenital (infantile) esotropia   [Manifests by 6 months of age, the angle of esodeviation is usually large (>40–50 prism diopters) and equal at distance and near fixation. Refractive error is usually normal for age (slightly hyperopic). Amblyopia is often present in those who do not cross-fixate. The patient may have family history of the condition, and often develops latent nystagmus and dissociated vertical deviation.]

- Accommodative esotropia   (Convergent misalignment of the eyes associated with activation of the accommodative reflex. Average age of onset is 2.5 years.)

    Subtypes

    1. Refractive accommodative esotropia   [These children are hyperopic (farsighted) in the range of +3.00 to +10.00 diopters. The measured angle of esodeviation is usually moderate (20–30 prism diopters) and is equal at distance and near fixation. Full hyperopic correction eliminates the esodeviation. The accommodative convergence/accommodation ratio (AC/A) is normal. Amblyopia is common.]

2. Nonrefractive accommodative esotropia   [The measured angle of esodeviation is greater at near fixation than at distance fixation. The refractive error is similar to that of normal children of similar age (slightly hyperopic). The AC/A ratio is high. Amblyopia is common.]

3. Partial or decompensated accommodative esotropia   (Refractive and nonrefractive accommodative esotropias that demonstate a significant reduction in the esodeviation when given full hyperopic correction, but still have a residual esodeviation. The residual esodeviation is the nonaccommodative component. This condition often occurs when there is a delay between the onset of the accommodative esotropia and the use of full hyperopic correction.)

- Sensory deprivation esotropia   [An esodeviation that occurs in a patient with a monocular or binocular lesion or a condition that prevents good vision. (e.g., corneal opacity; cataract; retinal scars, inflammations, tumors; optic neuropathy, anisometropia).]

- Divergence insufficiency   (A convergent ocular misalignment that is greater at distance fixation than at near fixation. This is a diagnosis of exclusion and must be differentiated from divergence paralysis, which can be associated with pontine tumors, neurologic trauma, and other conditions.)

B. Incomitant esodeviations   [The measured angle of esodeviation varies with the direction of gaze at distance fixation (see "Strabismus Syndromes," Section 9.5, and "Isolated Sixth-Nerve Palsy," Section 11.7).]

Differential Diagnosis
- Pseudoesotropia   (The eyes appear esotropic; however, there is no ocular misalignment detected during cover-uncover testing. Usually, the child has a wide nasal bridge, prominent epicanthal folds, or a small interpupillary distance.)

See "Strabismus Syndromes," Section 9.5.

Work-up
1. History: When were the eyes first noted to be "crossed"? Any old photographs? Constant or intermittent? Straightened by glasses? Trauma?
2. Visual acuity of each eye separately, with correction and pinhole, to evaluate for amblyopia.
3. Ocular motility examination; observe for restricted movements.
4. Measure the distance deviation in all fields of gaze and the near deviation in the primary position (straight ahead) using prisms. See Appendix 2.
5. Manifest and cycloplegic refractions.
6. Pupillary, slit-lamp, and fundus examinations; look for causes of sensory deprivation.
7. If divergence insufficiency or paralysis is present, a head CT scan (axial

and coronal views) or an MRI and a neurological evaluation are necessary to rule out an intracranial mass lesion.

8. If abduction is limited, and the esodeviation is incomitant, then observe for characteristics of strabismus syndromes (Section 9.5) or isolated sixth-nerve palsy (Section 11.7) and work-up as appropriate.

Treatment

In *all* cases, correct refractive errors of > + 2.00 to + 3.00 diopters, and treat any amblyopia by patching the better-seeing eye (see "Amblyopia," Section 9.6).

- Congenital esotropia: When equal vision is obtained in the two eyes, corrective muscle surgery is usually performed.
- Accommodative esotropia:
  1. If the patient is younger than 5–6 years of age, correct the hyperopia with the full cycloplegic refraction.
  2. If the patient is older than age 5–6 years of age, push plus lenses during the manifest (noncycloplegic) refraction until distance vision blurs, and give the most plus lenses without blurring distance vision.
  3. If the patient's eyes are straight at distance with full correction, but still esotropic at near distance (high AC/A ratio), then consider bifocals to straighten the eyes at near distance. (An "executive"-style bifocal with a + 2.50 to + 3.00 diopter add, the top of the bifocal segment crossing the lower pupillary border, is usually used.)

❖ **Note** *Glasses for accommodative esotropia need to be worn full-time.*

- Nonaccommodative esotropia and decompensated accommodative esotropia: Muscle surgery is usually performed to correct any significant esotropia that remains when glasses are worn.
- Sensory-deprivation esotropia:
  1. Attempt to correct the cause of poor vision.
  2. Give the full cycloplegic correction.
  3. Muscle surgery to correct the esotropia is usually cosmetic.
  4. All patients with very poor vision in one eye need to wear protective glasses (e.g., polycarbonate lenses) at all times.

❖ **Note** *In children younger than 9–11 years of age, a trial of patching to correct any superimposed amblyopia is usually attempted.*

Follow-up

At each visit, evaluate for amblyopia and measure the degree of deviation with prisms (with glasses worn if the patient has a pair).

- If amblyopia is present, see Section 9.6 for management and follow-up guidelines.

- If amblyopia is not present, the child is reevaluated in 3–6 weeks after a new prescription is given or in 1–6 months if no changes are made and the eyes are straight.
- When a residual esotropia is present while the patient wears glasses, an attempt is made to add more plus power to the current prescription. Children younger than 6 years of age should receive a new cycloplegic refraction; plus lenses are pushed without cycloplegia in older children. The maximum additional plus lens that does not blur distance vision is prescribed. If the eyes cannot be straightened with more plus power, then a decompensated accommodative esotropia has developed (see above).
- Hyperopia (farsightedness) often decreases slowly after 5–7 years of age, and the strength of the glasses may need to be reduced so as not to blur distance vision on manifest refraction. If the strength of the glasses must be reduced to improve visual acuity and the esotropia returns, then this is a decompensated accommodative esotropia (see above).

9.4 EXODEVIATIONS IN CHILDREN

Critical Signs

Either eye is constantly or intermittently turned outward (i.e., "wall-eyed"). On the cover-uncover test, when the fixating eye is covered, the uncovered eye turns inward to fixate (See Appendix 2).

Other Signs

Amblyopia, overaction of the superior or inferior oblique muscles (producing an "A" or a "V" pattern), vertical deviation.

Types

- Intermittent exotropia   (The most common type of exodeviation in children. Onset is usually from infancy to age 4 years, and it is often, but not always, progressive in frequency. Amblyopia is rare.)

    Phases:
    Phase I
    One eye turns out at distance fixation, spontaneously or when it is covered.
    Primarily occurs when the patient is fatigued, sick, or not concentrating.
    The eyes become straight within 1–2 blinks of the cover being removed.
    The eyes are straight at near fixation. Patient often has diplopia and squints to relieve symptoms.

Phase 2
Increasing frequency of exotropia at distance fixation.
Exotropia begins to occur at near fixation.
Phase 3
There is a constant exotropia at distance and near fixations.

- Sensory-deprivation exotropia   (An eye that does not see well, for any reason, turns outward.)
- Duane's syndrome, type 2   (Limitation of adduction of one eye, with globe retraction and narrowing of the palpebral fissure on attempted adduction. Rarely bilateral.)
- Third-nerve palsy   (Limitation of eye movement superiorly, medially, and inferiorly, usually with ptosis. See Section 11.5.)
- Orbital disease (e.g., tumor, orbital pseudotumor)   (Proptosis and restriction of ocular motility are usually evident. See Section 7.1.)
- Myasthenia gravis   [Ptosis and limitation of eye movement can vary throughout the day, positive edrophonium chloride (e.g., Tensilon) test. See Section 11.10.]
- Convergence insufficiency   (Usually occurs in patients older than 10 years of age. Blurred near vision, headaches when reading. An exodeviation at near fixation, but straight at distance fixation. Must be differentiated from convergence paralysis. See Section 15.6.)

Differential Diagnosis
- Pseudoexotropia   (The patient appears to have an exodeviation, but no movement is noted on cover-uncover testing despite good vision in each eye. A wide interpupillary distance or temporal dragging of the macula from retinopathy of prematurity, toxocariasis, or other retinal disorders may be responsible.)

Work-up
1. Evaluate visual acuity of each eye, with correction and pinhole, to evaluate for amblyopia.
2. Perform motility examination; observing for restricted eye movements or signs of Duane's syndrome.
3. Measure the exodeviation in all fields of gaze at distance and in primary position (straight ahead) at near, using prisms (see Appendix 2).
4. Check for proptosis with Hertel exophthalmometry.
5. Perform pupillary, slit-lamp, and fundus examinations; check for causes of sensory deprivation.
6. Manifest and cycloplegic refractions.
7. Consider an edrophonium chloride (e.g., Tensilon Chloride) test when myasthenia gravis is suspected.
8. Consider a CT scan (axial and coronal views) and/or an MRI of the orbit and brain, as needed.

Treatment

In *all* cases, correct significant refractive errors and treat amblyopia (see Section 9.6).

- Intermittent exotropia:
  Phase 1: Follow patient closely.
  Phase 2: Muscle surgery may be indicated to maintain normal binocular vision.
  Phase 3: Muscle surgery is often considered at this point. Bifixation and peripheral fusion can occassionally be attained.

- Sensory-deprivation exotropia:
  1. Correct the underlying cause, if possible.
  2. Treat any amblyopia.
  3. Muscle surgery may be performed for manifest exotropia.
  4. When one eye has very poor vision, protective glasses (e.g., polycarbonate lenses) should be worn at all times to protect the good eye.

- Duane's syndrome: Consider muscle surgery if an abnormal head position is present.
- Third-nerve palsy: See Section 11.5.
- Convergence insufficiency: See Section 15.6.

Follow-up
- If amblyopia is being treated, see Section 9.6.
- If no amblyopia is present, then reexamine every 4–6 months. The parents and patient are told to return sooner if the deviation increases or becomes more frequent.

9.5 STRABISMUS SYNDROMES

Motility disorders that demonstrate typical features of a particular syndrome. Specific entities include the following:

Syndromes
- Duane's syndrome (A motility disorder characterized by limited abduction, limited adduction, or both. The globe retracts and the eyelid fissure narrows on attempted adduction. Amblyopia may occur. Rarely associated with Goldenhar's syndrome and deafness.)
  Type 1: Limited abduction, most common.

Type 2: Limited adduction.

Type 3: Limited abduction and adduction.

- Brown's syndrome   (A motility disorder characterized by limitation of elevation of the adducted eye. Elevation in abduction is relatively normal. Typically, eyes are straight in primary gaze. May be congenital or acquired secondary to trauma, surgery, or inflammation, especially in the area of the trochlea. Bilateral in 10% of patients.)
- Nystagmus blockage syndrome   (An esotropia associated with nystagmus, which begins in early infancy. The nystagmus is reduced when the fixing eye is adducted and increased when the fixing eye is abducted. When one eye is occluded, a head turn toward the uncovered eye develops.)
- Double-elevator palsy   (Limitation of elevation in all fields of gaze. There may be hypotropia of the paretic eye when the nonparetic eye fixates. Ptosis or pseudoptosis may be present in primary gaze. The child may assume a chin-up position to maintain fusion in downgaze.)
- Möbius' syndrome   (Unilateral or bilateral esotropia, with inability to abduct the eye or eyes. Unilateral or bilateral, partial or complete facial nerve palsy may be present. Other cranial nerve palsies may also occur.)

Work-up

1. History: Age of onset? History of trauma? History of other ocular or systemic diseases?
2. Complete ophthalmic examination; observe alignment in primary position and in all fields of gaze. Note if head-turn is present. Observe for nystagmus. Determine if amblyopia is present.
3. Complete physical examination, including cranial nerve evaluation and complete neurologic examination.
4. Radiologic studies (e.g., MRI or CT scan) may be indicated for acquired, atypical, and/or progressive motility disturbances.

Treatment

1. No treatment is usually indicated unless a significant head-turn or chin-up position exists, or a significant horizontal or vertical deviation exists in primary gaze.
2. Treat any amblyopia (see Section 9.6).
3. Correct any significant refractive errors.
4. Surgery, when indicated, is dependent on the particular motility disorder, extraocular muscle function, and the degree of head-turn.

Follow-up

Follow-up is dependent on the condition or conditions being treated (e.g., amblyopia).

9.6 AMBLYOPIA

Symptoms

Decreased vision in one eye.[1] A history of patching, strabismus, and/or muscle surgery as a child may be elicited.

Critical Sign

Poorer vision in one eye that is not improved with refraction and not entirely explained by an organic lesion. The decrease in vision develops during the first decade of life and does not deteriorate thereafter.

Other Signs

Crowding phenomenon (individual letters can be read better than a whole line). A neutral density filter significantly reduces vision in organic disease, but generally does not in pure amblyopia.

❖ **Note** *Amblyopia, even when severe, rarely causes a significant relative afferent pupillary defect.*

Etiology

- Anisometropia   (A difference in refractive error between the two eyes.)
- Strabismus   (The eyes are not straight. Vision is worse in the nonfixating eye. Strabismus can lead to, or be the result of, amblyopia.)
- Occlusion   [Ptosis—congenital or secondary (e.g., eyelid hemangioma) or iatrogenic (e.g., patching).]
- Organic   [Media opacity (e.g., cataract, corneal scar, persistent hyperplastic primary vitreous, retinal or macular lesion).]

Work-up

1. History: Eye problem in childhood, particularly misaligned eyes? Patching or muscle surgery as a child?
2. Complete ocular examination to rule out an organic cause for the reduced vision. Carefully check the pupils, optic disc, and macula.
3. Cover-uncover test to evaluate eye alignment (see Appendix 2).
4. Cycloplegic refraction.

Treatment/Follow-up

A. Patients <9–11 years of age:

1. Spectacle correction if significant anisometropia is present.

---

[1]Amblyopia occasionally occurs bilaterally as a result of bilateral visual deprivation (e.g., congenital cataracts, high refractive errors.)

2. Full-time patching (e.g., Coverlet or Opticlude eye patch) over the eye with better vision for one week per year of age (e.g., 3 weeks for a 3-year-old), followed by a repeat eye examination.

3. Continue patching as above until the vision is equalized, or if vision does not improve after three compliant cycles of patching. If a recurrence of amblyopia is likely, then part-time patching (e.g., 2–6 hours/day) is used until the child reaches 9–11 years of age.

4. In noncompliant patients, consider placing atropine 0.5–1% tid into the better eye to reduce its vision. This may succeed only if the vision of the better-seeing eye is reduced below that of the poorer-seeing eye.

5. If occlusion amblyopia (i.e., a decrease in vision in the patched eye) develops, patch the eye with the better vision for a short period of time (e.g., 1 day per year of age), and repeat the examination.

6. In strabismic amblyopia, delay strabismus surgery until the vision in the two eyes is equal, or maximal vision has been obtained in the amblyopic eye.

B. Patients older than 11 years of age:
No treatment is useful. Protective glasses (e.g., polycarbonate lenses) should be worn at all times if only one eye has good vision.

❖ **Notes**
1. *Pirate patches and patches worn over glasses are less effective than patches that are placed directly over the eye and adhere to the skin.*
2. *When a patch causes periorbital erythema and irritation, have the patient's parent apply tincture of benzoin to the skin before applying the patch. The patch can often be removed with less irritation if a warm-water compress is placed on the patch for several minutes before removal.*

9.7 CONGENITAL CATARACT

Presentation
A white fundus reflex (leukocoria) or abnormal eye movements (nystagmus) in one or both eyes. Infants with bilateral cataracts may be noted to be visually inattentive.

Critical Sign
Opacity of the lens (see types, below).

Other Signs
Eye misalignment (strabismus), nystagmus, or a blunted red reflex may be present. In patients with a monocular cataract, the involved eye is often smaller. A cataract alone does not cause a relative afferent pupillary defect.

Types of Cataracts
A. Polar   (Opacity of the lens capsule and adjacent cortex. May be anterior or posterior.)
B. Zonular (lamellar)   (Small white opacities, usually in a concentric zone around the nucleus. Bilateral.)
C. Lenitcular   (Opacity involves the lens nucleus or a zonular band outside of the lens nucleus.)
D. Sutural   (Y-shaped or inverted Y-shaped cataracts in the central area of the lens. Rarely affect vision.)
E. Capsular   (Opacification of the most anterior portion of the lens, the lens capsule. Generally does not affect vision.)

Etiology
- Idiopathic
- Galactosemia   (Cataract may be the sole manifestation when galactokinase deficiency is responsible. A deficiency of galactose-1-phosphate uridyl transferase may produce mental retardation and symptomatic cirrhosis along with cataracts. The typical oil-droplet opacity may or may not be seen.)
- Persistent hyperplastic primary vitreous (PHPV)   (Unilateral. The involved eye is usually slightly smaller than the normal fellow eye. Examination after pupil dilatation may reveal a plaque of fibrovascular tissue behind the lens with elongated ciliary processes extending to it. Progression of the lens opacity often leads to angle-closure glaucoma.)
- Rubella   (Nuclear cataract, "salt-and-pepper" chorioretinitis, iritis, a smaller involved eye than the normal contralateral eye, and sometimes glaucoma. Associated hearing defects and heart abnormalities are common.)
- Lowe's syndrome (oculocerebrorenal syndrome)   (Opaque lens, congenital glaucoma, renal disease, and mental retardation. X-linked recessive. Patient's mothers may have small white opacities within their lens cortices.)
- Others   (Hereditary, chromosomal disorders, systemic syndromes, other intrauterine infections, trauma, drugs, other metabolic abnormalities.)

Differential Diagnosis
See "Leukocoria," Section 9.1.

Work-up
1. History: Maternal illness or drug ingestion during pregnancy? Systemic or ocular disease in the infant or child? Radiation exposure or trauma? Family history of congenital cataracts?
2. Visual assessment of each eye alone if possible, using illiterate E's, pictures, or by following small toys or a light.
3. Ocular examination: Attempt to determine the visual significance of the cataract. Evaluate the size and location of the cataract and whether the retina can be seen with a direct ophthalmoscope when looking through an

undilated pupil. A portable slit lamp is helpful when available, as is a retinoscope (a blunted retinoscopic reflex suggests the cataract is visually significant). Check for signs of associated glaucoma (e.g., large corneal diameter, corneal edema, breaks in Descemet's membrane) and examine the retina for pathology, if possible.

❖ **Note** *Cataracts 3 mm in diameter or larger usually affect vision.*

4. Cycloplegic refraction.
5. B-scan ultrasonography is necessary when the fundus view is obscured.
6. Medical examination by a pediatrician looking for associated abnormalities.
7. Red blood cell (RBC) galactokinase activity (galactokinase levels) with or without RBC galactose-1-phosphate-uridyltransferase activity to rule out galactosemia.
8. Other tests as suggested by the systemic or ocular examination:
   a. Blood: Calcium and phosphorus levels (hypocalcemia, hypoparathyroidism), glucose levels (hypoglycemia, diabetes mellitus).
   b. Urine: Sodium nitroprusside test (homocystinuria), blood and protein quantitation (Alport's syndrome), amino acid content (Lowe's syndrome), copper level (Wilson's disease).
   c. Antibody titers (rubella, other infectious agents).

❖ **Note** *The chance that one of these conditions is present in a healthy child is small.*

Treatment
1. Referral to a pediatrician to correct any underlying disorder (e.g., galactosemia requires dietary restriction of milk and other galactose-containing products).
2. Treat associated ocular diseases (e.g., glaucoma, see "Congenital Glaucoma," Section 9.10).
3. Treat amblyopia in children younger than 9–11 years of age (see "Amblyopia," Section 9.6).
4. Cataract extraction, usually within days to weeks of discovery, is performed in the following circumstances:
   a. Vision is obstructed, and the eye's visual development is at risk.
   b. The lens is responsible for intraocular disease (e.g., lens-related glaucoma, uveitis).
   c. Cataract progression threatens the health of the eye (e.g., in PHPV).

❖ **Note** *Unlike adult cataracts, significant delay in treating congenital cataracts may lead to irreversible amblyopia.*

5. A mydriatic agent (e.g., phenylephrine 2.5% tid or homatropine 2% tid) may be used as a temporizing measure, allowing peripheral light rays to

pass around the lens opacity and reach the retina. This rarely is successful on a long-term basis.

Follow-up

Young infants that do not undergo surgery are followed closely for cataract progression and amblyopia. Older children without amblyopia are less likely to develop it unless the cataract progresses; they are followed on a 6–12 month basis.

❖ **Note** *Children with rubella must be isolated from pregnant women.*

9.8 OPHTHALMIA NEONATORUM
(Newborn Conjunctivitis)

Critical Sign

Purulent, mucopurulent, or mucoid discharge from one or both eyes in the first month of life, with diffuse conjunctival injection.

Other Signs

Eyelid edema, chemosis.

Etiology

- Chemical   [Seen within a few hours of instilling a prophylactic agent (e.g., silver nitrate), lasts no more than 24–36 hours.]
- *Chlamydia trachomatis*   [May see basophilic intracytoplasmic inclusion bodies in conjunctival epithelial cells, polymorphonuclear leukocytes (polys), or lymphocytes on Giemsa stain.]
- *Neisseria gonorrhea*   (May see gram-negative diplococci in polys on Gram's stain.)
- Bacteria   (Staphylococci, streptococci, and gram-negative species may be seen on Gram's stain)
- Herpes simplex virus   (May have typical herpetic vesicles on the eyelid margins, can see multinucleated giant cells on Giemsa stain.)

Differential Diagnosis

- Dacryocystitis   (Swelling and erythema of the inner canthus. Purulent discharge may be expressed from the punctum by rolling a finger from the lacrimal sac to the punctum. Nasal conjunctival injection may be present, but diffuse injection is typically not present.)
- Nasolacrimal duct obstruction   (Tearing, may have a mild mucopurulent

discharge from the punctum, minimal-to-no conjunctival injection or eyelid swelling.)

Work-up

1. History: Previous veneral disease in the mother? Were cervical cultures performed during pregnancy? If so, obtain the results.
2. Ocular examination with a penlight and then a blue light after fluorescein instillation; look for corneal involvement.
3. Conjunctival scrapings for three slides: Gram's stain, Giemsa stain, and one slide to be held in reserve.
   Technique: Irrigate the discharge out of the fornices, place a drop of topical anesthetic (e.g., proparacaine) in the eye, and scrape the palpebral conjunctiva of the lower eyelid with a flamed-sterilized spatula after it cools off. Place the scrapings on the slides.
4. Conjunctival cultures for blood and chocolate agars (and Thayer-Martin cultures in patients highly suspicious for gonorrhea). Chocolate agar should be placed in an atmosphere of 2–10% carbon dioxide after being plated.
   Technique: Reanesthetize the eye if necessary. Moisten a calcium alginate swab (a cotton-tipped applicator is a less-desirable alternative) with liquid broth media, and vigorously rub it along the inferior palpebral conjunctiva. Plate it directly on the culture dish. Repeat the procedure for additional cultures.
5. Viral culture: Moisten another cotton-tipped applicator and roll it along the palpebral conjunctiva. Break off the end of the applicator and place it into the viral transport medium.
6. Scrape the conjunctiva for the chlamydial immunofluorescent antibody test.

Treatment

Initial therapy is based on the results of the Gram's and Giemsa stains, if they can be examined immediately. Therapy is then modified accourding to the culture results and the clinical response.

A. No information from stains, no particular organism suspected: Erythromycin ointment qid plus erythromycin syrup 50 mg/kg/day[2] for 2–3 weeks.
B. Suspect chemical (e.g., silver nitrate) toxicity: No treatment. Reevaluate in 24 hours.
C. Suspect chlamydia: Erythromycin syrup 50 mg/kg/day[2] for 2–3 weeks, plus erythromycin or sulfacetamide ointment qid.
   If confirmed by culture or immunofluorescent stain, treat the mother and her sexual partner or partners with one of the following:

---

[2]Erythromycin syrup is divided into 4 doses daily and placed into the baby's formula.

Tetracycline 250–500 mg po qid or doxycycline 100 mg po bid for 7 days (for men and mothers who are neither breast-feeding nor pregnant) or

Erythromycin 250–500 mg po qid for 7 days (for breast-feeding or pregnant women).

❖ **Note** *Inadequately treated chlamydial conjunctivitis in a neonate can lead to chlamydial pneumonia.*

D. Suspect *Neisseria gonorrhea:* Treatment is not well established. We favor the following:

1. Hospitalize and evaluate for disseminated gonococcal infection with careful physical examination (especially of joints). Blood and cerebrospinal fluid cultures are obtained if a culture-proven infection is present.

2. Ceftriaxone 25–50 mg/kg/day IV each day for 7 days. If the condition is improving, the IV antibiotic can be changed to an oral antibiotic (e.g., penicillin VK or cefaclor, depending on the patient sensitivity) to complete a 7-day course. In penicillin- or cephalosporin-allergic patients, an infectious disease consult is obtained.

3. Bacitracin ointment qid.

4. Topical saline lavage to remove any discharge qid.

5. Scopolamine 0.25% tid, if the cornea is involved.

6. All neonates with gonorrhea should also be treated for chlamydia with erythromycin syrup 50 mg/kg/day[3] × 14 days.

❖ **Note** *If confirmed by culture, the mother and her sexual partner or partners should be treated in accordance with the sensitivity results for 7 days. Additionally, chlamydia should be treated as outlined above.*

E. Gram-positive bacteria on Gram's stain, with no suspicion of gonorrhea and no corneal involvement: Erythromycin ointment qid for two weeks.

F. Gram-negative bacteria on Gram's stain, but no suspicion of gonorrhea, and no corneal involvement: Gentamicin ointment qid for 2 weeks.

G. Bacteria on Gram's stain and corneal involvement: Hospitalize, work-up, and treat as for "Infectious Corneal Infiltrate/Ulcer," Section 4.12.

H. Suspect herpes simplex virus: Vidarabine 3% ointment (e.g., Vira-A) 5 times per day or trifluorothymidine 1% drops (e.g., Viroptic) q 2 h for 1 week, then cut dosage in half for 1 week. Consider systemic acyclovir with pediatric consultation.

Follow-up

Initially, examine daily as an inpatient or outpatient. If the condition worsens (e.g., corneal involvement develops), reculture and hospitalize. As mentioned

---

[3]Erythromycin syrup is divided into 4 doses daily and placed into the baby's formula.

above, therapy is tailored according to the clinical response and the culture results. The frequency of follow-up visits may be reduced once improvement is clearly demonstrated.

References

Ullman S, Roussel TJ, Forster RK. Gonococcal keratoconjunctivitis. *Surv Ophthalmol* 32:199, 1987.

9.9 CONGENITAL NASOLACRIMAL DUCT OBSTRUCTION

Presentation
Persistent tearing, chronic low-grade discharge, matting of the eyelids.

Critical Signs
Wet-looking eye (tears flowing over the eyelid margin); may have crusting on the eyelashes (predominantly medially), and reflux of mucoid or mucopurulent material from the punctum when pressure is applied to the area over the lacrimal sac, where the lower eyelid abuts the nose.

Other Signs
Erythema (irritation) of the surrounding skin; redness and swelling of the medial canthus. Preseptal cellulitis can develop from dacryocystitis.

❖ **Note** *Nasolacrimal duct obstruction may be associated with an otitis or pharyngitis.*

Etiology
Usually the result of an imperforate membrane at the distal end of the nasolacrimal duct.

Differential Diagnosis
- Conjunctivitis   (Red eye, discharge. Usually acute. Follicles or papillae may or may not be present on the inferior tarsal conjunctiva. Tearing is usually not chronic.)
- Congenital anomalies of the upper lacrimal drainage system   (Atresia of the lacrimal puncta or canaliculus.)
- Mucocele of the lacrimal sac   (Bluish, cystic, nontender mass located just

below the medial canthal angle. Caused by both a distal and a proximal obstruction of the nasolacrimal apparatus.)
- Other causes of tearing (Entropion/trichiasis, corneal defects, foreign body under the upper eyelid, congenital glaucoma.)

Work-up
1. Slit-lamp or penlight examination to rule out other causes of tearing. Make sure the corneal diameter is not large, and ruptures in Descemet's membrane are not present (congenital glaucoma).
2. Palpate over the lacrimal sac; observe for any mucoid or mucopurulent discharge from the punctum.
3. Measure intraocular pressure if congenital glaucoma is suspected; Schiötz tonometry is often easiest in a child.

Treatment
1. Digital massage 2–4 times per day [The mother is taught to place her index finger over the child's common canaliculus (inner corner of the eye) and to stroke downward slowly, several times in succession.]
2. Consider erythromycin ointment bid for 1 week if a significant mucopurulent discharge is present.
3. Warm compresses 2–4 times per day are used to keep the eyelids clean when a discharge is present.
4. In the presence of acute dacryocystitis, a systemic antibiotic is needed (see "Darcyocystitis," Section 6.8).

The majority of cases will open spontaneously with this regimen by 1 year of age. If this is not the case:

5. Nasolacrimal duct probing is performed at 13 months of age (Some physicians will probe children younger than 12 months of age; we generally do not.) The majority of obstructions will be corrected after the initial probing; others may require repeat probings. If patency is not established after three probings, then consider placing sialastic tubing in the nasolacrimal duct and leave it in place for weeks to months.

❖ **Note** *Children who develop recurrent or persistent infections of the lacrimal drainage apparatus despite antibiotics may need to be probed earlier than 13 months of age.*

Follow-up
Acute dacryocystitis should be treated as soon as possible and the patient followed every day until significant improvement is noted; all other patients can be followed by monthly phone calls (the child returns if the situation becomes worse or if the parents are unsure).

Reference

Nelson LB, Calhoun JK, Menduke H. Medical management of congenital nasolacrimal duct obstruction. *Pediatrics* 76:172, 1985.

9.10 CONGENITAL GLAUCOMA

Presentation

Photophobia, tearing, or eyelid squeezing (blepharospasm), most commonly in an infant; red eye may be present.

Critical Signs

Enlarged globe and corneal diameter (horizontal corneal diameter >12 mm before 1 year of age is suspicious), corneal edema, increased intraocular pressure (IOP), increased cup/disc ratio, commonly bilateral.

Other Signs

Linear tears in Descemet's membrane of the cornea, usually running horizontally or concentric to the limbus; corneal stromal scarring; conjunctival injection; myopic shift in refractive error.

Etiology

- Primary congenital glaucoma   (Not associated with other ocular or systemic disorders.)
- Developmental anterior segment abnormality (Axenfeld's anomaly, Rieger's anomaly/syndrome, Peter's anomaly, others)   (Bilateral. Abnormalities of the cornea, iris, and anterior-chamber angle.)
- Lowe's syndrome (oculocerebrorenal syndrome)   (Cataract, glaucoma, and renal disease; X-linked recessive.)
- Rubella (Glaucoma, cataracts, "salt-and-pepper" chorioretinopathy, hearing and cardiac defects.)
- Phakomatoses   (Sturge-Weber, neurofibromatosis, others.)
- Others   (Aniridia, homocystinuria, persistent hyperplastic primary vitreous, etc.)

Differential Diagnosis

- Congenital megalocornea (Large corneal diameter without corneal edema. IOP and cup/disc ratio are normal.)
- High myopia (A large corneal diameter may be found along with a large

eye; however, a highly myopic refractive error, tilted optic discs with adjacent myopic crescents, normal corneal thickness, and normal IOP are also found.)

- Birth trauma (May produce tears in Descement's membrane and corneal edema; however, the tears are typically vertical or oblique in orientation and the corneal diameter is normal. Birth trauma is generally unilateral and may often be obtained from the history.)
- Congenital hereditary endothelial dystrophy (Bilateral corneal edema at birth with a normal corneal diameter and normal IOP.)
- Mucopolysaccharidoses and cystinosis (Some inborn errors of metabolism produce cloudy corneas, but the corneal diameter and IOP are normal.)
- Nasolacrimal duct obstruction (Tearing, sometimes with a mild mucopurulent discharge from the punctum. The cornea is clear and not enlarged. The IOP is normal.)

Work-up
1. History: Other systemic abnormalities? Infection during pregnancy? Birth trauma? Family history of congenital glaucoma?
2. Ocular examination, including a visual acuity assessment of each eye separately (can the child fixate and follow?), a penlight examination to detect corneal enlargement and haziness, and a refraction. IOP measurement is attempted, and a dilated fundus examination is performed to evaluate the optic disc and retina. A hand-held portable slit lamp is sometimes used in uncertain cases to look for tears in Descemet's membrane and corneal edema.
3. Gonioscopy may be attempted in cooperative children who are not expected to undergo examination under anesthesia.
4. Examination under anesthesia is performed in suspicious cases and in those in whom surgical treatment is planned. The horizontal corneal diameter and IOP are measured; retinoscopy, gonioscopy, and ophthalmoscopy are performed. Ultrasound is often employed to measure axial length.

❖ **Note** *IOP may be lowered substantially by general anesthesia, particularly halothane; an IOP of 20 mm Hg or greater under halothane anesthesia is suggestive of glaucoma. An exception is ketamine hydrochloride, which may increase IOP. In general, IOP is measured as soon as possible after general anesthesia is induced to achieve as accurate a measurement as possible.*

Treatment
Definitive treatment is usually surgical. Medical therapy is temporary and is started initially, pending surgery.

A. Medical (Any or all of the following may be used.)
1. Topical beta-blocker (e.g., levobunolol 0.25–0.5% bid or timolol 0.25–0.5% bid).

2. Carbonic anhydrase inhibitor (e.g., acetazolamide 5 mg/kg po q 6 h).
3. Epinephrine compound (e.g., dipivefrin 0.1% bid).

❖ **Note** *Miotics are rarely effective in controlling and may raise IOP, but they sometimes are used to constrict the pupil in preparation for a surgical goniotomy.*

B. Surgical
First choice   Goniotomy (incising the trabecular meshwork with a blade under gonioscopic visualization) or trabeculotomy (opening Schlemm's canal into the anterior chamber). These procedures are often repeated if they are unsuccessful at first attempt.
Other   Trabeculectomy.

❖ **Note** *Amblyopia may be superimposed upon glaucoma and should be treated by patching (see Section 9.6).*

Follow-up
Repeat examinations, under anesthesia when needed, are necessary to follow corneal diameter, IOP, cup/disc ratio, and axial length. These patients need to be followed throughout life to monitor for progression.

9.11 DEVELOPMENTAL ANTERIOR SEGMENT AND LENS ANOMALIES

Unilateral or bilateral congenital abnormalities of the cornea, iris, anterior-chamber angle, and lens. Specific entities include the following:

• Megalocornea   (A nonprogressive corneal enlargement. The horizontal corneal diameter is >12 mm in the newborn. There are two types:
  1. Simple megalocornea: bilateral, clear corneas of normal thickness; autosomal dominant.
  2. Anterior megalophthalmos: Bilateral; associated with abnormalities of the iris, angle, and lens; may be associated with glaucoma; X-linked recessive.)
• Microcornea   [Horizontal corneal diameter <11 mm. May be isolated or associated with nanophthalmos (a small globe that is otherwise anatomi-

cally normal) and microphthalmos (a small globe with multiple anomalies).]

- Posterior embryotoxon (A prominent, anteriorly displaced Schwalbe's ring. A normal variant.)
- Axenfeld's anomaly (Posterior embryotoxon associated with iris strands that span the angle to insert into the prominent Schwalbe's ring. Fifty percent of patients develop glaucoma. Autosomal dominant or sporadic.)
- Rieger's anomaly (Axenfeld's anomaly plus iris thinning and abnormally shaped and displaced pupils. Sixty percent of patients develop glaucoma. Autosomal dominant or sporadic.)
- Rieger's syndrome (Rieger's anomaly associated with dental, craniofacial, and sketal abnormalities. May be associated with short stature secondary to growth hormone deficiency, cardiac defects, deafness, and mental retardation. Autosomal dominant or sporadic.)
- Peter's anomaly (Central corneal opacity, usually with iris strands that extend from the iris border to the margin of the corneal defect. The lens may be clear and normally positioned; cataractous and displaced anteriorly, making the anterior chamber shallow; or adherent to the corneal defect.)
- Microspherophakia (The lens is small and spherical in configuration. The lens can subluxate into the anterior chamber, causing a secondary glaucoma.)
- Anterior and posterior lenticonus (An anterior or posterior ectasia of the lens surface. Often associated with cataract. Usually unilateral.)
- Ectopia lentis (Simple ectopia lentis typically consist of bilateral, usually superior, lens displacement. Glaucoma may occur. Autosomal dominant.)
- Ectopia lentis et pupillae (Lens displacement associated with pupillary displacement in the opposite direction. Glaucoma may occur. Autosomal recessive.)
- Aniridia (Bilateral, near-total abscence of the iris. The pupil appears to occupy the entire area of the cornea. Glaucoma, foveal hypoplasia with poor vision, nystagmus, and corneal pannus can occur. At least two inheritance patterns are known to exist:
  1. Autosomal dominant in two thirds of patients. This type is not associated with Wilms' tumor.
  2. Sporadic in one third of patients. Twenty-five percent of children with sporadic aniridia will develop Wilms' tumor.)

Work-up

1. History: Family history of ocular disease? Associated systemic abnormalities?
2. Complete ophthalmic examination, including gonioscopy of the anterior-chamber angle and intraocular pressure (IOP) determination (may require examination under anesthesia).

3. Complete physical examination by a pediatrician or family physician with blood pressure determination (may be elevated with renal abnormalities).
4. Chromosomal karyotype in patients with sporadic cases of aniridia. (There is an increased incidence of Wilms' tumor in patients with a deletion of the short arm of chromosome 11.)
5. Renal ultrasound and possibly intravenous pyelography in patients with sporadic aniridia.

Treatment
1. Correct refractive errors and treat amblyopia if present (see Section 9.6). Children with unilateral structural abnormalities often have improved visual acuity after amylyopia therapy.
2. Treat glaucoma if present. Beta-blockers and carbonic anhydrase inhibitors are often more effective than pilocarpine and epinephrine compounds (see "Primary Open-Angle Glaucoma," Section 10.1). Surgery is often used initially (see "Congenital Glaucoma," Section 9.10).
3. Consider cataract extraction if a significant cataract exists and a corneal transplant if a dense corneal opacity exists.
4. Genetic counseling.
5. Systemic abnormalities (e.g., Wilms' tumor) are managed by pediatric specialists.

Follow-up
1. Ophthalmic examination every 6–12 months throughout life, checking for increased IOP and other signs of glaucoma.
2. If amblyopia exists, then follow-up may need to be more frequent (see Section 9.6)
3. Renal ultrasound every 3–6 months in children with sporadic aniridia until the age of 4–5 years.
4. Periodic physical examinations by a pediatrician, including blood pressure determination, until the age of 4–5 years in children with sporadic aniridia.

9.12 THE BLIND INFANT

An infant whose visual skills are far below those expected (e.g., an inability to fix on and follow objects after several months of age) may have an obvious or inconspicuous ocular or neuro-ophthalmic disorder. Obvious causes include bilateral central corneal opacities, congenital cataracts, or infectious retinal problems with macular scarring. The following are conditions that may not be obvious on clinical examination.

I. Conditions that *usually* produce a searching nystagmus:
   A. Pupils react poorly to light:
   - Leber's congenital amaurosis [May have a normal-appearing fundus initially or pigmentary retinal changes that progress to a retinitis pigmentosa–like picture. Narrowing of the retinal vessels and optic disc pallor may be present early. The electroretinogram (ERG) is markedly abnormal or flat. Autosomal recessive.]
   - Optic nerve hypoplasia [A small optic disc that can be difficult to detect when bilateral (compare disc to vessels). If unilateral, may go unnoticed until later in life. When present, a "double ring" sign (a pigmented ring at the inner and outer edge of peripapillary atrophy) is diagnostic. Usually idiopathic but can be a result of maternal diabetes or quinine, phenytoin, alcohol, or LSD use.]
   - Achromatopsia (Rod monochromatism) (Normal fundus, but photopic ERG is markedly attenuated or nonrecordable. Scotopic ERG is normal.)

❖ **Note** *Optic-nerve hypoplasia is associated with septo-optic dysplasia (de Morsier syndrome), which includes midline abnormalities of the brain and growth, thyroid, and other tropic hormone deficiencies. Growth retardation, seizures as a result of hypoglycemia, and diabetes insipidus may develop.*

   - Congenital optic atrophy (Rare. Pale, normal-sized optic disc, often associated with mental retardation or cerebral palsy. Normal ERG. Autosomal recessive.)
   B. Pupils react briskly to light:
   - Infantile nystagmus (Some patients with this condition have a severe visual deficit. The iris is normal. It may be accompanied by face turn, head nodding, or both.)
   - Albinism with delayed maturation (Patients often have iris transillumination defects and foveal hypoplasia.)
II. No nystagmus present and pupils react normally to light:
   - Diffuse cerebral dysfunction (Infants do not respond to sound or touch and are neurologically abnormal. Vision may slowly improve with time.)
   - Delayed maturation of the visual system (Normal response to sound and touch, and neurologically normal. The ERG is normal, and vision usually develops between 4 and 12 months of age.)
   - Extreme refractive error (Diagnosed on cycloplegic refraction.)

Work-up
1. History: Premature? Normal development and growth? Maternal infection, diabetes, or drug use during pregnancy? Family history of eye disease?
2. Evaluate the infant's ability to fixate on an object and follow it with each eye individually (patch one eye and then the other).

3. Pupillary examination.
4. Look carefully for nystagmus.
5. Penlight examination of the anterior segment; check especially for iris transillumination defects.
6. Dilated retinal and optic nerve evaluation.
7. Cycloplegic refraction.
8. ERG, especially if the cause of poor vision is not known.
9. Consider a CT scan and/or MRI of the brain.
10. Consider a sweep visual evoked potential (VEP) for vision measurement.
11. Consider eye movement recordings to evaluate the nystagmus wave form, if available.

Treatment

1. Correct refractive errors and treat known or suspected amblyopia.
2. Parental counseling is necessary in all of the above conditions with respect to the infant's visual potential.
3. Information concerning educational services for the visually handicapped or blind may be helpful.
4. Genetic counseling.
5. Children who have small stature, a history of failure to thrive, or developmental delay should be referred for pediatric endocrine evaluation. A CT scan (axial and coronal views) and/or an MRI of the brain may be obtained, especially if a neuro-ophthalmic condition exists.
6. The child's pediatrician should be informed of the child's condition and instructed to refer the patient for an endocrine evaluation if growth or development becomes delayed in children with optic-nerve hypoplasia.

GLAUCOMA

10.1 PRIMARY OPEN-ANGLE GLAUCOMA (POAG)

Symptoms

Usually asymptomatic until the late stages, at which point decreased peripheral or central vision may be noted.

Critical Signs

1. A large or enlarging cup/disc ratio, often with asymmetry between the two eyes.
2. Visual field defects, commonly nasal, paracentral, or extending in an arcuate distribution from the blind spot nasally.
3. Elevated intraocular pressure (IOP), generally >22 mm Hg.
4. The anterior-chamber angle is open on gonioscopy, and peripheral anterior synechiae are not present.

Other Signs

The rim of the optic cup may be notched, the cup may be elongated vertically, and nerve fiber layer loss may be apparent. Large daily fluctuations in IOP (such that single IOP measurements may be misleading), absence of corneal edema, and a white, uninflamed eye are characteristic.

Risk Factors

Glaucoma in the contralateral eye, family history of blindness or visual loss as a result of glaucoma, diabetes or hypertension (systemic vascular disease), black race, myopia, age.

The Wills Eye Manual: Office and Emergency Room Diagnosis and Treatment of Eye Diseases, Second Edition, edited by R. Douglas Cullom, Jr., M.D., and Benjamin Chang, M.D. © 1994 J. B. Lippincott Company.

Differential Diagnosis
- Low-tension glaucoma   (Findings of POAG, but IOP consistently not elevated.)
- Chronic angle-closure glaucoma   (Findings of POAG, but peripheral anterior synechiae are present on gonioscopy, closing part of the anterior-chamber angle. Patients with chronic angle-closure glaucoma do not typically develop the sudden, painful, acute rise in IOP seen with acute angle-closure glaucoma. It may be superimposed upon POAG.)
- Secondary open-angle glaucoma   [Lens-induced, inflammatory, exfoliative, pigmentary, steroid-induced, developmental anterior-segment abnormalities, angle recession, traumatic (direct injury from blood or debris), iridocorneal endothelial (ICE) syndrome, glaucoma related to increased episcleral venous pressure (e.g., Sturge-Weber syndrome, carotid-cavernous fistula), glaucoma related to intraocular tumors or other ocular conditions. See specific sections for more detailed information.]
- Optic atrophy   (Chiasmal tumors, syphilis, ischemic optic neuropathy, drugs, retinal vascular or degenerative disease, others. IOP is not elevated in these conditions, unless a secondary glaucoma is also present. These conditions are differentiated by more pallor of optic nerve than cupping and characteristic visual field loss. If cupping is present, the rim is typically pale as well as cupped.)

Work-up
1. History: Known glaucoma or ocular disease? Family history of glaucoma? Previous trauma, red or inflamed eye, or chronic steroid use? Medical problems, specifically diabetes, hypertension, asthma, congestive heart failure, heart block, renal stones, or allergies?
2. Ocular examination, with special attention to IOP, gonioscopic evaluation of the anterior-chamber angle, and optic-disc assessment with a slit-lamp and a 60-diopter, Hruby, or fundus contact lens.
3. Stereo photographs of the optic discs are obtained in suspected or definite cases to facilitate recognition of optic-disc changes on future examinations.
4. Formal visual field examination, preferably automated (e.g., Humphrey, Octopus). Goldmann visual fields are obtained in patients who lack the visual ability or intelligence required for automated visual fields.
5. In atypical cases, a low-tension glaucoma work-up may be appropriate (see Section 10.2).

Treatment
The goal of therapy is to prevent further cupping and visual field loss by lowering IOP. There are no set rules as to when to institute therapy and what therapeutic modalities to use initially. The following guidelines may be used.

A. Patients with mildly elevated IOP (22–27 mm Hg), normal optic discs, and normal visual fields may be followed as "glaucoma suspects," their IOP and optic-nerve appearance monitored a few times per year, and their formal visual field rechecked yearly. Patients with risk factors for glaucoma, especially a positive family history, are sometimes given the option of treatment, particularly when the IOP is at the higher end of this range.

B. Patients with normal IOP but suspicious optic nerves and questionable or unreliable visual fields: Follow as in (A).

C. Patients with optic nerves suggestive of glaucoma, mild-to-moderate visual field changes consistent with glaucoma, and mild-to-moderately elevated IOP are generaly started on one antiglaucoma medication in one eye on a 3–6-week trial basis. The IOP level of the two eyes is rechecked after the 3–6-week period, preferably at the same time of the day as the initial check, comparing the levels of the treated and untreated eyes to their levels prior to treatment. A decision of whether to maintain or discontinue the trial drug is based on whether the treated eye's IOP declined a significant amount compared to the untreated, contralateral eye. If there is any hint of glaucoma in the untreated contralateral eye, both eyes should be treated with a drug shown to be effective in that patient.

D. Patients with IOP >27 mm Hg, regardless of the disc and field changes, are generally treated as in (C) to lower the risk of glaucomatous visual field loss.

E. Patients with marked optic-nerve cupping and a very high IOP upon presentation are treated aggressively with multiple antiglaucomatous medications initially, even prior to obtaining the visual field. A therapeutic trial is not performed if both eyes have advanced glaucoma and there is an impending risk of central visual loss. These patients are often followed more often than the typical 3–6-week interval to evaluate the effect of treatment. If the IOP is well controlled with multiple medications, one drug at a time may be stopped to determine its antiglaucomatous efficacy.

Medications

Drugs chosen for therapeutic trials must both lower IOP and be tolerable. Patients who experience unpleasant side effects will not be compliant with their medication.

TYPICAL FIRST-LINE THERAPY

Topical medication

1. Beta-blockers (e.g., levobunolol 0.25 0.5% each day or bid, timolol 0.25–0.5% bid, metipranolol 0.3% bid, or carteolol 1% bid), often effectively lower IOP, but cannot be given to patients with breathing problems (e.g., asthma), heart block, or congestive heart failure. Betaxolol qd or bid may be used cautiously in patients with emphysema and heart disease, if

permitted by the patient's internist. The pulse is usually checked prior to and after initiating therapy with these drugs.

2. Miotics (e.g., pilocarpine qid) are generally used in low strengths initially (e.g., 0.5–1%) and then built up to higher strengths (e.g., 4–6%). Commonly not tolerated in patients <40 years of age because of accommodative spasm. Strong miotics are generally contraindicated in patients with retinal holes and should be used cautiously in patients at risk for retinal detachment (e.g., high myopes, aphakes).

❖ **Note** *Pilocarpine is also available in a 4% gel used nightly or as an ocular insert replaced once a week; the latter is especially valuable in young patients.*

3. Epinephrine compounds (e.g., dipivefrin 0.1% bid or epinephrine 0.5–2% bid) rarely reduce IOP to the degree of the first two classes of drugs, but have very few side effects. They may cause cystoid macular edema in aphakic patients.

SECOND-LINE THERAPY

Generally reserved for patients who demonstrate progressive cupping or visual field loss on maximally tolerated topical medications. Topical medications are continued.

1. Oral carbonic anhydrase inhibitors (e.g., methazolamide 25–50 mg po 2–3 times per day, acetazolamide 250 mg po qid, or acetazolamide 500 mg sequel po bid) cannot be given to patients with a sulfa allergy and should be avoided or used cautiously in patients with a history of calcium renal stones. As these agents are also mild diuretics, potassium levels need to be monitored if the patient is taking other diuretic agents or digitalis. Side effects, such as nausea and confusion, are often intolerable. Rare, but severe, hematologic side effects have occurred.

2. Laser trabeculoplasty: Effectiveness is usually limited to 1–5 yrs. Side effects are few.

THIRD-LINE THERAPY

Glaucoma filtering surgery (e.g., trabeculectomy).

FOURTH-LINE THERAPY

Any of the following: Repeat filtering surgery with adjunct antifibrosis therapy (e.g., 5-FU or mitomycin C), shunt tube procedure (e.g., Schocket, Baerveldt, Molteno), YAG laser cyclophotocoagulation, cyclodialysis, cyclocryotherapy.

Follow-up

As mentioned above, patients are reexamined 3–6 weeks after starting a new medication to evaluate its efficacy; in severe glaucoma, the patient can be followed sooner. Once the IOP has been lowered substantially, patients are reevaluated in 3–6-month intervals for IOP and optic-nerve checks. Gonioscopy is performed yearly and after starting a new strength cholinergic agent (e.g., pilocarpine). Formal visual fields of the same type (e.g., Humphrey, Octopus) are rechecked every 6–12 months. Dilated retinal examinations should be performed yearly. If glaucomatous damage progresses, check patient compliance with medications before initiating additional therapy. The goal of additional therapy is to lower the IOP to a target pressure 25–30% beneath the range at which glaucomatous progression has occurred. This target pressure depends on the severity of disease and speed of progression, and it needs to be updated often.

See the Drug Glossary for additional drug information.

10.2 LOW-TENSION GLAUCOMA

Description
1. A large or enlarging cup/disc ratio, often with asymmetry between the two eyes.
2. Visual field defects, usually paracentral, nasal, or extending in an arcuate fashion from the blind spot to the nasal periphery.
3. Intraocular pressure (IOP) always ≤22 mm Hg.
4. Open angle seen on gonioscopy with no peripheral anterior synechiae.

Other Signs
Splinter hemorrhages at the edge of the cup, pallor of the optic nerve, nerve fiber–layer loss, acquired optic pit.

Differential Diagnosis
- Primary open-angle glaucoma   (IOP >22 mm Hg in the past, or at other times of the day. See Section 10.1.)
- Angle-closure glaucoma (Narrow angles usually bilaterally, peripheral anterior synechiae. Patients often have a history of acute episodes of pain, photophobia, and red eye. See Section 10.10.)
- Previous glaucomatous damage (e.g., from steroids, uveitis, glaucomatocyclitic crisis, trauma).
- Previous ischemic damage to the optic nerve (e.g., a previous hypotensive event or ischemic optic neuropathy) (A history of acute visual loss can often be elicited. Visual field defects may be identical to glaucoma or may be altitudinal. Cupping and visual field abnormalities do not usually progress, but the contralateral eye can become affected.)
- Hematologic disease (e.g., anemia or polycythemia vera)

- Syphilis [Positive FTA-ABS, may have a history or signs of prior iritis (e.g., synechiae), ghost vessels (blood vessels devoid of blood) in the cornea, or a salt-and-pepper appearance to the fundus. See Section 14.2.]
- Compressive optic neuropathy [Optic-nerve pallor greater than cupping, often from a tumor or aneurysm. Visual field defects are often atypical for glaucoma (i.e., show respect of vertical meridian).]
- Congenital nerve defect (e.g., myopic discs, colobomas, optic nerve pits, optic nerve drusen) (Cupping and visual field abnormalities do not usually progress.)

❖ **Note** *Low-tension glaucoma can develop as a consequence of any of the above. A compromised optic nerve may not tolerate IOP in the teens.*

Work-up

1. History: Acute episodes of eye pain or redness? Steroid use? Acute visual loss? Ocular trauma? Surgery, trauma, heart attack, or other event that may have caused a hypotensive episode?
2. Slit-lamp examination with IOP measurement.
3. Gonioscopy of the anterior-chamber angle.
4. Optic-nerve evaluation, preferably with a fundus contact, Hruby, or 60-diopter lens at the slit lamp.
5. Stereo optic disc photographs.
6. Visual field testing, preferably automated (e.g., Humphrey, Octopus).
7. Diurnal IOP curve (multiple IOP checks during the course of a day).
8. Complete blood count, ESR, RPR, FTA-ABS, with or without ANA.
9. CT scan (axial and coronal views) and/or MRI of the orbit and brain for atypical cases [e.g., unilateral cases, those in young patients, when visual field defects are uncharacteristic or are neurological (e.g., homonymous defects)] or when other neurological signs or symptoms are present.
10. Have the patient see their medical doctor for a complete cardiovascular evaluation.

Treatment/Follow-up

In general, the goal of treatment is to lower the IOP 25–30% below the level at which damage occurred. This is often as low as 10–12 mm Hg. See "Primary Open-Angle Glaucoma," Section 10.1, for a detailed treatment and follow-up regimen.

A. Treatment may be indicated for:
  1. Advanced optic-nerve cupping.
  2. A visual field defect threatening central vision, as determined by the visual field test.
  3. Glaucomatous cupping and field loss that cannot be accounted for by any disease other than low-tension glaucoma.

4. Progression of cupping and/or field loss unexlained by progression of another disease process (e.g., cataract).

B. Observation (e.g., IOP and optic-nerve evaulation every 3–4 months; visual field examination every 6–12 months) may be indicated in the following situations:

1. The diagnosis of glaucoma is in question (e.g., possible old nonarteritic ischemic optic neuropathy).

2. An explanation for the glaucomatous changes is available (e.g., previous prolonged use of steroids or a previous episode of hypoperfusion).

10.3 ANGLE-RECESSION GLAUCOMA

Symptoms

Usually asymptomatic until the late stages, at which point unilateral visual field or acuity loss may be noted. A history of trauma to the glaucomatous eye can usually be elicited, sometimes up to years prior to presentation.

Critical Signs

Glaucoma [large or enlarging cup/disc ratio, characteristic visual field loss, and/or elevated intraocular pressure (IOP)] in an eye with gonioscopic findings. These include an uneven iris insertion with an area of torn iris processes and posteriorly recessed iris to reveal a widened cilary band. In some cases, these findings and the angle recession extend for 360 degrees. Comparison with corresponding angle structures of the normal contralateral eye help in identification of recessed areas.

Other Signs

The scleral spur may appear abnormally white on gonioscopy because of the recessed angle; other signs of previous trauma may be present (e.g., cataract, iris sphincter tears).

Differential Diagnosis

See "Primary Open-Angle Glaucoma," Section 10.1.

Work-up

1. History: Trauma? Family history of glaucoma?
2. Slit-lamp examination, including IOP measurement.
3. Gonioscopy of the anterior-chamber angle.
4. Optic-nerve evaluation with a slit lamp and 60-diopter, Hruby, or fundus contact lens.

5. Stereo photographs of the optic discs for a baseline.

6. Formal visual field examination, preferably automated (e.g., Humphrey, Octopus) in cases suspicious for, or with definite, glaucoma.

Treatment

Similar to primary open-angle glaucoma (see Section 10.1), except miotics (e.g., pilocarpine) may be ineffective or even cause elevation of IOP as a result of a reduction of uveoscleral outflow. Argon laser trabeculoplasty is rarely effective in this condition.

Follow-up

Patients with angle recession without glaucoma are examined yearly. Those with glaucoma are examined according to the guidelines of "Primary Open-Angle Glaucoma," Section 10.1. Follow-up should carefully monitor both eyes, as there is a high incidence of delayed open-angle glaucoma in the uninvolved as well as the traumatized eye.

10.4 INFLAMMATORY OPEN-ANGLE GLAUCOMA

Symptoms

Pain, photophobia, decreased vision; symptoms may be minimal.

Critical Signs

Increased intraocular pressure (IOP), often unilateral with a significant amount of aqueous white blood cells and flare, open angle on gonioscopy.

Other Signs

Miotic pupil, peripheral anterior synechiae, keratic precipitates on the posterior corneal surface or trabecular meshwork, conjunctival injection, ciliary flush.

❖ **Note** *Acute IOP elevation is distinguished from chronic IOP elevation by the presence of corneal edema, pain, and the perception of halos around light.*

Etiology

- Anterior uveitis
- Intermediate and posterior uveitis
- Panuveitis
- Kerato-uveitis   (Corneal pathology present in addition to uveitis.)
- Following trauma or intraocular surgery.

Differential Diagnosis

- Glaucomatocyclitic crisis (Posner-Schlossman syndrome)   [Markedly elevated IOP (usually 40–60 mm Hg), open angle and absence of synechiae on gonioscopy, mild anterior-chamber reaction with few fine keratic precipitates, and minimal-to-no conjunctival injection. Unilateral with recurrent attacks. See Section 10.12.]
- Acute angle-closure glaucoma   (Angle closed in the involved eye and usually narrow in the contralateral eye, mid-dilated pupil that reacts poorly to light, iris bombé, corneal edema, mild anterior-chamber reaction without keratic precipitates. See Section 10.10.)
- Pigmentary glaucoma   (Acute rise in IOP, often after exercise or pupillary dilatation; *pigment* cells in the anterior chamber, on the trabecular meshwork, and along the posterior corneal surface. The angle is open, and radial iris transillumination defects are often present. See Section 10.6.)
- Neovascular glaucoma   (Iris and anterior chamber angle neovascularization are present. See Section 10.13.)
- Fuchs' heterochromic iridocyclitis   (Asymmetry of the iris color, mild iritis in the eye with the lighter-colored iris, usually unilateral, often associated with cataract, glaucoma, or both. Conjunctival injection and ciliary flush are minimal. See "Anterior Uveitis," Section 13.1.)

Work-up

1. History: Recent dilating drops or a systemic anticholinergic agent (suggests angle-closure glaucoma)? Previous attacks? Systemic disease (e.g., juvenile rheumatoid arthritis, ankylosing spondylitis, sarcoidosis, AIDS)? Previous corneal disease?
2. Slit-lamp examination: Assess the degree of conjunctival injection and aqueous cell and flare.
3. Measure IOP.
4. Gonioscopy of the anterior-chamber angle: Is the angle open? Synechiae present? Neovascular membrane present?
5. Evaluation of the optic nerve.

Treatment

1. Topical steroid (e.g., prednisolone acetate 1%) q 1–6 h, depending on the severity of the anterior-chamber cellular reaction.

❖ **Note** *Topical steroids are not used, or are used with extreme caution, in patients with an infectious process, particularly a fungal or herpes simplex infection.*

2. Mydriatic/cycloplegic (e.g., scopolamine 0.25% tid or atropine 1% tid)
3. Topical beta-blocker (e.g., timolol 0.5% bid or levobunolol 0.5% bid).

One or more of the following pressure-lowering agents can be used in addition to the above treatments, depending on the IOP and the status of the optic nerve:

4. Carbonic anhydrase inhibitor (e.g., methazolamide 25–50 mg po 2–3 times per day, or acetazolamide 250 mg po qid or 500 mg sequel po bid).
5. Topical epinephrine compound (e.g., epinephrine 0.5–2% bid or dipivefrin 0.1% bid).
6. Hyperosmotic agent when IOP is acutely elevated (e.g., mannitol 20% 1–2 g/kg IV over 45 minutes; a 500-cc bag of mannitol 20% contains 100 g of mannitol).
7. Manage the underlying problem.
8. When IOP remains dangerously elevated despite maximum medical therapy (a rare event), glaucoma filtering surgery with adjunct antifibrosis therapy may be indicated.

❖ **Note** *Miotics (e.g., pilocarpine) are contraindicated in inflammatory glaucoma.*

Follow-up
Patients are seen every 1–7 days at first. The higher the IOP and the greater the amount of glaucomatous damage already present (e.g., the larger the optic nerve cup), the more frequent the follow-up. Steroids are tapered as the inflammation subsides. Antiglaucoma medications are discontinued as IOP returns to normal. Steroid-response glaucoma should always be considered in unresponsive cases (see Section 10.5).

10.5 STEROID-RESPONSE GLAUCOMA

Critical Signs
Increased intraocular pressure (IOP) with steroid use, usually within a few weeks of starting topical (eye drops or skin cream), repository, or systemic steroids, although the IOP rise may develop from a few days to a few months after initiating therapy. The IOP usually returns to normal within days to weeks of discontinuing the steroid.

Other Signs
Signs of primary open-angle glaucoma may develop, including optic-nerve cupping and field loss in an eye with an open anterior-chamber angle.

❖ **Note** *Patients with primary open-angle glaucoma or a predisposition to develop glaucoma (i.e., positive family history, diabetes, and high myopia) are more likely to develop a steroid response and subsequent glaucoma.*

tion, it may be difficult to determine the cause of the increased IOP. See Section 10.4.)

- Neovascular glaucoma (Abnormal iris vessels, anterior-chamber angle vessels, or both may develop in the presence of ocular inflammation, producing open-angle and later, closed-angle glaucoma. See Section 10.13.)

Work-up

1. History: Duration of steroid use? Previous steroid use or an eye problem from steroid use? Glaucoma or family history of glaucoma? Diabetes?
2. Complete ocular examination: Evaluate the degree of ocular inflammation and determine whether iris neovascularization, angle neovascularization (by gonioscopy), or both is present. Measure IOP, and inspect the optic nerve.
3. Optic disc photographs and formal visual fields (e.g., Humphrey, Octopus) are obtained when the optic nerve appears damaged or when the duration of IOP elevation is prolonged or unknown.

Treatment

Any or all of the following may be necessary to reduce IOP.

1. Discontinue the steroid or reduce the frequency of its administration (steroids should not be discontinued abruptly, but rather tapered).
2. Reduce the concentration or dosage of the steroid (e.g., topical prednisolone acetate 1% can be changed to topical prednisolone acetate 0.12%).
3. Switch from a potent steroid with a greater propensity to produce a steroid response (e.g., prednisolone acetate) to one with a lesser propensity (e.g., fluorometholone).
4. Switch to a topical nonsteroidal antiinflammatory agent (i.e., diclofenac 0.1%).
5. Start antiglaucoma therapy. See "Inflammatory Open-Angle Glaucoma," Section 10.4, for medical therapy options.

❖ **Notes**

1. *When a high IOP is found in a patient on topical steroids for inflammatory glaucoma, it may be difficult to determine the cause of the increased IOP (i.e., whether it is the result of the inflammatory reaction or the steroids). If the inflammation is moderate to severe, we usually increase the steroids initially to reduce the inflammation while initiating antiglaucoma (e.g., topical beta-blocker) therapy. If the inflammation subsides, but IOP remains elevated, the glaucoma is assumed to be steroid-induced, and the treatment regimen above is followed.*
2. *When a dangerously high IOP that is uncontrollable with medication develops after a depot steroid injection, the steroid may need to be excised.*

10.6 PIGMENTARY GLAUCOMA

Symptoms

May be asymptomatic or the patient may experience episodes of blurred vision, eye pain, and colored halos around lights after exercise or pupillary dilatation. More common in young adult men. Usually bilateral.

Critical Signs

Midperipheral spokelike iris transillumination defects, dense homogeneous pigmentation of the trabecular meshwork for 360 degrees (seen on gonioscopy), and glaucoma [optic-nerve cupping, glaucomatous visual field loss, and/or increased intraocular pressure (IOP)]. The anterior-chamber angle is open.

Other Signs

A vertical pigment band on the corneal endothelium (Krukenberg's spindle); pigment deposition on the equatorial lens surface, on Schwalbe's line, and sometimes along the iris (which can produce iris heterochromia); myopia; and typically, large fluctuations in IOP. During IOP spikes, pigment cells may be seen floating within the anterior chamber and corneal edema may be present.

Differential Diagnosis

- Exfoliative glaucoma   (Trabecular meshwork pigmentation is black and more prominent inferiorly. Iris transillumination defects may be present, but they are near the pupillary margin and are usually less prominent. White flaky material may be seen on the pupillary border and anterior lens capsule. See Section 10.7.)
- Inflammatory open-angle glaucoma   (White blood cells and flare in the anterior chamber; typically no iris transillumination defects. Central corneal endothelial pigment deposits sometimes appear. See Section 10.4.)
- Iris melanoma   (Pigmentation of the angular structures accompanied by either a raised, pigmented lesion on the iris or a diffusely darkened iris. No iris transillumination defects. See Section 8.2.)

Work-up

1. History: Previous episodes of decreased vision or halos?
2. Slit-lamp examination, particularly checking for iris transillumination: Shine a small slit beam directly into the pupil to obtain a red reflex and search for transillumination defects. Scleral transillumination also works well.
3. Measure IOP.
4. Gonioscopy of the anterior-chamber angle.
5. Evaluate the optic-nerve.

6. Dilated retinal examination, with special attention to the periphery.
7. Stereo disc photographs.
8. Visual field examination, preferably automated (e.g., Humphrey, Octopus).

Treatment

Depends on the IOP, status of the optic nerve, visual field changes, and extent of the symptoms. A stepwise approach to control IOP is usually taken when mild-to-moderate glaucomatous changes are present. When advanced glaucoma is discovered on initial examination, maximal medical therapy may be instituted initially. (See "Primary Open-Angle Glaucoma," Section 10.1.)

1. Miotic agents (the theoretical first line of therapy because they minimize iridozonular contact, which produces pigmentary release into the anterior chamber). However, because most patients are young and myopic, miotic drops, with resultant fluctuation in myopia, may not be practical. In some cases, pilocarpine inserts (e.g., Ocuserts) used once per week or pilocarpine 4% gel qhs are tolerated.

❖ **Note** *Miotics should be used cautiously because of the risk of retinal detachmet in myopic patients.*

2. Other antiglaucoma medications (e.g., beta-blockers, epinerphrine compounds, carbonic anhydrase inhibitors) may be appropriate (see "Primary Open-Angle Glaucoma," Section 10.1).
3. Consider argon laser trabeculoplasty; these patients usually respond well.
4. Consider trabeculectomy when medical and laser therapy fail.
5. Laser peripheral iridectomy has been recommended but is still experimental.

Follow-up

Every 1–6 months, with a formal visual field test every 6–12 months, depending on the severity of the symptoms and the glaucoma.

❖ **Note** *Some patients have the "pigment dispersion syndrome" without glaucoma. These patients are at risk to develop glaucoma and are examined every 6–24 months.*

10.7 EXFOLIATIVE GLAUCOMA (PSEUDOEXFOLIATIVE GLAUCOMA)

Symptoms

Usually asymptomatic.

Critical Signs

White flaky material on the pupillary margin, anterior lens capsular changes (central zone of exfoliation material, often with rolled-up edges, middle clear zone, and a peripheral cloudy zone), and glaucoma [optic-nerve cupping, glaucomatous visual field loss, and/or increased intraocular pressure (IOP)].

Other Signs

Irregular black pigment deposition on the trabecular meshwork and along Schwalbe's line (Sampaolesi's line) seen on gonioscopy especially inferiorly. Bilateral, but often asymmetric. Incidence increases with age.

Differential Diagnosis

- Pigmentary glaucoma   (Pigmented trabecular meshwork accompanied by midperipheral iris transillumination defects. There may be a vertical pigment band on the corneal endothelium. See Section 10.6.)
- Capsular delamination (true exfoliation)   [Trauma, exposure to intense heat (e.g., glass blower), or severe uveitis can cause a thin membrane to peel off the anterior lens capsule. Glaucoma uncommon.]
- Primary amyloidosis   (Amyloid material can deposit along the pupillary margin or anterior lens capsule. Glaucoma can occur.)

Work-up

1. History: Occupational exposure to heat?
2. Slit-lamp examination with IOP measurement; often need to dilate the pupil to see the anterior lens capsular changes.
3. Gonioscopy of the anterior-chamber angle.
4. Optic-nerve evaluation.
5. Stereo disc photographs.
6. Visual field test, preferably automated (e.g., Humphrey, Octopus).

Treatment

1. For medical therapy, see "Primary Open-Angle Glaucoma," Section 10.1.
2. Consider argon laser trabeculoplasty, which has a higher initial success rate in exfoliative than in primary open-angle glaucoma).
3. Consider trabeculectomy when medical or laser therapy fails.

❖ **Note** *Cataract extraction does not eradicate the glaucoma. Cataract extraction may be complicated by weakened zonular fibers and synechiae between the iris and peripheral anterior lens capsule. The posterior capsule is easily ruptured.*

Follow-up

Every 1–3 months, depending on the severity of the glaucoma.

❖ **Note** *Many patients have exfoliation syndrome without glaucoma. These patients are reexamined every 6–12 months because they are at risk for glaucoma, but they are not treated unless glaucoma develops.*

10.8 PHACOLYTIC GLAUCOMA

Definition

Leakage of lens material from a cataract through an intact lens capsule leads to trabecular meshwork outflow obstruction.

Symptoms

Unilateral pain, decreased vision, tearing, photophobia.

Critical Signs

Markedly increased intraocular pressure (IOP), accompanied by iridescent particles and white material within the anterior chamber or on the anterior surface of the lens capsule. A hypermature (liquefied) or mature cataract is typical.

Other Signs

Corneal edema, anterior-chamber cells and significant flare, pseudohypopyon, and severe conjunctival injection. Gonioscopy reveals an open anterior-chamber angle.

Differential Diagnosis

All of the following can produce an acute rise in IOP to high levels, but none display iridescent particles and white material in the anterior chamber.

- Inflammatory glaucoma   (Acute increased IOP as a result of severe anterior uveitis. See Section 10.4.)
- Glaucomatocyclitic crisis   (Recurrent idiopathic attacks of increased IOP with an open anterior-chamber angle and mild iritis. See Section 10.12.)
- Acute angle-closure glaucoma   (Increased IOP as a result of sudden closure of the anterior-chamber angle, confirmed by gonioscopy. See Section 10.10.)
- Lens-particle glaucoma   ("Fluffed-up" lens material is seen in the anterior chamber; a history of traumatic lens damage or cataract extraction in the involved eye is characteristic. See Section 10.9.)
- Endophthalmitis   (History of recent surgery or trauma, pain can be severe. See Section 13.10.)

Work-up

1. History: Recent trauma or ocular surgery? Recurrent episodes? Uveitis in the past?
2. Slit-lamp examination: Look for iridescent or white particles as well as cells and flare within the anterior chamber. Evaluate for cataract and elevated IOP producing corneal edema.
3. Gonioscopy of the anterior-chamber angles of both eyes: Topical glycerin

may be placed on the cornea after topical anesthesia to clear it temporarily if it is edematous.

4. Retinal and optic-disc examination if possible: The degree of optic-nerve cupping helps to determine how long the elevated IOP may be tolerated.
5. If the diagnosis is in doubt, paracentesis can be performed to detect macrophages bloated with lens material on microscopic examination.
6. B-scan ultrasound prior to cataract extraction when there is no fundus view to rule out an intraocular tumor or retinal detachment.

Treatment

The goal of therapy is to lower the IOP and to reduce the inflammation. The cataract should be removed promptly (within several days).

1. Topical beta-blocker (e.g., levobunolol 0.25–0.5% or timolol 0.25–0.5% in one dose initially, and then bid).
2. Carbonic anhydrase inhibitor (e.g., acetazolamide 250-mg tablets po in one dose, then 250 mg po qid).
3. Topical cycloplegic (e.g., scopolamine 0.25% tid).
4. Topical steroid (e.g., prednisolone acetate 1% q 15 min for four doses, then q 1 h).
5. Hyperosmotic agent if necessary and no contraindications are present (e.g., mannitol 1–2 g/kg IV over 45 minutes; a 500-cc bag of mannitol 20% contains 100 g of mannitol).
6. Cataract extraction is performed after IOP is under control and the inflammation has been reduced. It is generally performed within 24–36 hours. If the IOP cannot be controlled medically, the patient may need hospitalization and urgent cataract extraction. Trabeculotomy is usually not necessary at the same time as cataract surgery.

Follow-up

If patients are not hospitalized, they should be reexamined the day following surgery. Patients are usually hospitalized after their cataract surgery so that their IOP can be monitored over the ensuing 24 hours. If the IOP returns to normal after the procedure, the patient should be rechecked within 1 week.

10.9 LENS-PARTICLE GLAUCOMA

Definition

Lens material, liberated by trauma or surgery, which obstructs aqueous outflow channels.

Symptoms

Pain, blurred vision, red eye, tearing, photophobia. History of recent ocular trauma or cataract surgery.

Critical Signs

White, fluffy pieces of lens cortical material in the anterior chamber, combined with increased intraocular pressure (IOP). A break in the lens capsule may be observed in post-traumatic cases.

Other Signs

Anterior-chamber cell and flare, conjunctival injection, or corneal edema. The anterior-chamber angle is open on gonioscopy.

Differential Diagnosis

See "Phacolytic Glaucoma," Section 10.8. In phacolytic glaucoma, the cataractous lens has not been extracted nor traumatized.

- Infectious endophthalmitis   (Unless lens cortical material can be unequivocally identified in the anterior chamber, and there is nothing atypical about the presentation, endophthalmitis must be ruled out.)
- Phacoanaphylactic endophthalmitis   (Follows trauma or intraocular surgery, producing anterior-chamber inflammation and sometimes a high IOP. The inflammation is often granulomatous, and fluffy lens material is not present in the anterior chamber.)

Work-up

1. History: Recent trauma or ocular surgery?
2. Slit-lamp examination: Search the anterior chamber for lens cortical material and measure the IOP.
3. Gonioscopy of the anterior-chamber angle.
4. Optic-nerve evaluation: The degree of optic-nerve cupping helps determine how long the elevated IOP can be tolerated.

Treatment

1. Topical beta-blocker (e.g., levobunolol 0.5% bid or timolol 0.25–1.5% bid).
2. Carbonic anhydrase inhibitor (e.g., methazolamide 25–50 mg po 2–3 times per day, or acetazolamide 250 mg po qid or 500 mg sequel po bid).
3. Topical cycloplegic (e.g., scopolamine 0.25% tid).
4. Topical steroid (e.g., prednisolone acetate 1% qid).
   - If IOP is markedly elevated (e.g., >45 mm Hg in a previously healthy eye or less in a patient with previous optic-nerve damage), a hyperosmotic agent is added to acutely lower the pressure (e.g., mannitol 1–2 g/kg IV over 45 minutes; a 500-cc bag of mannitol 20% contains 100 g of mannitol).

- If medical therapy fails to control the IOP, the residual lens material must be removed surgically.

Follow-up

Depending on the IOP and the health of the optic nerve, patients are reexamined in 1–7 days.

10.10 ACUTE ANGLE-CLOSURE GLAUCOMA

Symptoms

Pain, blurred vision, colored halos around lights, frontal headache, nausea and vomiting.

Critical Signs

Closed angle in the involved eye, acutely elevated intraocular pressure (IOP), corneal microcystic edema.

Other Signs

Conjunctival injection; fixed, mid-dilated pupil; shallow anterior chamber.

Etiology
- Pupillary block   [Anatomically predisposed in eyes with narrow anterior-chamber angle recess, anterior iris insertion of the iris root, or both; common in Asians and Eskimos and hyperopes. May be precipitated by topical mydriatics or rarely miotics, systemic anticholinergics (e.g., antihistamines or antipsychotics), or dim illumination (e.g., movie theater). Posterior synechiae from previous ocular inflammation also predisposes to pupillary block. The angle is narrow or occludable in the contralateral eye.]
- Angle crowding as a result of an abnormal iris configuration (e.g., plateau iris syndrome—angle closure occurs despite a patent peripheral iridectomy.)
- Neovascular or inflammatory membrane pulling the angle closed   (Abnormal misdirected blood vessels along the pupillary margin, the trabecular meshwork, or both are seen.)
- Mechanical closure of the angle secondary to anterior displacement of the lens-iris diaphragm:
    a. Lens-induced   [Pupillary block as a result of a large lens (phacomorphic).]
    b. Choroidal detachment (serous or hemorrhagic)   (Generally follows sur-

gery; diagnose by indirect ophthalmoscopy, B-scan ultrasonography or both.)

   c. Choroidal swelling following extensive retinal laser surgery or after placement of a tight encircling band in retinal detachment surgery

   d. Posterior segment tumor (e.g., choroidal or ciliary body melanoma)

   e. Malignant glaucoma (Aqueous misdirection.)

- Peripheral anterior synechiae (caused by uveitis, laser trabeculoplasty, iridocorneal endothelial syndrome, others.)

❖ **Note** *A secondary mechanical cause of angle-closure glaucoma should be suspected when contralateral eye's angle is wide open.*

Differential Diagnosis

Other causes of acute IOP rise, but with an open angle.

- Glaucomatocyclitic crisis (Posner-Schlossman syndrome) (Recurrent IOP spikes in one eye, mild cell and flare with or without fine keratic precipitates; the eye is generally not inflamed and not painful. See Section 10.12.)
- Inflammatory open-angle glaucoma (Moderate to severe anterior-chamber reaction. See Section 10.4.)
- Retrobulbar hemorrhage or inflammation (Proptosis and restriction of ocular motility.)
- Traumatic (hemolytic) glaucoma (History of trauma, red blood cells in the anterior chamber.)
- Pigmentary glaucoma (Pigment cells floating in the anterior chamber, often after exercise or pupillary dilatation; radial iris transillumination defects. See Section 10.6.)

Work-up

1. History: Family history? Retinal problem? Recent laser treatment or surgery? Medications?
2. Slit-lamp examination: Look for keratic precipitates, posterior synechiae, iris neovascularization, a swollen lens, anterior-chamber cells and flare or iridescent particles, and a shallow anterior chamber.
3. Measure IOP.
4. Gonioscopy of both anterior-chamber angles: It may be wise to initially avoid gonioscopy of the involved eye when there is a significant amount of corneal edema and the diagnosis is fairly well established; gonioscopy of an edematous cornea predisposes to a corneal abrasion. Gonioscopy of the involved eye after IOP is lowered is essential in determining whether the angle has opened and whether neovascularization is present.)

Treatment

Depends on severity and duration of attack. Use of medications with greater side-effects such as IV acetazolamide or osmotics is reserved for severe cases. See "Neovascular Glaucoma," Section 10.13, "Postoperative Glaucoma," Section 10.15, and "Malignant Glaucoma (Aqueous Misdirection), Section 10.16, for specific treatment of these conditions.

1. Attempt corneal compression with a gonioprism if the attack is of recent onset and no corneal edema is present; this may be of help in opening the angle and reducing the IOP.
2. Topical beta-blocker (e.g., levobunolol 0.5% or timolol 0.5%) in one dose.
3. Topical steroid (e.g., prednisolone acetate 1%) q 15–30 min for 4 doses, then hourly.
4. Carbonic anhydrase inhibitor (e.g., acetazolamide 250–500 mg IV or 2 250-mg tablets po, in one dose).
5. Osmotic agent (e.g., isosorbide 50–100 g po or mannitol 1–2 g/kg IV over 45 minutes; a 500-cc bag of mannitol 20% contains 100 g of mannitol).
6. Consider topical apraclonidine 0.1% × 1 for one dose.
7. When acute angle-closure glaucoma is the result of
   a. Phakic pupillary block or angle crowding: Pilocarpine 1–2% q 15 min for 2 doses and pilocarpine 0.5% in the contralateral eye for one dose.
   b. Aphakic or pseudophakic pupillary block or mechanical closure of the angle: Do *not* use pilocarpine. A mydriatic and cycloplegic agent (e.g., cyclopentolate 2% and phenylephrine 2.5% q 15 min for 4 doses) is used when laser or surgery is not initially employed because of corneal edema, inflammation, or both.
7. In cases of phacomorphic glaucoma, the lens urgently needs to be removed.

Recheck the IOP in 1 hour.

- If the IOP drops significantly *and* the angle is determined to be open by gonioscopy, definitive treatment is performed once the cornea is clear and the anterior chamber is quiet (see below). In most cases, this requires waiting 1–3 days for the inflammation to resolve. Patients are discharged on the following medications and followed daily.
  Prednisolone acetate 1% q 1–6 h, as needed.
  Acetazolamide 500 mg sequel po bid
  Topical beta-blocker (e.g., levobunolol 0.5% bid or timolol 0.5% bid)
  Pilocarpine 1–2% qid (in cases of phakic pupillary block or angle crowding)
  Pilocarpine 0.5% qid in the contralateral eye if the angle is narrow or occludable.

- If IOP is still elevated or the angle is still closed, medical treatment is continued or definitive treatment is implemented, despite ocular inflammation.

Definitive Treatment

A. *Pupillary block (all forms) or angle crowding*
1. Laser peripheral iridectomy (PI; argon or YAG) to the involved eye.
2. Laser PI to the contralateral eye if it is occludable. (Typically, only one eye is lasered in one sitting. If corneal edema prohibits laser in the involved eye at the time of initial treatment, the contralateral eye can be lasered first.)
3. Surgical iridectomy if a laser PI is not possible.
4. Consider a trabeculectomy when the IOP remains high despite an iridectomy and maximal medical treatment, especially in presence of significant optic-nerve cupping.

B. *Mechanical angle closure*
1. Consider argon laser gonioplasty to open the angle, particularly in cases that are the result of extensive retinal laser surgery, a tight encircling band from retinal detachment surgery, or nanophthalmos.
2. Consider goniosynechialysis for chronic angle closure less than 6 months in duration.
3. Treat the underlying problem.

Follow-up

After definitive treatment of one or both eyes, patients are reevaluated in weeks to months initially, and then less frequently. Visual fields (e.g., Humphrey, Octopus) and stereo disc photographs are obtained for baseline purposes.

❖ Notes

1. *The patient's cardiovascular status and electrolyte balance must be considered when contemplating osmotic agents, carbonic anhydrase inhibitors, and beta-blockers.*
2. *When mechanical angle-closure glaucoma is suspected, a B-scan ultrasound may be helpful in diagnosis.*
3. *If a repeat attack of angle closure occurs despite a patent iridectomy, a plateau iris syndrome may be present (see Section 10.11).*

10.11 PLATEAU IRIS

Symptoms

Usually asymptomatic, unless acute angle-closure glaucoma develops (decreased vision, throbbing pain, nausea, and vomiting; see Section 10.10).

Critical Signs

Flat iris plane and normal anterior-chamber depth centrally, convex peripheral iris with an anterior iris apposition seen on gonioscopy.

Other Signs

With acute angle-closure associated with a plateau iris, the axial anterior-chamber depth remains normal, but the peripheral iris bunches up to occlude the angle (see Section 10.10).

Types

Plateau iris configuration   Due to the anatomic configuration of the angle, these patients may develop acute angle-closure glaucoma from only a mild degree of pupillary block. These angle-closure attacks are cured by peripheral iridectomy (PI), because it relieves the pupillary block.

Plateau iris syndrome   A subset of the plateau iris configuration. The peripheral iris can bunch up in the anterior-chamber angle and obstruct aqueous outflow without any element of pupillary block. The diagnosis is made when angle-closure glaucoma occurs despite a patent PI.

Differential Diagnosis

- Acute angle-closure glaucoma associated with pupillary block   (The central anterior-chamber depth is decreased, and the entire iris has a convex appearance. See Section 10.10.)
- Malignant glaucoma   (Marked diffuse shallowing of the anterior chamber, often following cataract extraction or glaucoma surgery. See Section 10.16.)
- For other disorders, see "Acute Angle-Closure Glaucoma," Section 10.10.

Work-up

1. Slit-lamp examination: Specifically check for the presence of a patent PI and the critical signs listed previously.
2. Measure intraocular pressure (IOP).
3. Gonioscopy of both anterior-chamber angles.
4. Undilated optic-nerve evaluation.

❖ **Note** *If dilatation needs to be performed in a patient suspected of having a plateau iris, then warn the patient that this may provoke an acute angle-closure attack. Dilate with tropicamide 0.5% only. Recheck the IOP every few hours until the pupil returns to normal size. Have the patient notify you immediately if symptoms of acute angle-closure develop.*

Treatment

1. Treat acute angle-closure glaucoma medically if present (see Section 10.10).
2. A laser PI is performed within 1–2 days if the angle-closure attack can be

controlled medically. If the attack cannot be controlled, a laser or surgical PI may need to be done emergently.

3. One week after the laser PI, the eye should be dilated with a weak mydriatic (e.g., tropicamide 0.5%). If the IOP rises, plateau iris syndrome is diagnosed and should be treated with a weak miotic (e.g., pilocarpine 0.5–1% 3–4 times per day, chronically).

4. If angle-closure glaucoma develops despite a patent PI, then the plateau iris syndrome exists and should be treated with a weak miotic chronically as described previously.

5. Consider a laser gonioplasty (iridoplasty) in refractile cases or to break an acute attack not responsive to medical treatment and PI.

6. If the patient's IOP does respond to a laser PI (i.e., with plateau iris configuration, not syndrome by definition), then a prophylactic laser PI may be indicated in the contralateral eye within 1–2 weeks.

Follow-up

1. Following laser PI for an attack of acute angle-closure glaucoma, patients are reevaluated in 1 week, 1 month, and 3 months, then every 3–6 months. Examination should include IOP and gonioscopy at each visit; look for increasing angle closure. The PI should be examined for patency. In patients *not* receiving pilocarpine, periodic tests for the plateau iris syndrome should be performed with topical tropicamide 0.5%.

2. Patients suspected of having a plateau iris configuration who have never had an acute angle-closure attack are examined every 6 months. At each visit, IOP is measured and gonioscopy is performed; look for peripheral anterior synechiae formation and further narrowing of the anterior-chamber angle.

10.12 GLAUCOMATOCYCLITIC CRISIS
(Posner-Schlossman Syndrome)

Symptoms

Mild pain, decreased vision, observation of rainbows around lights. Often, a history of similar episodes is obtained. Usually unilateral in young to middle-aged patients.

Critical Signs

Markedly elevated intraocular pressure (IOP) (usually 40–60 mm Hg), open angle without synechiae on gonioscopy, minimal conjunctival injection (white eye), very mild anterior-chamber reaction (few aqueous cells and little flare).

Other Signs

Corneal epithelial edema, ciliary flush, pupillary constriction, iris hypochromia, few fine keratic precipitates on the corneal endothelium or trabecular meshwork.

Differential Diagnosis

- Inflammatory open-angle glaucoma   (Significant amount of aqueous cells and flare, conjunctival injection, and pain. Synechiae may be present. May be bilateral. See Section 10.4.)
- Acute angle-closure glaucoma   (Closed angle in the involved eye and usually a narrow angle in the contralateral eye; painful, conjunctival injection; corneal edema; patient may have history of recent dilatation with drops or use of systemic anticholinergic medication. See Section 10.10.)
- Pigmentary glaucoma   [Acute rise in IOP, often after exercise or pupillary dilatation, pigment cells in the anterior chamber, open angle, radial iris transillumination defects, vertically oriented pigmented cells on the posterior corneal surface (Krukenberg's spindle), and pigment in the trabecular meshwork seen on gonioscopy. See Section 10.6.]
- Neovascular glaucoma   (Iris and/or angle neovascularization is present. See Section 10.13.)
- Fuchs' heterochromic iridocyclitis   (Asymmetry of iris color, mild iritis in the eye with the lighter-colored iris, usually unilateral, often associated with cataract, glaucoma, or both. The rise in IOP is rarely as acute. See "Anterior Uveitis, Section 13.1.)
- Others   (e.g., Herpes simplex and herpes zoster keratouveitis.)

Work-up

1. History: Recent dilating drops, systemic anticholinergic agents, or exercise? Previous attacks? Corneal or systemic disease?
2. Slit-lamp examination: Assess the degree of conjunctival injection and aqueous cell and flare. Measure IOP.
3. Gonioscopy of the anterior-chamber angle: Angle open? Synechiae, neovascular membrane, or keratic precipitates present?
4. Optic-nerve evaluation.
5. Stereo optic disc photos and formal visual field testing.
6. Retinal examination: Vasculitis? Snowbanking of pars planitis?

Treatment

1. Topical beta-blocker (e.g., timolol 0.5% bid or levobunolol 0.5% bid).
2. Topical steroid (e.g., prednisolone acetate 1% qid).
3. Add a carbonic anhydrase inhibitor (e.g., methazolamide 25–50 mg po 2–3 times per day or acetazolamide 500 mg sequel po bid) if IOP is significantly elevated.
4. Hyperosmotic agents (e.g., mannitol 20% 1–2 g/kg IV over 45 minutes)

are used acutely when the IOP is determined to be dangerously high for the involved optic nerve. A 500-cc bag of mannitol 20% contains 100 g of mannitol.

5. Consider a cycloplegic agent (e.g., cyclopentolate 1% tid) if the patient is symptomatic.

Follow-up

Patients are seen every few days a first, then weekly until the episode resolves. Attacks usually subside within a few hours to a few weeks. No medical or surgical therapy is required between attacks. Steroids are tapered rapidly if they are used for 1 week or less, and slowly if they are used for longer. Note that both eyes are at risk of developing chronic open-angle glaucoma.

10.13 NEOVASCULAR GLAUCOMA

Symptoms

May be asymptomatic or patient may complain of pain, red eye, photophobia, and decreased vision.

Critical Signs

Stage 1   Abnormal, engorged, misdirected blood vessels along the pupillary margin, the trabecular meshwork, or both. No signs of glaucoma.

Stage 2   Stage 1 plus increased intraocular pressure (IOP) (open-angle neovascular glaucoma).

Stage 3   Partial or complete angle-closure glaucoma caused by a fibrovascular membrane covering the trabecular meshwork. Peripheral anterior synechiae and florid iris neovascularization are common.

Other Signs

Mild anterior-chamber cells and flare, conjunctival injection, corneal edema when an acute rise in IOP occurs, hyphema, eversion of the pupillary margin allowing visualization of the iris pigment epithelium (ectropion uvea), optic-nerve cupping, visual field loss.

Etiology

- Diabetic retinopathy
- Central retinal vein occlusion, particularly the ischemic type
- Central retinal artery occlusion
- Ocular ischemic syndrome (carotid occlusive disease)
- Others   (Branch retinal vein occlusion, chronic uveitis, chronic retinal

detachment, intraocular tumors, trauma, other ocular vascular disorders, and radiation therapy.)

Differential Diagnosis
- Inflammatory glaucoma　(Increased IOP, abundant anterior-chamber cells and marked flare, and dilated normal iris blood vessels may be seen. No neovascular vessels. Normal iris blood vessels run radially, have a sense of direction, and are usually symmetrical 360 degrees around the pupillary margin. The angle is open. See Section 10.4.)
- Primary acute angle-closure glaucoma　(No signs of new iris blood vessels. Usually a narrow angle in the contralateral eye. See Section 10.10.)

Work-up
1. History: Determine the underlying etiology.
2. Complete ocular examination, including IOP measurement and gonioscopic evaluation of the anterior-chamber angle to determine what degree of the angle is closed, if any. A dilated retinal evaluation is essential in determining the cause of the iris neovascularization.
3. Fluorescein angiogram as needed to identify an underlying retinal abnormality or in preparation for retinal laser treatment (panretinal photocoagulation).
4. Carotid noninvasive studies to rule out carotid disease when no retinal pathology can be found acountable for the neovascularization.
5. B-scan ultrasound is indicated when the retina cannot be visualized to rule out an intraocular tumor or retinal detachment.

Treatment
1. Control the IOP if it is elevated. Any or all of the following medications are used:
   a. Topical beta-blocker (e.g., levobunolol 0.5% bid or timolol 0.5% bid).
   b. Systemic carbonic anhydrase inhibitor (e.g., methazolamide 25–50 mg po 2–3 times per day or acetazolamide 500 mg po bid).
   c. Hyperosmotic agent (e.g., mannitol 20% 1–2 g/kg IV over 45 minutes). Note that a 500-cc bag of mannitol 20% contains 100 g of mannitol.

❖ **Note** *Miotics (e.g., pilocarpine) and epinephrine compounds are generally ineffective and are not often used.*

2. Reduce inflammation and pain: Topical steroid (e.g., prednisolone acetate 1% q 1–6 h) and a cycloplegic (e.g., atropine 1% tid). Atropine may lower IOP when the angle is closed by increasing uveoscleral outflow.
3. If retinal ischemia is thought to be responsible for the iris neovascularization, then treat with panretinal photocoagulation (PRP) if the retina can be visualized or panretinal cryoablation if it cannot be well seen. These

procedures are used if the angle is open or if the patient is going to have filtration surgery whether the angle is open or closed.

4. Goniophotocoagulation (laser photocoagulation of new vessels in the angle) may be used in addition to the previously described treatment in patients with significant angle neovascularization, but minimal-to-no angle closure. This procedure reduces risk of angle closure during the time interval required for the PRP to take effect (often several weeks).

5. Glaucoma filtration surgery (e.g., trabeculectomy) is often performed when the neovascularization is inactive and the IOP cannot be controlled with medical therapy. Shunt tube procedures or YAG laser cyclophotocoagulation are helpful to control IOP in patients with active neovascularization.

In eyes without useful vision, topical steroids and cycloplegics, beta-blockers, YAG-laser cyclophotocoagulation, cyclocryotherapy, retrobulbar alcohol injection, or enucleation may be required to reduce pain (see "The Blind, Painful Eye," Section 15.9).

6. Treat the underlying disorder; see the appropriate section.

Follow-up

The presence of iris neovascularization, especially when accompanied by high IOP, requires urgent therapeutic intervention, usually within 1–2 days. Angle closure can proceed relatively rapidly (within days to weeks).

❖ **Note** *Iris neovascularization without glaucoma is managed in a similar manner as to that described above; however, there is no need for antiglaucomatous therapy unless IOP rises.*

10.14 IRIDOCORNEAL ENDOTHELIAL (ICE) SYNDROME

Symptoms

Usually asymptomatic, but the patient may note an irregular iris appearance, blurred vision, or pain in one eye. Patients are typically young to middle-aged adults.

Critical Signs

Corneal endothelial changes (fine, hammered-metal appearance), peripheral anterior synechiae that often extend beyond Schwalbe's line, and iris alterations as follows:

Essential iris atrophy   Marked iris thinning often leading to iris holes and displacement and distortion of the pupil.

Chandler's syndrome   Mild iris thinning and pupil distortion. (The corneal changes are most marked in this variant.)

Cogan-Reese syndrome   Pigmented nodules on the iris surface, variable iris atrophy.

Other Signs

Corneal edema, increased intraocular pressure (IOP), optic-nerve cupping, or visual field loss. Typically unilateral, although mild changes consistent with this syndrome are sometimes found in the contralateral eye.

Differential Diagnosis

- Axenfeld-Rieger syndrome   [Prominent, anteriorly displaced Schwalbe's line (posterior embryotoxon), peripheral iris strands extending to Schwalbe's line, iris thinning with atrophic holes, may have dental, craniofacial and skeletal abnormalities. Bilateral and congenital. See Section 9.11.]
- Posterior polymorphous dystrophy   (Bilateral. Endothelial vesicles or bandlike lesions, occasionally associated with iridocorneal adhesions, corneal edema, and glaucoma. See Section 4.24.)
- Fuchs' endothelial dystrophy   (Bilateral corneal edema and endothelial guttata. The iris and anterior-chamber angle are normal. See Section 4.25.)
- Iris melanoma   (Pigmented iris lesion or lesions noted to enlarge over time. See Section 8.2.)

Work-up

1. Family history: ICE syndrome is not inherited; Axenfeld-Rieger syndrome and posterior polymorphous dystrophy are often autosomal dominant.
2. Slit-lamp examination: Assess the cornea and iris and measure IOP.
3. Gonioscopy of the anterior-chamber angle.
4. Optic-nerve examination, best with a Hruby, fundus contact, or 60-diopter lens.
5. Stereo disc photographs.
6. Visual field test, preferably automated (e.g., Humphrey, Octopus).

Treatment

No treatment is needed unless glaucoma or corneal edema is present, at which point one or more of the following treatments is used:

1. Antiglaucomatous medications for corneal edema or glaucoma (see "Primary Open-Angle Glaucoma," Section 10.1). The IOP may need to be lowered beneath a critical level to rid the cornea of edema. This critical level may become lower as the patient ages.

2. Hypertonic saline solutions (e.g., sodium chloride 5% drops qid and oint-ment qhs) to reduce corneal edema.
3. Consider trabeculectomy when medical therapy fails to maintain the IOP low enough to prevent corneal edema or progression of optic-nerve damage. (Argon laser trabeculoplasty and laser peripheral iridectomy are usually ineffective. Tube shunt procedures may be required for refractory cases.)
4. Consider a corneal transplant in cases of advanced chronic corneal edema in the presence of good IOP control.

Follow-up

Every 3–12 months, unless glaucoma is present, then every 1–3 months de-pending on the severity of the glaucoma.

10.15 POSTOPERATIVE GLAUCOMA

Early Postoperative Glaucoma

Intraocular pressure (IOP) tends to rise 6–7 hours postoperatively and generally returns to normal within 1 week. Etiologies include retained viscoelastic, hy-phema, pigment dispersion, and generalized inflammation. Most normal eyes can tolerate an IOP < 30 mm Hg for this short a duration. However, eyes with preexisting optic-nerve damage require antiglaucoma medications (e.g., levobu-nolol 0.5% bid, timolol 0.5% bid, or methazolamide 25–50 mg po 2–3 times per day) for any significant pressure rise. Any eye with an IOP > 30 mm Hg should likewise be treated. If inflammation is excessive, increase the topical steroid dose (see "Inflammatory Open-Angle Glaucoma," Section 10.4).

Aphakic/Pseudophakic Pupillary Block

Signs

Increased IOP, flat anterior chamber, absence of a patent peripheral iridectomy (PI).

Treatment

A. If the cornea is clear and the eye is not significantly inflamed, then a PI is performed, usually by laser.
B. If the cornea is hazy, the eye is inflamed, or a PI cannot be performed immediately, then:
   1. Mydriatic agent (e.g., cyclopentolate 2% and phenylephrine 2.5% q 15 min for 4 doses).

2. Carbonic anhydrase inhibitor (e.g., acetazolamide two 250-mg tablets po or 500 mg IV).
3. Topical beta-blocker (e.g., timolol 0.5%), one dose.
4. Consider a hyperosmotic agent (e.g., mannitol 1–2 g/kg IV over 45 minutes; a 500-cc bag of mannitol 20% contains 100 g of mannitol).
5. Topical steroid (e.g., prednisolone acetate 1% q 15–30 min for 4 doses).
6. PI, preferably laser, as soon as available and when the eye is less inflamed. If the cornea is edematous and cloudy, topical glycerin may be used to clear it temporarily.

Uveitis, Glaucoma, Hyphema (UGH) Syndrome

Signs

Anterior chamber cells and flare and increased IOP, often with a hyphema. Usually secondary to irritation from an anterior-chamber intraocular lens.

Treatment

1. Atropine 1% tid.
2. Topical steroid (e.g., prednisolone acetate 1% qid or more often if the uveitis is severe).
3. Carbonic anhydrase inhibitor (e.g., acetazolamide 250 mg po qid or 500 mg sequel po bid, or methazolamide 25–50 mg po 2–3 times per day).
4. Topical beta-blocker (e.g., timolol 0.5% bid or levobunolol 0.5% bid).
5. Consider argon laser treatment to control the hemorrhage if a bleeding site can be identified.
6. Consider surgical removal of the intraocular lens, especially if peripheral anterior synechiae are forming.

Malignant Glaucoma

See Section 10.16.

Steroid-Response Glaucoma

See Section 10.5.

Follow-up

Patients should generally not be sent out of the office or emergency room with an IOP > 35–40 mm Hg. If the patient is monocular or has significant optic-nerve damage, then the IOP should be even lower. For aphakic/pseudophakic pupillary block, be certain that the angle is open and the block is relieved (using gonioscopy). If the above criteria are met, the patient must be reevaluated in 1–7 days, depending on the particular situation.

10.16 MALIGNANT GLAUCOMA
(Aqueous Misdirection)

Symptoms

Pain, red eye, photophobia; often occurs after surgical treatment of angle-closure glaucoma or cataract extraction.

Critical Signs

Shallow or flat anterior chamber and elevated intraocular pressure (IOP) in the presence of a patent iridectomy and in the absence of a choroidal detachment.

Etiology

It is believed that aqueous is misdirected and accumulates within the vitreous, displacing the vitreous forward, and causing anterior ciliary body rotation and diffuse shallowing or flattening of the anterior chamber.

Differential Diagnosis

- Acute angle-closure glaucoma   (The anterior chamber is shallow, the angle is closed, the IOP is elevated, but a patent iridectomy is not present. See Section 10.10.)
- Choroidal detachment   (Shallow or flat anterior chamber, but the IOP is typically low. A choroidal detachment is seen on funduscopic examination or by B-scan ultrasound in most cases. See Section 12.21.)
- Suprachoroidal hemorrhage   (Shallow or flat anterior chamber, painful, often elevated IOP, but a choroidal detachment may be seen on funduscopic examination or B-scan ultrasound.)

Work-up

1. History: Previous eye surgery?
2. Slit-lamp examination: Determine if a patent iridectomy is present. Pupillary block is unlikely in the presence of a patent iridectomy, unless it is plugged with vitreous, totally bound down, or plateau iris syndrome is present.
3. Gonioscopy of the anterior-chamber angle.
4. Dilated retinal examination if a patent iridectomy is present and phakic angle closure is ruled out.
5. Consider B-scan ultrasound to rule out a choroidal detachment and suprachoroidal hemorrhage if they cannot be ruled out by ophthalmoscopy.

Treatment

1. If an iridectomy is not present or it is not certain whether an existing one is patent, pupillary block cannot be ruled out, and peripheral iridectomy

(PI) should be performed (see "Acute Angle-Closure Glaucoma," Section 10.10).

If signs of malignant glaucoma are still present with a patent iridectomy:

2. Atropine 1% and phenylephrine 2.5% qid topically.
3. Carbonic anhydrase inhibitor (e.g., acetazolamide 500 mg IV or two 250-mg tablets po, then 250 mg po qid).
4. Hyperosmotic agent (e.g., mannitol 20% 1–2 g/kg IV over 45 minutes; a 500-cc bag of mannitol 20% contains 100 g of mannitol).
5. Topical beta-blocker (e.g., timolol 0.5% bid or levobunolol 0.5% bid).
6. Consider topical apraclonidine 0.1% bid.

If the block is broken (the anterior chamber deepens and the IOP returns to normal), maintain atropine 1% once per day indefinitely.

If steps 1–6 are unsuccessful, consider one or more of the following:

7. YAG laser disruption of the anterior hyaloid face and posterior capsule if the patient is aphakic or pseudophakic.
8. Argon laser treatment of the ciliary processes.
9. Core vitrectomy and reformation of the anterior chamber.

❖ **Note** *A choroidal detachment may be present, yet undetectable. Therefore, a sclerotomy to drain a choroidal detachment may be advisable prior to vitrectomy.*

10. PI in the contralateral eye if the angle appears occludable; generally performed at a later date.

Follow-up
Variable, depending upon the therapeutic modality employed. PI is generally performed in an occludable contralateral eye 1 week after treatment of the involved eye.

Neuro-ophthalmology

11.1 Anisocoria

See Figure 11.1.

Definition
The two pupils are unequal in size.

Etiology

A. The abnormal pupil is constricted.
- Unilateral use of miotic eye drops (e.g., pilocarpine, green-top eye drops.)
- Iritis   (Eye pain, redness, and anterior-chamber cells and flare.)
- Horner's syndrome   (Mild ptosis is usually present on the side of the small pupil; positive cocaine test.)
- Argyll Robertson (syphilitic) pupil   (The pupil is irregular in shape, reacts poorly or not at all to light, but constricts normally during convergence. Although the disease is typically bilateral, a mild degree of anisocoria is often present; positive FTA-ABS.)
- Long-standing Adie's pupil   (The pupil is initially dilated, but over time may constrict. At the slit lamp, it can be seen to react slowly and irregularly to a bright light. It is supersensitive to pilocarpine 0.125% or methacholine 2.5%, constricting even further.)

B. The abnormal pupil is dilated.
- Iris sphincter muscle damage from trauma   (Torn pupillary margin or iris transillumination defects seen on slit-lamp examination.)
- Adie's tonic pupil   (The pupil is irregular, reacts minimally to light

The Wills Eye Manual: Office and Emergency Room Diagnosis and Treatment of Eye Diseases, Second Edition, edited by R. Douglas Cullom, Jr., M.D., and Benjamin Chang, M.D. © 1994 J.B. Lippincott Company.

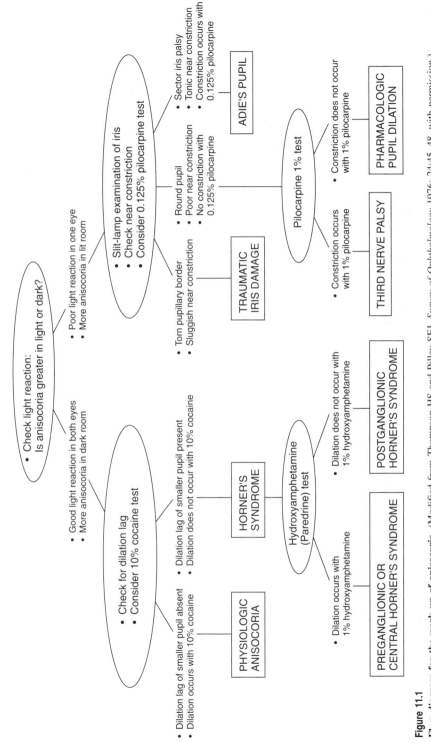

Figure 11.1

Flow diagram for the work-up of anisocoria. (Modified from Thompson HS and Pilley SEJ, *Survey of Ophthalmology* 1976; 24:45–48, with permission.)

and slowly to convergence, but is supersensitive to weak cholinergic agents such as pilocarpine 0.125% or methacholine 2.5%.)

- Third-nerve palsy   [Associated ptosis and extraocular muscle palsies. The pupil will not react to weak cholinergic agents, but will constrict to regular-strength miotic drops (e.g., pilocarpine 1%).]
- Unilateral use of a red-top dilating eye drop (e.g., atropine)   [If the drop has been instilled recently, the pupil will not react to pilocarpine 1% drops. If the effect of the drop is wearing off (e.g., atropine was used 1–2 weeks previously), the eye may be dilated and partly reactive to pilocarpine.]

C. Physiologic anisocoria   (Pupil size disparity is the same in light as in dark, and the pupils react normally to light. The size difference is usually, but not always ≤1 mm in diameter.)

Work-up

1. History: When was the anisocoria first noted? Any associated symptoms or signs? History of ocular trauma? Use of any eye drops or ointments? History of syphilis? History of decreased vision? Old photographs?
2. Ocular examination: Try to determine which is the abnormal pupil by observing the pupillary size. Younger patients tend to have pupillary diameters of 4–5 mm on average, whereas elderly patients often have slightly smaller pupils. If it is uncertain which is the abnormal pupil, compare pupil sizes in light and in dark. Anisocoria greater in light suggests the abnormal pupil is the larger pupil; anisocoria greater in dark suggests the abnormal pupil is the smaller pupil. Test the pupillary reaction to light. Test convergence if the light reaction is abnormal. Look for ptosis, evaluate ocular motility, and examine the pupillary margin with a slit lamp.

   - If the abnormal pupil is small, and anisocoria is thought to be worse in darkness, a diagnosis of Horner's syndrome may be confirmed by a cocaine test (see Section 11.2). In the presence of ptosis and unequivocal worsening of anisocoria in dim illumination, a cocaine test may be unnecessary because the diagnosis is made clinically.
   - If the abnormal pupil is large and there is no sphincter muscle damage, extraocular motility restriction, or ptosis consistent with a third-nerve palsy, the pupils may be tested with one drop of pilocarpine 0.125% or methacholine 2.5%. Within 10–15 minutes, an Adie's pupil will usually have constricted significantly more than the fellow pupil (see Section 11.4).

❖ **Note** *Soon after the development of an Adie's pupil, the pupil may be unreactive to a weak cholinergic agent.*

   - If the pupil does not constrict with pilocarpine 0.125% or methacholine 2.5% and/or pharmacologic dilatation is suspected, pilocarpine 1% is instilled in both eyes. A normal pupil constricts sooner and to a greater extent than the pharmacologically dilated pupil. An eye that recently received a strong mydriatic agent such as atropine usually will not constrict at all.

See "Horner's Syndrome," Section 11.2; "Argyll Robertson Pupil," Section 11.3; "Adie's Tonic Pupil," Section 11.4; and "Isolated Third-Nerve Palsy," Section 11.5, for more information regarding diagnosis and treatment.

11.2 HORNER'S SYNDROME

Symptoms
Droopy eyelid, pupil size disparity; often asymptomatic.

Critical Signs
Anisocoria that is greater in dim illumination (especially during the first few seconds the room light is dimmed) because of a small pupil that does not dilate as well as the normal, larger pupil; usually, mild ptosis and lower eyelid elevation occur on the same side as the small pupil.

Other Signs
All of the following may occur on the side affected by Horner's syndrome: Lower intraocular pressure, lighter iris color in congenital cases (iris heterochromia), loss of sweating ability (anhidrosis), increase in accommodation (older patients can be noted to hold their reading card closer in the Horner's eye). Light and near reactions are intact.

Differential Diagnosis
See "Anisocoria," Section 11.1.

Etiology
First-order neuron disorder   Stroke (e.g., vertebrobasilar artery insufficiency or infarct); tumor; rarely, severe osteoarthritis of the neck with bony spurs.
Second-order neuron disorder   Tumor (e.g., lung carcinoma, metastasis, thyroid adenoma, neurofibroma). Patients with arm pain should be suspected of having a Pancoast's tumor. In children, consider neuroblastoma, lymphoma, or metastasis.
Third-order neuron disorder   Headache syndrome (e.g., cluster migraine, Raeder's paratrigeminal syndrome), internal carotid dissection, herpes zoster virus, otitis media, and Tolosa-Hunt syndrome.
Congenital Horner's syndrome   Trauma (e.g., during delivery).

Work-up

1. If the diagnosis is uncertain, it may be confirmed with a cocaine test: One drop of cocaine 10% is placed into each eye and then repeated 1 minute later. Check the pupils in 15 minutes. If no change in pupillary size is noted, repeat one set of drops and recheck the pupils in another 15 minutes. A Horner's pupil dilates less well than the normal pupil.

2. Hydroxyamphetamine 1% (e.g., Paredrine) is used to distinguish a third-order neuron disorder from a first- and second-order neuron disorder: Place one drop of hydroxyamphetamine 1% into each eye, repeating the drop 1 minute later. Check the pupils in 30 minutes. Failure of the Horner's pupil to dilate to an equivalent degree as the fellow eye indicates a third-order neuron lesion.

❖ **Notes**

1. *Hydroxyamphetamine should not be administered within 24 hours of cocaine or they will interfere with each.other's action.*

2. *Both tests are thought to require an intact corneal epithelium and no prior eye drop administration for accurate results.*

3. Determine the duration of the Horner's syndrome from the patient's history and an examination of old photographs. New onset Horner's syndrome requires a more extensive diagnostic work-up. An old Horner's syndrome is more likely to be benign.

4. History: Headaches? Arm pain? Previous stroke? Previous surgery that may have damaged the sympathetic chain, including cardiac, thoracic, thyroid or neck surgery? History of head or neck trauma?

5. Physical examination (especially check for supraclavicular nodes, thyroid enlargement, or a neck mass).

Depending on the duration of Horner's syndrome and the results of the hydroxyamphetamine test, none or all of the following tests may be ordered. A more aggressive work-up is performed for new-onset Horner's syndromes, first- or second-order neuron disorders, and those with a history or physical examination that might indicate a tumor:

6. Chest x-ray with special views of the apex of the lung or CT scan of the chest.

7. CT scan (axial and coronal views) or MRI of the brain and neck.

8. Complete blood count with differential.

9. Lymph node biopsy when lymphadenopathy is present.

10. Carotid angiogram if carotid dissection suspected (especially with neck pain).

Treatment

1. Treat the underlying disorder if possible.

2. Ptosis surgery may be performed as needed.

Follow-up

Acute Horner's syndromes should be worked up as soon as possible to rule out life-threatening causes. Chronic Horner's syndromes can be evaluated with less urgency. With the exception of possible amblyopia in children, which only occurs when the eyelid covers the visual axis, there are no ocular complications that necessitate close follow-up.

11.3 ARGYLL ROBERTSON PUPIL

Symptoms

Usually asymptomatic.

Critical Signs

Small, irregular pupil that reacts poorly or not at all to light but constricts normally during convergence. By definition, vision is normal.

Other Signs

The pupil does not dilate well. Initially, it may be unilateral, but it becomes bilateral, although it may be asymmetric.

Etiology

Tertiary syphilis (positive FTA-ABS).

Differential Diagnosis

See "Anisocoria," Section 11.1.

Work-up

1. Test the pupillary reaction to light and convergence: To test the reaction of the pupil to convergence, patients are asked to look first at a distant target and then at their own finger, which the examiner holds in front of them and slowly brings in toward their face.
2. Slit-lamp examination: look for interstitial keratitis.
3. Dilated fundus examination: Search for chorioretinitis, papillitis, and uveitis.
4. FTA-ABS or MHA-TP, RPR or VDRL.
5. Consider a lumbar puncture if the diagnosis of syphilis is established (see Section 14.2).

Treatment

The decision to treat is based on whether active disease is present and whether the patient has been treated appropriately in the past. See "Acquired Syphilis," Section 14.2, for treatment indications and specific antibiotic therapy.

Follow-up

This is not an emergency, but a diagnostic work-up and determination of syphilitic activity should be undertaken within a few days of detecting an Argyll Robertson pupil.

11.4 ADIE'S TONIC PUPIL

Symptoms

Difference in the size of the pupils, blurred vision; may be asymptomatic.

Critical Signs

An irregularly dilated pupil exhibiting minimal or no reaction to light, slow constriction to convergence, and slow redilatation. It is typically unilateral and is found most often in young women. The pupil demonstrates supersensitivity to weak cholinergic agents (e.g., pilocarpine 0.125% or methacholine 2.5%).

Other Signs

It may develop acutely and may become bilateral. The pupil dilates normally to mydriatic agents. Deep tendon reflexes (knees and ankles) are often absent (Adie's syndrome). The involved pupil may become smaller than the normal pupil over time.

❖ **Note** *Supersensitivity may not be present soon after the development of an Adie's pupil and may need to be tested a few weeks later.*

Etiology

Idiopathic, orbital trauma or infection, herpes zoster infection, diabetes, autonomic neuropathies, Guillain-Barré syndrome, others.

Differential Diagnosis

See "Anisocoria," Section 11.1.

❖ **Note** *Parinaud's syndrome may produce bilateral mid-dilated pupils that react poorly to light but constrict normally during convergence. Eyelid retraction* *and paralysis of up-gaze with retraction nystagmus may additionally be pres-ent. A pinealoma or other midbrain abnormality needs to be ruled out by MRI.*

Work-up
See "Anisocoria," Section 11.1, for a general work-up when the diagnosis is uncertain.

1. Observe the suspect pupil with the slit lamp, shining a bright light on it. The Adie's pupil will contract slowly and irregularly.
2. Test for a supersensitive pupil: Have the patient fixate at distance and measure the pupil size of each eye. Instill one drop of methacholine 2.5% or pilocarpine 0.125% in each eye and recheck the pupil size in 10–15 minutes. Do not allow the patient to do near work during this interval. The tonic pupil constricts significantly more than the contralateral pupil in Adie's syndrome.

❖ **Note** *The methacholine/pilocarpine test may occasionally be positive in an Argyll Robertson pupil and in familial dysautonomia.*

3. If Adie's pupil and/or supersensitivity is present and the patient is younger than 1 year old, refer him or her to a pediatric neurologist to rule out familial dysautonomia (Riley-Day syndrome).

Treatment
Pilocarpine 0.125% bid–qid for cosmesis and to aid in accommodation, if desired.

Follow-up
If the diagnosis is established with certainty, follow-up is routine.

11.5 ISOLATED THIRD-NERVE PALSY

Symptoms
Double vision that disappears when one eye is closed; droopy eyelid, with or without pain.

Critical Signs
A. External ophthalmoplegia (i.e., motility status)
1. *Complete palsy*: Limitation of ocular movement in all fields of gaze except temporally.
2. *Incomplete palsy*: Partial limitation of ocular movement.

   3. *Superior-division pasly*: Ptosis and an inability to look up.
   4. *Inferior-division palsy*: Inability to look nasally or inferiorly; pupil is involved.
B. Internal ophthalmoplegia (i.e., pupil status)
   1. *Pupil-involved*: A fixed, dilated or minimally reactive pupil.
   2. *Pupil-spared*: Pupil not dilated and normally reactive to light.
   3. *Relative pupil-spared*: Pupil partially dilated and sluggishly reactive to light.

Other Signs

An exotropia or hypotropia. Aberrant regeneration [elevation of the upper eyelid with gaze down or nasally; sometimes pupil constriction (usually segmental) when looking up, down, or nasally].

❖ **Note** *Aberrant regeneration may occur spontaneously (primary regeneration), without a preceding third-nerve palsy. This is usually caused by a cavernous sinus tumor or aneurysm.*

Etiology

A. *Pupil-involved*
   More common   Aneurysm (particularly a posterior communicating artery aneurysm).
   Less common   Microvascular disease (typically a result of diabetes or hypertension), tumor, trauma, congenital.
   Rare   Uncal herniation, cavernous sinus mass lesion, orbital disease, herpes zoster, leukemia. In children, ophthalmoplegic migraine.
B. *Pupil-spared*
   More common   Microvascular disease.
   Less common   Cavernous sinus syndrome
C. *Relative pupil-spared:* Microvascular disease; less likely, aneurysm.
D. *Aberrant regeneration present:*   Trauma, aneurysm, tumor, congenital. *Not* microvascular.

Differential Diagnosis

- Myasthenia gravis   [Diurnal variation of symptoms and signs, pupil not involved, increased eyelid droop after sustained up-gaze, weak orbicularis oculi muscle, positive edrophonium chloride (e.g., Tensilon Chloride) test.]
- Thyroid eye disease   (Eyelid lag, stare, injection over the rectus muscles, proptosis, resistance on forced duction testing, abnormal CT scan of the orbits, no ptosis.)
- Chronic progressive external ophthalmoplegia   (Bilateral, slowly progressive ptosis and limitation of ocular motility, pupil spared, often no double vision.)

- Orbital inflammatory pseudotumor   (Pain and proptosis are usually present.)
- Midbrain lesion   (Inability to look up, down, or both; pupils react slowly to light and briskly to convergence; no ptosis; eyelid retraction and retraction nystagmus may or may not be present. Bilateral.)

Work-up

1. Complete ocular examination: Check for pupillary involvement, the directions of motility restriction (in both eyes), ptosis, a visual field defect (visual fields by confrontation), proptosis, resistance to retropulsion, and eyelid fatigue with sustained up-gaze. Look carefully for signs of aberrant regeneration (discussed previously).
2. Full neurological examination: Carefully assess the other cranial nerves on both sides. (The ipsilatral fourth nerve can be assessed by focusing with the slit lamp on a superior conjunctival blood vessel and asking the patient to look down and nasally. The eye should intort and the blood vessel should turn down and toward the nose.)
3. Edrophonium chloride (e.g., Tensilon Chloride) test when the pupil is not involved and myasthenia gravis is suspected (see Section 11.10).
4. *Immediate* CT scan of the brain (axial and coronal views) and/or MRI is indicated for:
   a. Pupil-involved (relatively or completely involved) third-nerve palsies.
   b. Pupil-spared third-nerve palsies in the following groups of patients:
      - Patients younger than 50 years of age (unless there is known long-standing diabetes or hypertension.)
      - Patients with incomplete third-nerve palsies (e.g., sparing of some muscle function), because this condition may be evolving into a pupil-involved third-nerve palsy.
      - Patients whose third-nerve palsy is of >3 months in duration, but has not improved.
      - Patients with an additional cranial-nerve or neurologic abnormality.
   c. All patients who develop aberrant regeneration, with the exception of regeneration following traumatic third-nerve palsies.

(A CT scan is generally not required in pupil-spared third-nerve palsies that do not fit the above criteria, especially when patients have known vasculopathic risk factors such as diabetes or hypertension.)

5. Complete blood count with differential in children.
6. Cerebral angiography is indicated for all patients older than 10 years of age with pupil-involved third-nerve palsies and whose MRI and/or CT scan is normal or shows a mass consistent with an aneurysm. This should be obtained as soon as possible.
7. Immediate ESR if giant cell arteritis is suspected (see Section 11.16).

Treatment
1. Treat the underlying abnormality or vasculopathic risk factors if present.
2. If the third-nerve palsy is causing double vision, a patch may be placed over the involved eye. Patching is generally not performed in children younger than 9–11 years of age due to the risk of amblyopia. Children should be monitored closely for the development of amblyopia in the deviated eye.

Follow-up
A. Pupil-involved third-nerve palsies: Immediate hospitalization and work-up as described above.
B. Pupil-spared third-nerve palsies: If new, observe for 5–7 days (after work-up described previously) for delayed pupil involvement, then recheck every 6 weeks. Patients should regain the function lost from their third-nerve palsy within 3 months. If the palsy does not reverse by this time or if an additional neurologic abnormality develops, an MRI is obtained.

11.6 ISOLATED FOURTH-NERVE PALSY

Symptoms
Binocular vertical diplopia (double vision that disappears when one eye is occluded; one image appears on top of or up and to the side of the second image with both eyes open), difficulty reading, sensation that objects appear tilted; may be asymptomatic.

Critical Signs
Deficient inferior movement of an eye when attempting to look down and in. The three-step test isolates a palsy of the superior oblique muscle (see the following discussion).

Other Signs
The involved eye is higher (hypertropic) when patient looks straight ahead. The hypertropia increases when looking in the direction of the uninvolved eye or tilting the head toward the ipsilateral shoulder. The patient often maintains a head tilt toward the contralateral shoulder to eliminate double vision.

Etiology
More common   Trauma; vascular infarct (often the result of underlying diabetes or hypertension); congenital, idiopathic, or demyelinating disease.
Rare   Tumor, hydrocephalus, giant cell arteritis, aneurysm.

Differential Diagnosis

All of the following may produce binocular vertical diplopia, hypertropia, or both.

- Myasthenia gravis   [Double vision worse toward the end of the day when fatigued, usually accompanied by ptosis, positive edrophonium chloride (e.g., Tensilon Chloride) test. See Section 11.10.]
- Thyroid eye disease   (May have proptosis, eyelid lag, stare, or injection over the involved rectus muscles. Positive forced duction test. See Section 7.2.)
- Orbital inflammatory pseudotumor   (Pain and proptosis are common. See Section 7.3.)
- Orbital trauma   (Can cause entrapment of the contralateral inferior rectus muscle.)
- Skew deviation   (The three-step test does not isolate a particular muscle. Rule out a posterior fossa lesion by CT scan or MRI of the brain if the previously described conditions are ruled out.)
- Vertical hypertropia   (One eye is higher than the other in all fields of gaze by a constant amount, no torsional component.)

Work-up

1. History: Onset and duration of the diplopia? Misaligned eyes or head tilt since early childhood? Trauma? Stroke?
2. Examine old photographs to determine whether the head tilt is long-standing, indicating an old or congenital fourth-nerve palsy.

❖ **Note** *A congenital fourth-nerve palsy can often be distinguished from an acquired fourth-nerve palsy by measuring the vertical fusional amplitudes. A patient with an acquired fourth-nerve palsy will have a normal vertical fusional amplitude of 1–3 prism diopters. On the other hand, a patient with a congenital fourth-nerve palsy has greater than 1–3 prism diopters (often up to 10–15 prism diopters) of fusional amplitude. This is detected using vertical prism bars. If a patient can fuse greater than 1–3 prism diopters, then the fourth-nerve palsy is probably congenital.*

3. Three-step test:
   Step 1   Determine which eye is deviated upward in primary gaze (looking straight ahead). This is best seen with the cover-uncover test (see Appendix 2). The higher eye comes down after being uncovered.
   Step 2   Determine whether the upward deviation is greater when the patient looks to the left or to the right.
   Step 3   Determine whether the upward deviation is greater when tilting the head to the left shoulder or right shoulder.
   As mentioned previously, patients with a superior oblique muscle paresis have a hyperdeviation that is worse when turning their elevated eye

nasally and when tilting their head toward the shoulder ipsilateral to the elevated eye.

Patients with a bilateral fourth-nerve palsy demonstrate hypertropia of the right eye when looking left, hypertropia of the left eye when looking right, and a V-pattern esotropia (the eyes cross more when looking down).

4. Perform the double Maddox rod test[1] if a bilateral fourth-nerve palsy is suspected.
5. Edrophonium chloride (e.g., Tensilon Chloride) test if myasthenia gravis is suspected (see "Myasthenia Gravis," Section 11.10).
6. Fasting blood sugar and/or glucose tolerance test.
7. MRI of the brain for:
   a. A fourth-nerve palsy accompanied by other cranial nerve or neurological abnormalities (i.e., not an isolated palsy).
   b. Children with an acquired fourth-nerve palsy.
   c. Adults with no vasculopathic risk factors.

Treatment

1. Treat the underlying disorder.
2. A patch may be placed over one eye or tape can be applied to one lens if the patient has symptomatic double vision. Patching is generally not performed in children younger than 9–11 years of age because of the risk of amblyopia.
3. Prisms in spectacles may be prescribed for small chronic hyperdeviations.
4. Surgery may be indicated for bothersome double vision in primary or reading position, for cosmetic purposes, or for a head tilt. We generally wait at least 6 months after the onset of the palsy, because many palsies resolve spontaneously.

Follow-up

Acquired fourth-nerve palsy   If the work-up is negative and no previous head tilt is observed in old photographs, reexamine the patient in 3 months, checking for the development of any new neurologic abnormality (CT scan or MRI of the brain would be indicated for any new development). Patients are instructed to return immediately if they notice a new deficit.

Congenital fourth-nerve palsy   As needed.

---

[1]A white Maddox rod is placed before one eye and a red Maddox rod is placed before the other eye in a trial frame, aligning the axes of each rod along the 90-degree vertical mark. While looking at a white light in the distance, the patient is asked if both the white and red lines seen through the Maddox rods are horizontal and parallel to each other (sometimes placing a six-prism diopter base-down in front of one eye helps the patient determine if the lines are parallel, but this should not be performed in the presence of a hypertropia). When the lines are not horizontal and parallel, the patient is asked to rotate the Maddox rod(s) until they are parallel. If he or she rotates the top of this vertical axis outward (away from the nose) for more than 10 degrees total for the two eyes, then a bilateral superior oblique muscle paresis exists.

11.7 ISOLATED SIXTH-NERVE PALSY

Symptoms

Binocular horizontal diplopia (double vision producing side-by-side images; single vision is restored when one eye is closed or covered), worse for distance than near, most pronounced in the direction of the paretic lateral rectus muscle.

Critical Sign

One eye does not turn outward (temporally).

Other Signs

No restriction on forced-duction testing. No significant proptosis.

Differential Diagnosis

All of the following may produce limitation of abduction.

- Thyroid eye disease   (Proptosis, injection of blood vessels over the restricted muscle, restriction on forced-duction testing. See Section 7.2.)
- Myasthenia gravis   [Symptoms worse towards the end of day when fatigued, orbicularis oculi weakness, ptosis may or may not be present, positive edrophonium chloride (e.g., Tensilon Chloride) test. See Section 11.10.]
- Orbital inflammatory pseudotumor   (Proptosis, pain, restriction on forced-duction testing. See Section 7.3.)
- Orbital trauma causing entrapment of the ipsilateral medial rectus   (Restriction on forced-duction testing.)
- Duane's syndrome, type 1   (Congenital; narrowing of the palpebral fissure and retraction of the globe on adduction.)
- Convergence spasm   (The pupils constrict on attempted abduction.)
- Möbius' syndrome   (Congenital; bilateral facial paralysis present.)

Etiology

ADULTS

More common   Vasculopathic (diabetes, hypertension, atherosclerosis), traumatic, idiopathic.

Less common   Increased intracranial pressure, giant cell arteritis, cavernous sinus mass (e.g., meningioma, aneurysm, metastasis), multiple sclerosis, sarcoidosis/vasculitis, postmyelography or lumbar puncture, stroke (usually not isolated).

CHILDREN

Benign postviral condition

Gradenigo's syndrome   (Petrositis causing sixth- and often seventh-nerve

involvement, with or without eighth- and fifth-nerve involvement on the same side.)
Pontine glioma
Trauma

Work-up

ADULTS

1. History: Do the symptoms fluctuate during the day? Past history of cancer, diabetes, or thyroid disease?
2. Complete neurologic and ophthalmic examinations; pay careful attention to the function of the other cranial nerves and the appearance of the optic disc. It is especially important to evaluate the fifth cranial nerve; corneal sensation (supplied by the first division) can be tested by touching a wisp of cotton or a tissue to the unanesthetized corneas.
3. Check blood pressure.
4. Fasting blood sugar and ESR (ESR is obtained only if the patient is older than 50–55 years of age).
5. MRI (axial and coronal views) of the brain is indicated if the sixth-nerve palsy is accompanied by any other neurologic or neuro-ophthalmic sign or by severe pain. Additionally, MRI should be obtained in any patient with a history of cancer.

CHILDREN

1. Complete ocular examination as described previously.
2. Neurologic examination, and otoscopic examination by a pediatrician.
3. MRI of the brain in all children.

Treatment

Any underlying problem revealed by the work-up is treated; otherwise, patients are managed by observation.

- In patients older than 9–11 years of age with bothersome diplopia, the paretic eye can be occluded with a patch or opaque glasses until the condition resolves. The nonparetic eye can be patched instead if its visual acuity is much worse.
- In patients younger than 9–11 years of age, patching is avoided. These patients are monitored closely for the development of amblyopia (see Section 9.6).

Follow-up

Reexamine every 6 weeks following the onset of the palsy until it resolves. MRI of the head is indicated if:

- Any neurologic or neuro-ophthalmic signs or symptoms develop during the follow-up period.
- The abduction deficit increases
- The isolated sixth-nerve palsy does not resolve in 3–6 months.

11.8 ISOLATED SEVENTH-NERVE PALSY

Symptoms

Weakness or paralysis of one side of the face, inability to close one eye, excessive drooling. May have decreased taste, hyperacusis, decreased or increased tearing.

Critical Signs

Weakness or paralysis of the facial musculature on one side.

- *Central*: Weakness or paralysis of lower facial musculature. (Upper eyelid closure and forehead wrinkling intact.)
- *Peripheral*: Weakness or paralysis of upper and lower facial musculature.

Other Signs

Flattened nasolabial fold, droop of corner of the mouth, ectropion, or lagophthalmos. May have ipsilateral decreased taste on anterior two thirds of tongue, decreased basic tear production, or hyperacusis. May have an injected eye with a corneal epithelial defect.

Synkinesis Simultaneous movement of muscles supplied by different branches of the facial nerve or simultaneous stimulation of visceral efferent fibers of facial nerve [e.g., corner of mouth contracts when eye closes, excessive lacrimation when patient eats (crocodile tears)]. Usually implies chronicity.

Etiology

CENTRAL LESIONS

1. Cortical   [Loss of voluntary facial movement; emotional facial movement sometimes intact. May also have ipsilateral hemiparesis. Lesion of motor cortex or internal capsule contralateral to facial palsy (e.g., vasculopathic or tumor).]
2. Extrapyramidal   [Loss of emotional facial movement; volitional facial movement intact. Not a true facial paralysis (e.g., parkinsonism, tumor, vascular lesion of basal ganglia).]

3. Brain stem   [Often ipsilateral sixth-nerve palsy, contralateral hemiparesis, cerebellar signs (e.g., multiple sclerosis, infarction, tumor) may or may not be present.]

PERIPHERAL LESIONS

1. Cerebellopontine angle (CPA) masses   [Gradually progressive onset, although sometimes acute. May have facial pain or twitching. May have eighth-nerve dysfunction including hearing loss, vertigo, or ataxia (e.g., acoustic schwannoma, facial neuroma, meningioma, cholesteatoma, metastasis).]
2. Trauma
   - Temporal bone fracture   [History of head trauma. May have Battle's sign (ecchymoses over mastoid), cerebrospinal fluid otorrhea, hearing loss, vertigo, or vestibular nystagmus.)
   - Other   [Accidental or iatrogenic (e.g., facial laceration, local anesthetic block, parotid or mastoid surgery).]
3. Otitis
   - Acute otis media
   - Chronic suppurative otitis media
   - Malignant external otitis   (Pseudomonas infection in diabetic or elderly patients. Begins in external auditory canal but may progress to osteomyelitis, meningitis, or abscess.)
4. Ramsey-Hunt syndrome (herpes zoster cephalicus)   (Viral prodrome followed by ear pain, vesicles on pinna, external auditory canal, tongue, face, or neck. Progresses over 10 days. Patient may have sensorineural hearing loss or vertigo.)
5. Guillain-Barré syndrome   (Viral syndrome followed by progressive motor weakness or paralysis and/or cranial-nerve palsies. Often areflexic. Patient may have bilateral facial palsies.)
6. Lyme disease   (Patient may have rash, fever, fatigue, arthralgias, myalgias, nausea. There may or may not be a history of tick bite.)
7. Sarcoidosis   (Patient may have a history of uveitis or lymphadenopathy. May have bilateral facial palsies.)
8. Parotid neoplasm   (Slowly progressive paralysis of all or portion of facial musculature. Parotid mass with facial pain.)
9. Metastasis   [History of primary tumor (e.g., breast, lung, prostate) with multiple cranial-nerve palsies in rapid succession. Can be the result of basilar skull metastasis or carcinomatous meningitis.]
10. Bell's palsy   (A diagnosis of exclusion. May have viral prodrome followed by ear pain, facial numbness, decreased tearing or taste. Facial palsy may be complete or incomplete and progress over 10 days. May be bilateral or recurrent. May or may not have family history of the disease.)
11. Others   (Diabetes mellitus, botulism, human immunodeficiency virus,

syphilis, Epstein-Barr virus, acute porphyrias, nasopharyngeal carcinoma, collagen-vascular disease)

Work-up

1. History: Onset and duration of facial weakness? First bout or recurrence? Facial or ear pain? Trauma? Stroke? Recent infection? Hearing loss, tinnitus, dizziness, or vertigo? History of cancer?
2. Complete neurologic examination: Determine if facial palsy is central or peripheral, complete or incomplete. Assess taste with bitter or sweet solution on anterior two thirds of tongue on affected side. Carefully assess other cranial nerves, especially the fifth, sixth, and seventh. Look for motor weakness, cerebellar signs.
3. Complete ocular examination: Check ocular motility and look for nystagmus. Check orbicularis strength bilaterally, degree of ectropion, and Bell's phenomenon. Examine cornea carefully for signs of exposure (superficial punctate keratitis, abrasion, ulcer). Do Schirmer's test to assess basic tear production.
4. Otolaryngologic examination: Examine ear and oropharynx for vesicles, masses, or other lesions. Palpate parotid for mass or lymphadenopathy. Check hearing.
5. CT scan if history of trauma to rule out basilar skull fracture. Axial and coronal cuts with attention to temporal bone.
6. MRI or CT scan of brain if any other associated neurologic signs or with history of cancer. If sixth-nerve involvement, pay attention to brain stem. If eighth-nerve involvement, pay attention to CPA. If multiple cranial nerves involved, pay attention to base of skull.
7. Chest x-ray and angiotensin converting enzyme level if high index of suspicion for sarcoid.
8. Lyme titer, Epstein-Barr virus titer, RPR, HIV, complete blood test with differential if one of these infections is suspected.
9. Rheumatoid factor, ESR, ANA, antineutrophil cytoplasmic antibody if collagen-vascular disease suspected.
10. Echocardiogram, Holter monitor, carotid noninvasives studies in patients with a history of a stroke, to determine source.
11. Lumbar puncture (LP) three times in patients with history of primary neoplasm to rule out carcinomatous meningitis.

Treatment/Follow-up

1. Cerebrovascular accident: If patient presents within 72 hours of onset, admit to hospital for observation.
2. CPA masses, temperal bone fracture, nerve laceration: Refer to neurosurgeon.
3. Otitis: Refer to ear, nose, and throat specialist.

4. Ramsey-Hunt syndrome: Acyclovir 800 mg 5 times per day for 7–10 days in patients with no history of renal insufficiency who are seen within 72 hours of onset.

5. Guillain-Barré syndrome: Refer to neurologist. May require hospitalization for progressive motor weakness or respiratory distress.

6. Lyme disease: Refer to an infectious disease specialist. May need LP. Treat with oral doxycycline or penicillin or IV ceftriaxone.

7. Sarcoidosis: Order MRI to evaluate central nervous system sarcoidosis. Consider LP. Refer to a neurologist. May require oral prednisone for systemic or central nervous system disease.

8. Metastatic disease: Systemic chemotherapy, radiation, or both may be required.

9. Bell's palsy: Any treatment is controversial; 86% of patients recover completely without treatment. Options include:
   a. Observation.
   b. Facial massage or electrical stimulation of facial musculature.
   c. Steroids (consider in patients who present with complete palsy. Oral prednisone 60 mg daily for 4 days, tapering to 5 mg daily over 10 days).
   d. Surgical decompression of facial nerve (refer to ear, nose, and throat specialist).

Follow all patients at 1 and 3 months, or more frequently if corneal complications arise (see the following discussion).

If no recovery in 3 months, order MRI of brain.

TREATMENT OF OCULAR COMPLICATIONS OF FACIAL PALSY

1. Minimal-to-mild exposure keratitis: Artificial tears qid with lubricating ointment qhs.

2. Mild-to-moderate exposure keratitis: Preservative-free artificial tears every 1–2 hours, moisture chamber during the day with lubricating ointment, or tape tarsorrhaphy qhs. Consider a permanent tarsorrhaphy.

3. Moderate-to-severe exposure keratitis: Temporary or permanent tarsorrhaphy, gold weight on upper eyelid, or eyelid spring.

TREATMENT OF NONRESOLVING FACIAL PALSY (COMPLETE WORK-UP NEGATIVE):

In patients who strongly desire facial reanimation, consider referral to neurosurgeon or plastic surgeon for facial nerve graft, cranial nerve reanastamosis, or temporalis muscle transposition surgery.

REFERENCE

May M, Klein SR. Differential diagnosis of facial nerve palsy. *Otolaryngol Clin North Am* 7(2):613, 1991.

11.9 CAVERNOUS SINUS/SUPERIOR ORBITAL FISSURE SYNDROME
(Multiple Ocular Motor Nerve Palsies)

Symptoms

Double vision, eyelid droop, facial pain or numbness.

Critical Signs

Limitation of eye movement corresponding to any combination of a third-, fourth-, or sixth-nerve palsy on one side; facial pain and/or numbness corresponding to one or more branches of the fifth cranial nerve; a droopy eyelid and a small pupil (Horner's syndrome); the pupil may also be dilated if the third cranial nerve is involved. All signs involve the same side of the face when one cavernous sinus/superior orbital fissure is involved.

Other Signs

Proptosis may be present when the superior orbital fissure is involved.

Etiology

- Arteriovenous fistula (carotid-cavernous or dural-cavernous) (Exophthalmos and chemosis; dilated episcleral and conjuctival blood vessels; often a bruit, which may be heard by the patient and sometimes by the physician during ocular ausculation. Intraocular pressure may be elevated. Abnormal pulsations of the globe are often present, but difficult to observe. CT scan or MRI shows an enlarged superior ophthalmic vein.)
- Cavernous sinus thrombosis (Proptosis, chemosis, and eyelid edema. Usually bilateral. Fever, nausea, vomiting, and an altered level of consciousness often develop. Commonly the result of spread of infection from the face, mouth, throat, sinus, or orbit. Less commonly noninfectious, resulting from trauma or surgery.)
- Metastatic tumors to the cavernous sinus (e.g., breast, lung, lymphoma)
- Perineural spread of a periocular skin malignancy (e.g., squamous cell carcinoma) (Resected tumors may invade the cavernous sinus years after resection.)
- Pituitary apoplexy (Acute onset of the critical signs listed previously; often bilateral with severe headache, decreased vision, and possibly bilateral temporal heminanopsia or blindness. An enlarged sella turcica or a sellar mass, usually with acute hemorrhage, is seen on CT scan or MRI of the brain.)
- Intracavernous aneurysm (Usually unruptured. If aneurysm does rupture, the signs of a carotid-cavernous fistula develop.)

- Mucormycosis (Must be suspected in all diabetics, particularly those in ketoacidosis, and any debilitated or immunocompromised individual with multiple cranial-nerve palsies, with or without proptosis. Onset is typically acute. Nasal discharge of blood may be present, and nasal examination may reveal a black, crusty material. This condition is life-threatening.)
- Herpes zoster (Patients with the typical zoster rash may develop ocular motor nerve palsies as well as a mid-dilated pupil that reacts better to convergence than light.)
- Tolosa-Hunt syndrome (Acute inflammation of the superior orbital fissure or anterior cavernous sinus. Orbital pain often precedes restriction of eye movements. Recurrent episodes are common. This is a diagnosis of exclusion.)
- Others (Meningioma, sphenoid sinus carcinoma, mucocele, or infections.)

Differential Diagnosis
- Myasthenia gravis [Eyelid droop and limitation of eye movements, especially when fatigued; weakness of the orbicularis oculi muscle; positive edrophonium chloride (e.g., Tensilon Chloride) test. No pupillary abnormality, no pain, no proptosis.]
- Chronic progressive external ophthalmoplegia (Slowly progressive, painless, bilateral limitation of eye movements with ptosis. The pupils are normal, and the orbicularis oculi muscles are usually weak.)
- Orbital lesions (e.g., tumor, thyroid disease, pseudotumor) [Proptosis and resistance to retropulsion are usually present, in addition to motility restriction. Forced-duction tests are abnormal (see Appendix 5). May have an afferent pupillary defect if the optic nerve is involved.]
- Brain stem disease (Tumors and vascular lesions of the brain stem can produce multiple ocular motor nerve palsies. MRI of the brain is best for making this diagnosis.)
- Carcinomatous meningitis (Diffuse seeding of the leptomeninges by metastatic tumor cells can produce a rapidly sequential bilateral cranial-nerve disorder. Diagnosis is made by lumbar punctures $\times$ 3, if first 2 are negative.)
- Nasopharyngeal carcinoma (Most commonly affects the sixth cranial nerve, but the second, third, fourth, and fifth cranial nerves may be involved as well. Typically, one cranial nerve after another is affected by invasion of the base of the skull. The patient may have cervical lymphadenopathy, nasal obstruction, ear pain or popping caused by serous otitis media or blockage of the eustachian tube, weight loss, or exophthalmos.)
- Parinaud's syndrome (dorsal midbrain syndrome) (Deficient upward gaze, retraction-convergence nystagmus on attempted upward gaze, can have mid-dilated pupils that react better to convergence than to light; some patients have accompanying deficient downgaze.)

- Progressive supranuclear palsy (Vertical limitation of eye movements; initially, downward gaze restriction, dementia and rigidity of the neck and trunk. All eye movements are eventually lost.)
- Rare [Myotonic dystrophy, the bulbar variant of the Guillian-Barré syndrome (Miller-Fisher variant), intracranial sarcoidosis, others.]

Work-up

1. History: Diabetes? Prior cancer (including skin cancer)? Weight loss? Ocular bruit? Recent infection? Severe headache? Diurnal variation of symptoms?
2. Ophthalmic examination: Pay special attention to pupils, extraocular motility, Hertel exophthalmometry, and resistance to retropulsion.
3. Examine the periocular skin for malignant lesions.
4. CT scan (axial and coronal views) and/or MRI of the sinuses, orbit, and brain.
5. Consider color Doppler imaging if arteriovenous fistula is suspected.

If the CT scan and MRI are normal, consider any or all of the following:

6. Lumbar puncture ($\times$ 3, if first 2 are negative) to rule out carcinomatous meningitis in patients with a history of primary carcinoma.
7. Nasopharyngeal examination with or without a blind nasopharyngeal biopsy to rule out nasopharyngeal carcinoma.
8. Lymph node biopsy when lymphadenopathy is present.
9. Complete blood count with differential, ESR, ANA, rheumatoid factor to rule out infection, malignancy, and systemic vasculitis. Antineutrophilic cytoplasmic antibody if Wegener's granulomatosis is suspected.
10. Cerebral arteriogram is rarely required to rule out an aneurysm or arteriovenous fistula because most of these are seen by CT scan or MRI.

If cavernous sinus thrombosis is being considered, obtain blood cultures 2–3 times and culture the presumed primary source of the infection.

Treatment/Follow-up

ARTERIOVENOUS FISTULA

1. Many dural fistulas will close spontaneously or after arteriography. Others may require neurosurgical or interventional neuroradiologic techniques.
2. Treat secondary glaucoma with a topical beta-blocker (e.g., timolol 0.25–0.5% bid or levobunolol 0.25–0.5% bid) with or without a carbonic anhydrase inhibitor (e.g., methazolamide 50 mg po bid). Drugs that increase outflow facility (e.g., epinephrine and pilocarpine) are generally not as effective because the intraocular pressure is increased as a result of increased episcleral venous pressure.

CAVERNOUS SINUS THROMBOSIS

1. For possible infectious cases (usually caused by *Staphylococcus aureus*), hospitalize the patient and treat with intravenous antibiotics for several weeks:
   Nafcillin 1–2 g IV q 4 h or cefazolin 1 g IV q 8 h (alternatively, vancomycin 1 g IV q 12 h if the patient is penicillin allergic)
   Ceftazidime 1–2 g IV q 8 h
   Blood culture results usually dictate later therapy.
2. Intravenous fluid replacement is usually required.
3. For aseptic cavernous sinus thrombosis, consider systemic anticoagulation (heparin followed by warfarin) or aspirin 600 mg po daily. Systemic anticoagulation therapy may require collaboration with a medical internist.
4. Exposure keratopathy needs to be treated with lubricating ointment tid and qhs (e.g., Refresh PM). See Section 4.4.
5. Treat glaucoma as described previously for arteriovenous fistulas.

METASTIC DISEASE TO THE CAVERNOUS SINUS

Often requires systemic chemotherapy (if a primary is found) with or without radiation therapy to the metastasis.

PITUITARY APOPLEXY

Refer emergently to neurospecialist for surgical consideration.

INTRACAVERNOUS ANEURYSM

Refer to a neuro-specialist for arteriogram, only if treatment is contemplated.

MUCORMYCOSIS

1. Hospitalize and treat the underlying disorder.
2. Consultation with a medical, infectious disease specialist, an ear, nose, and throat specialist, or both may be helpful.
3. Surgical debridement of all necrotic tissue with irrigation of the involved sinuses with amphotericin B is usually necessary.
4. Amphotericin B 0.25–0.30 mg/kg IV in D5W slowly over 3–6 hours on the first day, 0.5 mg/kg IV on the second day, then 45–50 mg IV daily. The duration of treatment is determined by the clinical condition.
5. Blood urea nitrogen and creatinine levels are obtained every other day; watch for renal compromise.

TOLOSA-HUNT SYNDROME

Prednisone 100 mg po daily; taper rapidly as the pain subsides. If pain persists despite steroid therapy, reinvestigation may be necessary to rule out other disorders.

REFERENCES

Kohn R, Hepler R. Management of limited rhino-orbital mucormycosis without exenteration. *Ophthalmology* 92: 1440, 1985.
Levine SR, Twyman RE, Gilman S. The role of anticoagulation in cavernous sinus thrombosis. *Neurology* 38:517, 1988.

11.10 MYASTHENIA GRAVIS

Symptoms
Droopy eyelid and/or double vision that is worse toward the end of the day or when the individual is fatigued; may have weakness of facial muscles, proximal limb muscles, difficulty swallowing or breathing.

Critical Signs
Worsening of eyelid droop with sustained upgaze or double vision with continued eye movements, weakness of the orbicularis muscle on the affected side (cannot close the eyelid as forcefully as on the unaffected side), no pupillary abnormalities.

Other Signs
Can have complete limitation of ocular movements.

Etiology
Autoimmune disease sometimes triggered by an underlying thymoma, thyroid disease, or infection.

Differential Diagnosis
- Eaton-Lambert syndrome   (A myasthenia-like condition that is caused by a carcinoma located elsewhere in the body. Isolated eye signs do *not* occur in this condition, although eye signs may accompany systemic signs of weakness. Unlike myasthenia, muscle strength increases after exercise. Electromyography distinguishes between the two conditions. Specifically, look for lung cancer.)
- Myasthenia-like syndrome due to medication (e.g., penicillamine, aminoglycosides)
- Chronic progressive external ophthalmoplegia (CPEO)   [No diurnal variation of symptoms or relation to fatigue; usually a negative edrophonium chloride (e.g., Tensilon Chloride) test, but not always.]
- Kearns-Sayre syndrome   (CPEO and retinal pigmentary degeneration in a young person; heart block develops a few years later. See Section 11.11.)

- Third-nerve palsy (Pupil may be involved, no orbicularis weakness, no fatigability, no diurnal variation.)
- Horner's syndrome (Miosis accompanies the ptosis. Pupil does not dilate well in darkness.)
- Levator muscle dehiscence or disinsertion (High eyelid crease on the side of the droopy eyelid, no variability of eyelid droop, no orbicularis weakness.)
- Thyroid eye disease (No ptosis. May have eyelid retraction or eyelid lag, may or may not have exophthalmos, no diurnal variation of double vision.)
- Orbital inflammatory pseudotumor (Proptosis, pain with ocular movements, inflammation.)
- Myotonic dystrophy (May have ptosis and rarely, gaze restriction. After a handshake, these patients are often unable to release their grip.)

Work-up

1. History: Do the signs fluctuate with the time of the day and fatigue? Any systemic weakness? Difficulty swallowing, chewing, or breathing? Medications?
2. Have the patient focus on your finger in upgaze for one minute. Observe whether the eyelid droops more than expected.
3. Test for double vision in upgaze (hold the eyelid back so each eye can see your finger.)
4. Assess orbicularis function by asking the patient to squeeze the eyelids shut while you attempt to force them open.
5. Test pupillary function.
6. Blood test for acetylcholine-receptor antibodies.
7. Edrophonium chloride (e.g., Tensilon Chloride) test to confirm the diagnosis:
    a. Inject Tensilon 0.2 ml IV. Observe for 1 minute. If an improvement in eyelid droop or double vision (whichever was present initially) is noted, the test is positive and may be stopped at this point. If no improvement nor untoward reaction to the medication develops, continue.
    b. Tensilon 0.4 ml IV. Observe for 30 seconds for a response or side-effect. If neither develops, proceed.
    c. Tensilon 0.4 ml IV. If no improvement is noted within two additional minutes, the test is negative.

Improvement within the stated time period is diagnostic of myasthenia gravis (rarely a patient with CPEO, an intracavernous tumor, or some other rare disorder will have a false-positive result). A negative test does *not* exclude myasthenia.

❖ **Note** *Cholinergic crisis, syncopal episode, and respiratory arrest, although rare, may be precipitated by a Tensilon Chloride test. Treatment includes atropine 0.4 mg IV while monitoring vital signs.*

8. Check swallowing function.
9. Thryoid function tests (T3, T4, TSH).
10. CT scan of the chest to rule out thymoma.
11. Consider ANA, rheumatoid factor, and other tests to rule out other autoimmune disease.

Treatment

Consider collaborating with a neurologist or medical physician familiar with this disease.

1. If the patient is having difficulty swallowing or breathing, hospitalization with consideration for plasmapheresis and/or ventilatory support may be indicated.
2. If the condition is mild and not disturbing to the patient, therapy need not be instituted (the patient may patch one eye as needed).
3. If the condition is disturbing or more than mild, an oral anticholinesterase agent (e.g., pyridostigmine 60 mg po qid) should be given. The dosage must be adjusted according to the response. (Patients rarely benefit from greater than 120 mg po q 3 h of pyridostigmine.) Overdosage may produce cholinergic crisis.
4. If symptoms persit, consider systemic steroids. (There is no uniform agreement concerning the dosage. One way is to start with prednisone 20 mg po daily, increasing the dose slowly until the patient is receiving 100 mg/day. These patients are monitored in the hospital for several days when the steroids are started if they have systemic myasthenia.)
5. Immunosuppressive therapy may be helpful.
6. Treat any underlying thyroid disease or infection.
7. Surgical removal of a thymoma is usually performed. Thymectomy on patients without a thymoma occasionally helps.

Follow-up

If systemic symptoms are present or the ocular involvement is acute, patients need to be followed closely at first (every 1–4 days) until improvement is demonstrated. Patients who have had their isolated ocular abnormality for an extended time period (e.g., months) need not be seen again for weeks (assuming no worsening of the condition develops). Pateints should always be warned to return immediately if swallowing or breathing difficulties arise.

❖ **Note** *Myasthenia should be looked for in newborns of myasthenic mothers. Poor sucking reflex, ptosis, or an ocular motility disturbance may be seen.*

11.11 CHRONIC PROGRESSIVE EXTERNAL OPHTHALMOPLEGIA (CPEO)

Symptoms

Gradual onset of a droopy eyelid, double vision, and other muscle weakness may or may not be present; ocular involvement is usually bilateral; there is no diurnal variation; there may be a positive family history.

Critical Signs

Ptosis, limitation of ocular motility (sometimes complete limitation), normal pupils.

Other Signs

Weak orbicularis oculi muscles, weakness of limb and facial muscles, exposure keratopathy.

Differential Diagnosis

See "Myasthenia Gravis," Section 11.10, for a complete list. The following are four syndromes that need to be ruled out when CPEO is diagnosed. All of them may have CPEO as part of their clinical picture:

- Kearns-Sayre syndrome   (Onset before age 20 years, retinal pigmentary degeneration with a salt-and-pepper appearance, heart block that generally occurs years after the ocular signs and may cause sudden death. There is usually no double vision. Other signs may include hearing loss, mental retardation, cerebellar signs, short stature, delayed puberty, nephropathy, vestibular abnormalities, elevated cerebrospinal fluid protein, and characteristic findings on muscle biopsy. Inheritance pattern is maternal mitochondrial DNA.)
- Abetalipoproteinemia (Bassen-Kornzweig syndrome)   (Retinal pigmentary degeneration similary to retinitis pigmentosa, diarrhea, ataxia, and other neurologic signs, acanthocytosis of red blood cells seen on peripheral blood smear, increased cerebrospinal fluid protein. See "Retinitis Pigmentosa," Section 12.24, for treatment.)
- Refsum's disease   (Retinitis pigmentosa and increased blood phytanic acid level. May have polyneuropathy, ataxia, hearing loss, anosmia, others. See "Retinitis Pigmentosa," Section 12.24, for treatment.)
- Ocular pharyngeal dystrophy   (Difficulty swallowing, sometimes leading to aspiration of food; may have autosomal dominant inheritance.)

Work-up

1. Careful history: determine the rate of onset (gradual versus sudden, as in cranial-nerve disease).
2. Family history.
3. Examine the pupils and ocular motility carefully.
4. Test orbicularis oculi strength.
5. Fundus examination: Look for diffuse pigmentary changes.
6. Check swallowing function.
7. Edrophonium chloride (e.g., Tensilon Chloride) test to rule-out myasthenia gravis (see Section 11.10).

❖ **Note** *Sometimes patients with CPEO are supersensitive to Tensilon Chloride.*

8. Consider electromyography for a more definitive diagnosis.
9. Consider a lumbar puncture if Kearns-Sayre syndrome is a possibility.
10. Yearly electrocardiograms by a cardiologist if Kearns-Sayre syndrome is a possibility.
11. Lipoprotein electrophoresis and peripheral blood smear to check for acanthocytes if abetalipoproteinemia is suspected.
12. Serum phytanic acid level if Refsum's disease is suspected.

Treatment

There is no proven cure as of yet for CPEO. The following treatments will help:

1. Treat exposure keratopathy with lubricants at night (e.g., Refresh PM ointment) and artificial tears during the day (e.g., Refresh 4–8 times per day). See "Exposure Keratopathy," Section 4.4, for additional treatments.
2. Base-down prisms within reading glasses may help reading when downward gaze is restricted.
3. In Kearns-Sayre syndrome, a pacemaker may be required.
4. In ocular pharyngeal dystrophy, dysphagia and aspirations may require cricopharyngeal surgery.
5. In severe ptosis, consider surgical repair, but watch for worsening exposure keratopathy.
6. Genetic counseling.

Follow-up

Depends on ocular and systemic findings.

11.12 INTERNUCLEAR OPHTHALMOPLEGIA (INO)

Symptoms

Blurry vision or double vision that disappears when one eye is occluded.

Critical Signs

Weakness or paralysis of inward (nasal) eye movement with nystagmus of the opposite eye when it attempts to look outward temporally.

Other Signs

A skew deviation (either eye is turned upward, but the three-step test cannot isolate a specific muscle, see "Isolated Fourth-Nerve Palsy," Section 11.6), and upbeat nystagmus in upgaze when INO is bilateral. The involved eye can sometimes turn in when attempting to read (intact convergence). Unilateral or bilateral. Bilateral disease can give an exotropia.

Etiology

- Multiple sclerosis (more common in young patients)
- Ischemic vascular disease of the brain stem (more common in elderly patients)
- Brain stem mass lesion (e.g., tumor)

Differential Diagnosis

(Weakness of inward eye movement.)

- Myasthenia gravis   [May closely mimic INO; however, ptosis and orbicularis oculi weakness are common. Nystagmus of INO is faster; myasthenia gravis is more gaze paretic. Symptoms worsen toward the end of the day when the patient is fatigued. An edrophonium chloride (e.g., Tenisilon Chloride) test is usually positive.]
- Orbital disease (e.g., tumor, thyroid disease, inflammatory pseudotumor)   (Proptosis, globe displacement, or pain may be present additionally. Nystagmus is usually not present. Orbital CT scan is abnormal.)

Work-up

1. History: Age? Are symptoms always present or do they only occur toward the end of the day when fatigued? Previous episode of optic neuritis, urinary incontinence, numbness or paralysis of an extremity, or another unexplained neurologic event (multiple sclerosis)?
2. Complete ocular examination, including a careful evaluation of eye movement.

❖ **Note** *Ocular motility can appear full, but a muscle weakness can be detected by observing slower saccadic eye movement in the involved eye compared with the contralateral eye. The ability of the right eye to look medially is assessed by holding one of the fingers of the examiner's left hand lateral to the patient's right eye. The patient is asked to first look at the examiner's finger and then at the examiner's nose. If a right INO is present, the right eye will show slower eye movement from the finger to the nose than the left* *eye. The left eye may be tested in a similar fashion, by holding a finger from the examiner's right hand lateral to the patient's left eye.*

3. Edrophonium chloride (e.g., Tensilon Chloride) test when the diagnosis of myasthenia gravis cannot be ruled out (see Section 11.10).
4. MRI of the brain stem and midbrain.

Treatment/Follow-up
- Patients with the diagnosis of a stroke within 72 hours of the acute onset of symptoms are admitted to the hospital for neurological evaluation and obervation.
- Otherwise, patients are managed by physicians familiar with the underlying disease.

11.13 PAPILLEDEMA

Definition
Optic disc swelling produced by increased intracranial pressure.

Symptoms
Episodes of transient, often bilateral, visual loss (lasting seconds) often precipitated by changes in posture; headache; double vision; nausea; vomiting; and rarely, a decrease in visual acuity (a mild decrease in visual acuity can occur in the acute setting if associated with a macular disturbance). Visual field defects and severe loss of central visual acuity can occur with chronic papilledema.

Critical Signs
Bilaterally swollen, hyperemic discs (in early papilledema, disc swelling may be asymmetric) with blurring of the disc margin, often obscuring the blood vessels. The nerve-fiber layer is also usually involved.

Other Signs
Papillary or peripapillary retinal hemorrhages (often flame-shaped); loss of venous pulsations (note that 20% of the normal population do not have venous pulsations); dilated, tortuous retinal veins; normal pupillary response and color vision; an enlarged physiologic blind spot by formal visual field testing.

As chronic papilledema progresses to optic atrophy, the hemorrhages and cotton-wool spots resolve, peripapillary gliosis and narrowing of the peripapillary retinal vessels occur, and optociliary shunt vessels may develop on the disc. Loss of color vision, central visual acuity, and peripheral visual field, especially inferonasally, also occur.

❖ **Note** *A unilateral or bilateral sixth-nerve palsy may also result from increased intracranial pressure.*

Etiology
- Primary and metastatic intracranial tumors
- Aqueductal stenosis producing hydrocephalus
- Pseudotumor cerebri (Often occurs in young, overweight females. See Section 11.14.)
- Subdural and epidural hematomas (From trauma.)
- Subarachnoid hemorrhage (Severe headache, may have preretinal hemorrhages.)
- Arteriovenous malformation
- Brain abscess (Often produces high fever.)
- Meningitis [Fever, stiff neck, headache (e.g., syphilis, tuberculosis, Lyme disease, bacterial).]
- Encephalitis (Often produces mental status abnormalities.)
- Sagittal sinus thrombosis

Differential Diagnosis
(Other causes of disc swelling.)

- Pseudopapilledema (e.g., optic disc drusen or congenitally anomalous disc) (Not true disc swelling. Vessels overlying the disc are not obscured, the disc is not hyperemic, and the surrounding nerve-fiber layer is normal. Spontaneous venous pulsations are often present. Buried drusen may be seen.)
- Papillitis (An afferent pupillary defect and decreased color vision are often present, white blood cells are seen in the posterior vitreous, pain occurs with eye movement, decreased visual acuity occurs in most cases, usually unilateral. See "Optic Neuritis," Section 11.15.)
- Malignant hypertensive retinopathy (Blood pressure extremely high, narrowed arterioles. May have arteriovenous crossing changes. Hemorrhages with or without cotton-wool spots extend to the peripheral retina.)
- Central retinal vein occlusion (Hemorrhages extend far beyond the peripapillary area, dilated and tortuous veins, generally unilateral, acute loss of vision in most cases.)
- Ischemic optic neuropathy (Disc swelling is pale, not hyperemic; initially unilateral with sudden, sometimes severe, visual loss.)
- Optic-disc vasculitis (Unilateral disc swelling in a young patient. There may be flame-shaped hemorrhages in the periphery.)
- Infiltration of the optic disc (e.g., sarcoid or tuberculous granuloma, leukemia, metastasis, other inflammatory disease or tumor) (Other ocular or

systemic abnormalities may be present. The disc may have an irregular outline. Usually unilateral.)

- Leber's optic neuropathy   (Usually occurs in men in the second to third decade of life; initially unilateral but rapidly bilateral; rapid, progressive visual loss; disc swelling associated with peripapillary telangiectasias. Optic atrophy later develops.)
- Orbital optic-nerve tumors   (Unilateral disc swelling, may or may not have proptosis.)
- Diabetic papillitis   (Disc edema in a young, type 1 diabetic; usually bilateral. May have moderate-to-severe retinopathy.)
- Grave's ophthalmopathy   (May have a history of thyroid dysfunction. May have lid lag or retraction, ocular misalignment, proptosis, elevated intraocular pressure, and resistance to retropulsion.)
- Uveitis (e.g., syphilis or sarcoidosis)   (May produce pain or photophobia. May have injection, keratic precipitates, anterior chamber cell and flare, posterior synechiae and vitreous cells.)

❖ **Note** *Optic-disc swelling in a patient with a history of leukemia is often a visually threatening sign of leukemic infiltration of the optic nerve. Immediate radiation therapy is usually required to preserve vision.*

Work-up
1. History and physical examination, including blood pressure measurement.
2. Ocular examination, including a pupillary and color vision (using color plates) assessment, posterior vitreous evaluation to check for white blood cells, and a dilated fundus examination using indirect ophthalmoscopy. The optic disc is best examined with a slit lamp and Hruby, fundus contact, or 60-diopter lens.
3. Emergent CT scan (axial and cornal views) and/or MRI of the head and orbit.
4. Lumbar puncture if the CT and/or MRI do not reveal the cause of the papilledema. Consider blood tests for thyroid disease, diabetes, and anemia.

Treatment
Treatment should be directed at the underlying cause of the elevated intracranial pressure.

11.14 PSEUDOTUMOR CEREBRI
(Idiopathic Intracranial Hypertension)

Symptoms
Headache (usually worse in the morning), transient episodes of visual loss (typically lasting seconds) often precipitated by changes in posture, double vision

(objects appear side by side; the double vision resolves when one eye is covered), tinnitus, dizziness, nausea, or vomiting. Occurs predominantly in women.

Critical Signs

By definition, a patient with pseudotumor cerebri will display the following symptoms:

1. Increased intracranial pressure with papilledema.
2. Normal head CT scan or MRI.
3. Normal cerebral spinal fluid composition.

Other Signs

See "Papilledema," Section 11.13. As with other causes of papilledema, may have unilateral or bilateral sixth-nerve palsy.

Etiology

Associated factors include obesity, pregnancy, and various medications, including oral contraceptives, tetracycline, nalidixic acid, and vitamin A. Systemic steroid withdrawal may also be causative.

Differential Diagnosis

See "Papilledema," Section 11.13.

Work-up

1. History: Inquire specifically about medications.
2. Ocular examination, including pupillary and intraocular pressure assessment, color vision test (color plates), and optic-nerve evaluation.
3. Systemic examination, including blood pressure and temperature.
4. MRI of the orbit and brain. Any patient who presents with papilledema needs to be imaged immediately. If normal, the patient should have a thorough neuro-ophthalmologic evaluation, including a lumbar puncture, to rule out other causes of papilledema and to determine the opening pressure (see Section 11.13).
5. Visual field test (e.g., Octopus, Humphrey, Goldmann, or other).

Treatment

Pseudotumor cerebri may be a self-limited process. Treatment is indicated in the following situations:

1. Severe intractable headache.
2. Evidence of progressive visual acuity or visual field loss.

Methods of treatment include the following:

1. Weight loss if overweight.

2. Diuretics (e.g., acetazolamide 250 mg po qid initially, building up to 500 mg qid if tolerated).
3. Discontinuation of any causative medication.

If treatment by these methods is unsuccessful, one of the following may be tried:

4. Systemic steroids (controversial).
5. Optic-nerve sheath decompression surgery (our choice).
6. Lumbo-peritoneal shunt.

❖ **Note** *Elevated intraocular pressure often needs to be treated aggressively.*

Follow-up
Every 2–3 weeks initially, monitor for visual loss, especially visual field loss; then every 4–6 weeks, depending on the response to treatment.

11.15 OPTIC NEURITIS

Symptoms
Loss of vision deteriorating over hours (rarely) to days (most commonly), with the nadir about 1 week after onset. Visual loss may be subtle or profound.

- Usually unilateral, but may be bilateral.
- Age typically 18–45 years.
- Orbital pain, especially with eye movement.
- Acquired loss of color vision.
- Reduced perception of light intensity.
- Occasionally Uhtoff's sign (visual deficit with exercise or increase in body temperature).
- May have neurologic symptoms or an antecedent viral syndrome (e.g., upper respiratory, gastrointestinal).

Critical Signs
Relative afferent pupillary defect (RAPD) in unilateral or asymmetric cases; decreased color vision; central, cecocentral, arcuate, or altitudinal visual field defects.

Other Signs
Swollen disc with or without peripapillary flame-shaped hemorrhages (papillitis—most commonly seen in children and young adults) or a normal disc

(retrobulbar optic neuritis—more common in adults). Posterior vitreous cells may be observed.

Etiology
- Idiopathic
- Multiple sclerosis
- Childhood infections (e.g., measles, mumps, chicken pox)
- Other viral infections (e.g., mononucleosis, herpes zoster, encephalitis)
- Contiguous inflammation of the meninges, orbit, or sinuses
- Granulomatous inflammations (e.g., tuberculosis, syphilis, sarcoidosis, cryptococcus)
- Intraocular inflammations

Differential Diagnosis
- Ischemic optic neuropathy (ION) (Visual loss is sudden, no pain with ocular motility, optic nerve swelling tends to be pale. Visual field defects are most commonly inferior altitudinal. In ION caused by giant cell arteritis, patients are older than 55 years of age. In nonarteritic ION, patients are typically 40–60 years of age. See Section 11.16 and 11.17.)
- Acute papilledema (Bilateral disc edema, no decreased color vision, no decreased visual acuity, no pain with ocular motility, no vitreous cells. Spontaneous venous pulsations are almost always absent. An enlarged blind spot is often noted on visual field testing. See Section 11.13.)
- Severe systemic hypertension (Bilateral disc edema, elevated blood pressure, flame-shaped retinal hemorrhages, and cotton-wool spots.)
- Orbital tumor compressing the optic nerve (Unilateral, often proptosis or restriction of extraocular motility is evident; there are no vitreous cells even when disc swelling is present.)
- Intracranial mass compressing the afferent visual pathway (Normal disc, positive afferent pupillary defect, decreased color vision, mass evident on CT scan or MRI of the brain.)
- Leber's optic neuropathy (Usually occurs in men in the second or third decade of life, may or may not have positive family history, rapid visual loss of one and then the other eye within days to months, may have peripapillary telangiectasias. Disc swelling is followed by optic atrophy.)
- Toxic or metabolic optic neuropathy [Progressive painless bilateral visual loss, may be secondary to alcohol, malnutrition, various toxins (e.g., ethambutol, chloroquine, isoniazid, chlorpropamide, heavy metals), anemia, and others.]

Work-up
1. History: Determine the patient's age and the rapidity of onset of the visual loss. Previous episode? Pain with eye movement?
2. Complete ophthalmic and neurologic examinations, including pupillary

assessment, color vision evaluation with color plates, evaluation of the vitreous for cells, and dilated retinal examination with optic-nerve assessment.

3. Check blood pressure.
4. Visual field test, preferably automated (e.g., Octopus, Humphrey).
5. For atypical cases (e.g., out of typical age range, no pain with eye movement), consider the following: CBC, RPR, FTA-ABS, $+/-$ ANA, $+/1$ ESR, MRI of the orbits and brain.

Treatment
If patient seen acutely:

A. If vision 20/40 or better: Observation is indicated.
B. If vision 20/50 or worse:
    1. Observation, or
    2. IV methylprednisolone 250 mg IV given over 30 minutes q 6 h for 12 doses, followed by prednisone 1 mg/kg/day po for 11 days, then 20 mg for one day, then 15 mg qod for doses.

Do not use oral prednisone as primary treatment because of increased risk of recurrences.

❖ Notes
1. *See medical glossary for a systemic steroid work-up.*
2. *An anti-ulcer medication (e.g., ranitidine 150 mg po bid) is given along with steroids.*

Follow-up
In general, examine the patient every 1–3 months. Patients being treated with steroids need to be followed more closely because of the risk of intraocular pressure rise.

REFERENCE

Beck R, Cleary PA, Anderson MM et al. A randomized controlled trial of corticosteroids in the treatment of acute optic neuritis. *N Engl J Med* 326:581, 1992.

11.16 ARTERITIC ISCHEMIC OPTIC NEUROPATHY
[Giant Cell Arteritis (GCA)]

Symptoms
Sudden, painless, nonprogressive visual loss; initially unilateral, but may rapidly become bilateral; occurs in patients older than 50 years of age; antecedent

or simultaneous headache, jaw claudication (pain with chewing), scalp tenderness (tenderness with hair combing), proximal muscle and joint aches (polymyalgia rheumatica), anorexia, weight loss, or fever may occur.

Critical Signs

Afferent pupillary defect; devastating visual loss (often counting fingers or worse); pale, swollen disc, often with flame-shaped hemorrhages. Later, optic atrophy occurs as the edema resolves. The ESR may be markedly elevated.

Other Signs

Visual field defect (commonly altitudinal or involving the central field); a palpable, tender, and nonpulsatile temporal artery; a central retinal artery occlusion or a cranial-nerve palsy (especially a sixth-nerve palsy) may occur.

Differential Diagnosis

- Nonarteritic ischemic optic neuropathy   (Patients may be younger, usually have less severe visual loss, do not have the accompanying symptoms listed previously, and usually have normal ESRs. See Section 11.17.)
- Inflammatory optic neuritis (papillitis)   (Affects a younger age group, typically less severe and less sudden onset of visual loss, pain with eye movements, optic-disc swelling is more hemorrhagic, posterior vitreous cells are often present, no symptoms of GCA. See Section 11.15.)
- Compressive optic nerve tumor   (Slowly progressive visual loss, few-to-no symptoms in common with GCA.)
- Central retinal vein occlusion   (Severe visual loss may be accompanied by an afferent pupillary defect and disc swelling, but the retina shows diffuse retinal hemorrhages extending out to the periphery. See Section 12.3.)
- Central retinal artery occlusion   (Sudden, painless, severe visual loss with an afferent pupillary defect, but the disc is not swollen, and retinal edema with a cherry-red spot is frequently observed. See Section 12.1.)

Work-up

1. History: Attempt to elicit the symptoms above. Age is critical.
2. Complete ocular examination, particularly pupillary assessment, color plates, dilated retinal examination to rule out retinal causes of severe visual loss, and optic-nerve evaluation.
3. Immediate ESR (Westergren is the most reliable method). A guideline for top normal ESRs: men = 0.5 × age, women = 0.5 × (age + 10).
4. Perform a temporal artery biopsy if GCA is suspected from the symptoms, signs, or ESR. The ESR may not be elevated.

❖ **Note** *The biopsy should be performed within 1 week after starting systemic steroids, but a positive result may be seen up to 1 month later. Biopsy is* *especially important in patients in whom steroids are relatively contraindicated (e.g., diabetics).*

5. Consider ocular pneumoplethysmography (OPG), if available, as an aid in diagnosis.

Treatment

Systemic steroids should be given immediately once GCA is suspected. We give methylprednisolone 250 mg IV q 6 h for 12 doses in the hospital, and then switch to prednisone 80–100 mg po daily. A temporal artery biopsy specimen is obtained while the patient is in the hospital.

- If the temporal artery biopsy is positive for GCA, then the patient needs to be maintained on prednisone 80–100 mg po daily.
- If the biopsy is negative on an adequate (2-cm) section, then the likelihood of GCA is small. However, in highly suspicious cases, biopsy of the contralateral artery is performed. Steroids are usually discontinued when the disease is not found in adequate biopsy specimens.

❖ **Notes**

1. *Without steroids (and occasionally on adequate steroids), the contralateral eye can become involved within 24 hours.*
2. *A histamine₂-blocker (e.g., ranitidine 150 mg po bid) or another anti-ulcer medication is given along with the steroids.*
3. *See medical glossary for systemic steroid work-up.*

Follow-up

Patients suspected of having GCA need to be evaluated and treated emergently. After the diagnosis is confirmed by biopsy, the initial oral steroid dosage is maintained for 2–4 weeks until the symptoms reverse and ESRs normalize. The dosage is then tapered slowly, repeating the ESRs with each dosage change or monthly to ensure that the new steroid dosage is enough to suppress the disease. If the ESR increases or symptoms return, the dosage must be increased. Treatment should last at least 3–6 months and sometimes for 1 year or more. The smallest dose that suppresses the disease is used.

11.17 NONARTERITIC ISCHEMIC OPTIC NEUROPATHY (ION)

Symptoms

Sudden, painless, nonprogressive visual loss of moderate degree, initially unilateral, but may become bilateral. Typically occurs in patients 40–60 years of age.

Critical Signs

Afferent pupillary defect, pale disc swelling often involving only a segment of the disc, flame-shaped hemorrhages, normal ESR.

1. Nonprogressive ION: Sudden initial decrease in visual acuity and visual field, which stabilizes.
2. Progressive ION: Sudden initial decrease in visual acuity and visual field followed by a second decrease in acuity or field days to weeks later.

Other Signs

Reduced color vision, altitudinal or central visual field defect, optic atrophy after the edema resolves.

Etiology

Idiopathic. (Arteriosclerosis, diabetes, and hypertension are thought to be causative, but this has never been proven.)

Differential Diagnosis

See "Arteritic Ischemic Optic Neuropathy," Section 11.16.

Work-up

Same as "Arteritic Ischemic Optic Neuropathy," Section 11.16. A medical evaluation by an internist is also obtained to rule out cardiovascular disease, diabetes, and hypertension.

Treatment

1. Nonprogressive ION: Observation.
2. Progressive ION: Optic nerve sheath decompression (ONSD) may be considered.

❖ **Note** *Ischemic optic neuropathy decompression trial is underway to determine the effect of ONSD on all forms of ION.*

Follow-up

One month.

REFERENCE

Sergott RC, Cohen MS, Bosley TM et al. Optic nerve decompression may improve the progressive form of NAION. *Arch Opththalmol* 107:1743, 1989.

11.18 MISCELLANEOUS OPTIC NEUROPATHIES

Toxic/Metabolic Optic Neuropathy

Symptoms

Painless, progressive, bilateral loss of vision.

Critical Signs

Bilateral cecocentral or central visual field defects, signs of alcoholism or poor nutrition.

Other Signs

Visual acuity of 20/50–20/200, reduced color vision, temporal disc pallor, optic atrophy or normal-appearing disc.

Etiology

- Tobacco/alcohol abuse
- Severe malnutrition with thiamine (vitamin B_1) deficiency
- Pernicious anemia   (Usually due to a problem with vitamin B_{12} absorption.)
- Toxic   [Often from chloramphenicol, ethambutol, isoniazid, digitalis, chloroquine, streptomycin, chlorpropamide, ethclorvynol (e.g., Placidyl), disulfiram (e.g., Antabuse), and lead.]

Work-up

1. History: Drug or substance abuse? Medications? Diet?
2. Complete ocular examination, including pupillary evaluation, color testing with color plates, and optic-nerve examination.
3. Formal visual field test (e.g., Goldmann).
4. Complete blood count.
5. Serum vitamin B_1, B_{12} and folate level (consider a gastrointestinal consult for possible Schilling's test if the vitamin B_{12} level is low).
6. Consider a heavy metal (i.e., lead, thallium) screen.
7. Consider blood test for Leber's hereditary optic neuropathy (clinical presentation of Leber's neuropathy may mimic toxic/metabolic optic neuropathy).

Treatment

1. Thiamine 100 mg po bid.
2. Folate 1.0 mg po daily.
3. Multivitamin tablet daily.
4. Eliminate any causative agent (e.g., alcohol, medication).
5. Vitamin B_{12} 1000 ug IM every month for pernicious anemia (usually coordinated by the patient's internist).

Follow-up

Every month at first, then every 6–12 months.

Compressive Optic Neuropathy

Symptoms

Slowly progressive visual loss, although occasionally acute or noticed acutely.

Critical Signs

Central visual field defect, relative afferent pupillary defect.

Other Signs

The optic nerve can be normal, pale, or occasionally, swollen; proptosis; optociliary shunt vessels (small vessels around the disc that shunt blood from the retinal to the choroidal venous circulation).

Etiology

- Optic-nerve glioma   (Patients usually younger than 20 years of age, often associated with neurofibromatosis.)
- Optic-nerve meningioma   [Usually affects adult women. Orbital imaging may show an optic-nerve mass, diffuse optic-nerve thickening, or a railroad-track sign (increased contrast of the periphery of the nerve).]
- Any intraorbital mass (e.g., hemangioma, schwannoma)

Work-up

All patients with progressive visual loss and optic-nerve dysfunction should have CT scan (coronal and axial views) or MRI of the orbit and brain.

Treatment/Follow-up

Depends on the etiology. Treatments of optic-nerve glioma and meningioma are controversial. These lesions are often followed unless there is evidence of intracranial involvement, at which point surgical excision may be indicated.

Leber's Optic Neuropathy

Symptoms

Rapidly progressive visual loss of one and then the other eye within days to months of each other, painless.

Critical Signs

Mild swelling of optic disc progessing over weeks to optic atrophy; small telangiectatic blood vessels near the disc that do not leak on IV fluorescein angiography, usually occurs in young men 15–30 years of age, and less commonly in females in their second to third decade of life.

Other Signs
Visual acuity 20/200 to counting fingers, cecocentral visual field defect.

Transmission
By mitochondrial DNA, so it is transmitted by females to all of offspring. However, 50–70% of sons and 10%–15% of daughters manifest the disease. All daughters are carriers and none of the sons can transmit the disease.

Work-up
Send blood for known Leber's mutations.

Treatment
No effective treatment is available. Genetic counseling should be offered. A cardiology consult may be indicated as patients have a higher incidence of cardiac conduction defects.

REFERENCE

Singh G, Lott MT, and Wallace DC. A mitochondrial DNA mutation as a cause of Leber's hereditary optic neuropathy. *N Engl J Med* 320:1300, 1989.

Dominant Optic Neuropathy

Mid-to-moderate bilateral visual loss (20/40–20/200) usually presenting about age 4–8 years, slow progression, temporal disc pallor, cecocentral visual field defect, tritanopic (blue-yellow) color defect on Farnsworth-Munsell 100-hue test, strong family history, no nystagmus.

Complicated Hereditary Optic Atrophy

Bilateral optic atrophy with spinocerebellar degenerations (e.g., Friedreich's, Marie's, Behr's), polyneuropathy (e.g., Charcot-Marie-Tooth), or inborn errors of metabolism.

Radiation Optic Neuropathy

Delayed effect (usually 1–5 years) after radiation therapy to the eye, orbit, sinus, nasopharynx, and occasionally brain with acute or gradual stepwise visual loss. Disc swelling, retinopathy, or both may or may not be present.

11.19 NYSTAGMUS

Nystagmus may be congenital or acquired.

Symptoms
Asymptomatic unless acquired after 8 years of age, at which point the environment may be noted to oscillate horizontally, vertically, or torsionally, or vision may seem blurred or unstable.

Critical Signs
Repetitive oscillations of the eye horizontally, vertically, or torsionally.

Jerk nystagmus: The eye slowly drifts in one direction (slow phase) and then abruptly returns to its original position (fast phase), only to drift again and repeat the cycle.
Pendular nystagmus: Drift occurs in two phases of equal speed, giving a smooth back-and-forth movement of the eye.

A. Congenital

1. Infantile

Onset at age 2–3 months, with wide, swinging eye movements. At age 4–6 months, small pendular eye movements are added, and at age 6–12 monts, jerk nystagmus and a null point (a position of gaze where the nystagmus is minimized) develop. Compensatory head nodding develops at any point up to age 20 years. Infantile nystagmus is usually horizontal and typically dampens with convergence. May have a latent component.

Etiology
- Idiopathic
- Albinism   (Iris transillumination defects and foveal hypoplasia are common.)
- Aniridia   (Bilateral, near-total absence of iris from birth.)
- Leber's congenital amaurosis   (Markedly abnormal or flat electroretinogram.)
- Others   (Bilateral optic-nerve hypoplasia, bilateral congenital cataracts, rod monochromatism, optic-nerve or macular disease)

Differential Diagnosis
- Opsoclonus   (Repetitive, irregular, multidirectional eye movements associated with cerebellar or brain stem disease, postviral encephalitis, visceral carcinoma, or neuroblastoma.)

- Spasmus nutans   (Head nodding and head turn with vertical, horizontal, or torsional nystagmus appearing between 6 months and 3 years of age and resolving between 2 and 8 years of age. Unilateral or bilateral. Glioma of the optic chiasm may produce an identical clinical picture and needs to be ruled out with MRI.
- Latent Nystagmus   (See the following.)
- Nystagmus blockage syndrome   (See the following.)

Work-up

1. History: Age of onset? Head nodding? Known ocular or systemic abnormalities? Medications? Family history?
2. Complete ocular examination: Carefully observe the eye movements, check for iris transillumination, and inspect the optic disc and macula for disease.
3. Consider obtaining an eye-movement recording if the diagnosis of infantile nystagmus is uncertain.
4. When opsoclonus cannot be ruled out, obtain a urinary vanillylmandelic acid and consider an abdominal CT scan to rule out neuroblastoma and visceral carcinoma.
5. In selected cases and in all cases of suspected spasmus nutans, a CT scan or MRI of the brain (axial and coronal views) may be obtained to rule out organic pathology.

Treatment

1. Maximize vision by refraction.
2. Treat amblyopia if indicated.
3. If small face turn: Prescribe prism in glasses with base in direction of face turn.
4. If large face turn: Consider muscle surgery.

2. Latent Nystagmus

a. *Latent nystagmus*: Occurs only when one eye is viewing. Fast phase of nystagmus beats toward viewing eye.
b. *Manifest latent nystagmus*: Occurs in children with strabismus or decreased vision in one eye. Nonfixating or poorly seeing eye acts as an occluded eye.

❖ **Note** *When testing visual acuity in one eye, fog (i.e., add plus lenses in front of) rather than cover the opposite eye.*

Treatment

1. Maximize vision by refraction.
2. Treat amblyopia if indicated.
3. Consider muscle surgery if symptomatic strabismus exists.

3. Nystagmus Blockage Syndrome (NBS)

Any nystagmus that decreases when fixating eye is in adduction and demonstrates an esotropia to dampen the nystagmus.

Treatment

For large face turn, consider muscle surgery.

B. Acquired

Etiology

Visual loss (e.g., dense cataract, trauma, cone dystrophy)   (Usually monocular and vertical nystagmus.)

Toxic/metabolic (e.g., alcohol intoxication, lithium, barbituates, phenytoin, salicylates, benzodiazepines, phencyclidine, other anticonvulsants or sedatives, Wernicke's encephalopathy, thiamine deficiency)

CNS disorders [e.g, thalamic hemorrhage, tumor, stroke, trauma, multiple sclerosis (MS)]

Nonphysiologic   (Voluntary, rapid, horizontal, small oscillatory movements of the eyes that usually can not be sustained more than 30 seconds without fatigue.)

Types with Localizing Neuroanatomic Significance

- See-saw   (One eye rises and intorts while the other descends and extorts. Most commonly, the lesion involves the chiasm and/or third ventricle. May have a bitemporal hemianopia secondary to a parasellar mass. Rarely, congenital.)
- Convergence retraction   (Convergencelike eye movements are accompanied by retraction of the globe into the orbit when the patient attempts to look up. There is limitation of upward gaze, eyelid retraction, and large, unreactive pupils. Papilledema may be present. Usually, a pineal gland tumor or other midbrain abnormality is responsible.)
- Upbeat   (The fast phase of the nystagmus is up. Most commonly, the lesion involves the brain stem or vermis of the cerebellum when the nystagmus is present in primary position. If the nystagmus is only present in upgaze, the most likely etiology is drug effect.)
- Rebound   (Triggered by changing directions of gaze. The fast phase is in the diretion of gaze, but fatigue occurs with sustained gaze, and the fast phase then changes direction. When gaze is returned to primary position, the fast phase increases in the direction the eye takes in returning to the primary position. Most commonly, the lesion involves the cerebellum.)
- Gaze-evoked   (Not present when the individual looks straight, but appears as the eyes look to the side. Nystagmus increases when looking in direction

of fast phase. Slow frequency. Most commonly the result of alcohol intoxication, sedatives, cerebellar or brain stem disease.)
- Downbeat   [The fast pahse of nystagmus is down. Most commonly, the lesion is at the cervicomedullary junction (e.g., Arnold-Chiari malformation).]
- Periodic alternating   [Fast eye movements are in one direction (with head turn) for 60–90 seconds, and then reverse direction for 60–90 seconds. The cycle repeats continuously. May be congenital, or rarely, the result of blindness. Acquired forms not caused by blindness are most commonly the result of lesions of the cervicomedullary junction.]
- Vestibular   [Horizontal or horizontal rotary nystagmus. May be accompanied by vertigo, tinnitus, or deafness. May be due to dysfunction of vestibular end organ (inner-ear disease), eighth cranial nerve, or eighth-nerve nucleus in brain stem. Destructive lesions produce fast phases opposite to affected end organ or nerve. Irritative lesions produce fast phase in the same direction as the affected end organ. Vestibular nystagmus associated with interstitial keratitis is called Cogan's syndrome.)

Differential Diagnosis
- Superior oblique myokymia   (Small, unilateral, vertical and torsional movements of one eye can be seen with a slit lamp or ophthalmoscope. Symptoms and signs are more pronounced when the involved eye looks inferonasally. Usually benign, resolving spontaneously. Can be treated with carbamazepine 200 mg po tid. A medical consult for hematologic evaluation prior to carbamazepine use and periodic evaluation during therapy are recommended.)
- Opsoclonus   (Rapid, chaotic conjugate saccades. Etiology in children is neuroblastoma or encephalitis. In adults, it can be seen with drug intoxication or following infarction.)
- Myoclonus   [Pendular oscillation associated with contraction of nonocular muscles (e.g., palate, tongue, facial muscles). Involves olive nucleus in medulla.]

Work-up
1. History: Nystagmus, strabismus, or amblyopia in infancy? Oscillopsia? Drug or alcohol use? Vertigo? Episodes of weakness, numbness, or decreased vision in the past (MS)?
2. Family history: Nystagmus? Albinism? Eye disorder?
3. Complete ocular examination: Pay close attention to the eye movements. Slit-lamp or optic-disc observation may be helpful in subtle cases. Iris transillumination should be performed to rule out albinism.
4. Obtain an eye-movement recording when congenital nystagmus is being considered.
5. Visual field examination, particularly with see-saw nystagmus.

6. Consider a drug/toxin/dietary screen of the urine, serum, or both.
7. CT scan or MRI as needed. (Make sure the scan carefully evaluates the area that most commonly causes the particular nystagmus.)

❖ **Note** *The cervicomedullary junction and cerebellum are best evaluated with MRI.*

Treatment

The underlying etiology must be treated. The nystagmus of periodic alternating nystagmus may respond to baclofen. Baclofen is given in three divided doses, starting with a total daily dose of 15 mg po and increasing by 15 mg every 3 days until a desired therapeutic effect is obtained. Do not exceed 80 mg/day. If there is no improvement with the maximum tolerated dose, the dosage should be tapered slowly. Baclofen is not recommended for use in children. Severe disabling nystagmus can be treated with retrobulbar injections of botulinum toxin.

Follow-up

A work-up should be instituted as soon as possible to rule out a central nervous system abnormality.

11.20 VERTEBROBASILAR ARTERY INSUFFICIENCY

Symptoms

Transient bilateral blurred vision lasting from a few seconds to a few minutes, sometimes accompanied by flashing lights. Ataxia, vertigo, dysarthria or dysphasia, and hemiparesis or hemisensory loss may accompany the visual symptoms. History of drop attacks (the patient suddenly falls to the ground without warning or loss of consciousness). Recurrent attacks are common.

Signs

Normal ocular examination.

Differential Diagnosis

(Causes of transient visual loss.)

- Papilledema (Bilateral visual loss lasts 5–15 seconds. See Section 11.13.)
- Migraine (Visual loss from 10–45 minutes, often with history of migraine

or car sickness, or a family history of migraine. May or may not be followed by a headache.)

- Amaurosis fugax   (Monocular, usually lasts minutes, appears as if a curtain drops down in front of the eye.)
- Giant cell arteritis (GCA)   (Can cause transient visual loss in patients older than 50 years of age. Usually associated with temporal headache, scalp tenderness, pain with chewing, weight loss, fever, and anorexia.)

Work-up
1. History: Associated symptoms of vertebrobasilar insufficiency? History of car sickness or migraine? Symptoms of GCA?
2. Dilated fundus examination: Look for retinal emboli or papilledema.
3. Blood pressure in each arm: Look for the subclavian steal syndrome.
4. Cardiac auscultation to rule out arrhythmia.
5. Electrocardiogram and Holter monitor for 24 hours: Look for sick sinus syndrome, ventricular ectopy.
6. Consider carotid noninvasive flow studies.
7. Complete blood count to rule out anemia and polycythemia, with or without ESR if giant cell arteritis is suspected.
8. Consider cervical spine x-rays to rule out compressive cervical spine disease if arthritis of the neck is present.

Treatment
1. Aspirin 80 mg po daily.
2. Control hypertension, diabetes, and hyperlipidemia if present, as per medical internist.
3. Reduce fat and cholesterol intake; stop smoking.
4. Correct any underlying problem revealed by the work-up.

Follow-up
One week to check test results.

11.21 CORTICAL BLINDNESS

Symptoms
Bilateral complete or severe loss of vision. Patients may deny they are blind (Anton's syndrome).

Critical Signs
Markedly decreased vision and visual field in both eyes (sometimes no light perception) with normal pupillary responses.

Etiology

Most common Bilateral occipital lobe infarctions

Rare Neoplasms (e.g., metastases and meningiomas)

Work-up

1. Test vision with a near card (sometimes patients with bilateral occipital lobe infarcts appear completely blind, but actually have a very small residual visual field and are unable to locate a distant eye chart.)
2. Complete ocular and neurological examinations.
3. Rule out functional visual loss by appropriate testing (see "Nonphysiologic Visual Loss," Section 11.22).
4. Cardiac auscultation to rule out arrhythmia.
5. Check blood pressure.
6. MRI of the brain.
7. Complete blood count to rule out polycythemia in cases of stroke.
8. Refer to a neurologist or internist for evaluation of stroke risk factors.

Treatment

1. Patients diagnosed with a stroke within 72 hours of the onset of symptoms are admitted to the hospital for neurological evaluation and observation.
2. If possible, treat the underlying condition.
3. Arrange for services to help the patient function at home and in the environment.

Follow-up

As per the internist or neurologist.

11.22 NONPHYSIOLOGIC VISUAL LOSS

Symptoms

Loss of vision. Malingerers frequently are involved with an insurance claim or are looking for some other form of financial gain. Hysterics truly believe they have lost vision.

Critical Signs

No ocular or neuro-ophthalmic findings that would account for the decreased vision. Normal pupillary light reaction.

Differential Diagnosis

The following must be considered in anyone with a normal neuro-ophthalmic examination:

- Amblyopia [Poor vision in one eye since childhood, rarely both eyes. Patient often has strabismus (eye misalignment best seen with a cover test) or anisometropia (one eye is usually more far-sighted, astigmatic, or very near-sighted). May have a history of eye patching as a child. Vision is no worse than counting fingers, especially in the temporal periphery of an amblyopic eye.]

- Cortical blindness   (Bilateral complete or severe visual loss with normal pupils. MRI of the brain shows bilateral occipital lobe infarcts in most cases.)
- Retrobulbar optic neuritis   (Afferent pupillary defect may be present.)
- Cone-rod dystrophy   [Positive family history, decreased color vision, abnormal dark adaptation studies and electroretinogram (ERG).]]
- Chiasmal tumor   (Visual loss may precede optic atrophy. Pupils usually react sluggishly to light, and an afferent pupillary defect is usually present. Visual fields are abnormal.)

Work-up

(Fooling the malingerer or hysteric into seeing better than he or she admits to seeing). The following tests may be used to deceive a patient with nonphysiologic visual loss. U, may be used to test patients feigning unilateral decreased vision; B, may be used to test patients feigning bilateral vision loss.

PATIENTS CLAIMING NO LIGHT PERCEPTION

Determine whether each pupil reacts to light (U): When one eye has no light perception, its pupil will not react to light. The pupil should *not* appear dilated unless the patient has bilateral no light perception or third-nerve involvement.

PATIENTS CLAIMING HAND-MOTION TO NO LIGHT PERCEPTION

1. Test for an afferent pupillary defect (U): A defect should be present in unilateral visual loss to this degree. If not, the diagnosis of nonphysiologic visual loss is made.
2. Mirror test (U or B): If the patient claims unilateral visual loss, cover the better seeing eye with a patch; otherwise leave both uncovered. Ask the patient to hold eyes still and slowly move a large mirror from side to side in front of the eyes, holding it beyond the patient's range of hand-motion vision). If the eyes move, the patient can see better than hand motion.
3. Optokinetic test (U or B): Patch the uninvolved eye when unilateral visual loss is claimed. Ask the patient to look straight ahead, and slowly move an optokinetic tape in front of the eyes (or rotate an optokinetic drum). If nystagmus can be elicited, vision is better than hand motion.

PATIENTS CLAIMING 20/40–20/400 VISION

1. Visual acuity testing (U or B): Start with the 20/10 line and ask the patient to read it. When the patient claims incompetence, look amazed and then offer reassurance. Inform the patient you will go to a larger line and show

the 20/15 line. Again, force the patient to work to see this line. Slowly proceed up the chart, asking the patient to read each line as you pass it (including the three or four 20/20 lines). Make the patient feel incompetent. By the time the 20/30 or 20/40 lines are reached, the patient may in fact read one or two letters correctly. The visual acuity can then be recorded.

2. Fog test (U): For example, in a patient feigning visual loss on the right. If patient wears glasses, dial patient's correction into phoropter, if not dial in plano. Add +4.00 to the left. Put patient in phoropter with both eyes open. Tell patient to use both eyes to read each line, starting at the 20/15 line and working up the chart slowly as described previously. Record visual acuity (this should be visual acuity of the right eye). Close phoropter over the right eye. Ask patient to read the same line as before; work up the chart until patient is able to read line. Record visual acuity (this should be visual acuity of the left eye with +4.00 fog).

3. Retest visual acuity in the "poorly seeing eye" at 10 feet from the chart (U or B): Vision should be twice as good (e.g., a patient with 20/100 vision at 20 feet should read 20/50 at 10 feet). If it is better than expected, record the better vision. If it worse, the patient has nonphysiologic visual loss.

4. Test near vision (U or B): If normal near vision can be documented, nonphysiologic visual loss or myopia has been documented.

5. Visual field testing (U or B): Goldmann visual field tests often reveal inconsistent responses and nonphysiologic field losses.

CHILDREN

1. Tell the child that there is an eye abnormality, but the strong drops about to be administered will cure it. Dilate the child's eyes (e.g., topicamide 1%), and retest the visual acuity in 40 minutes. Children, as well as adults, sometimes need a "way out."

2. Test as above.

Treatment

Patients are usually told that no ocular abnormality can be found that accounts for their decreased vision. Hysterical patients often benefit from being told that everything is going to be all right and that their vision can be expected to return to normal by their next visit. Psychiatric referral is sometimes indicated.

Follow-up

If nonphysiologic visual loss is highly suspected but cannot be proven, reexamine in 1–2 weeks. Consider obtaining an ERG, a fluorescein angiogram, and/or a CT scan or MRI of the brain. If functional visual loss can be documented, have the patient return as needed.

❖ **Note** *Always try to determine the patient's vision and document your findings.*

RETINA

12.1 CENTRAL RETINAL ARTERY OCCLUSION (CRAO)

Symptoms

Unilateral, painless, acute loss of vision (counting fingers to light perception in 90% of eyes) occurring over seconds; may have a history of amaurosis fugax.

Critical Signs

Superficial opacification or whitening of the retina in the posterior pole and a cherry-red spot in the center of the macula.

Other Signs

A marked afferent pupillary defect; narrowed retinal arterioles; boxcarring, or segmentation of the blood column, in the arterioles. Occasionally, retinal arteriolar emboli or cilioretinal artery sparing of the foveola is evident. If vision acuity is light perception or worse, strongly suspect ophthalmic artery occlusion.

Differential Diagnosis

- Acute ophthalmic artery occlusion   (Usually no cherry-red spot in the foveola; the entire retina appears whitened. The treatment is the same as for CRAO.)
- Inadvertent intraocular injection of gentamicin   (Recent injection.)
- Arteritic ischemic optic neuropathy   (Age ≥55 years, acute severe visual loss, history of temporal headache with scalp tenderness, jaw claudication, muscle pains, weakness, weight loss, a significant afferent pupillary defect, pale optic disc swelling, and a markedly elevated ESR are typical. See Section 11.16.)

The Wills Eye Manual: Office and Emergency Room Diagnosis and Treatment of Eye Diseases, Second Edition, edited by R. Douglas Cullom, Jr., M.D., and Benjamin Chang, M.D. © 1994 J. B. Lippincott Company.

- Other causes of a cherry-red spot (e.g., Tay-Sachs or other storage diseases) (Present in early life, other systemic manifestations, usually bilateral.)

Etiology

- Embolus (especially carotid or cardiac)
- Thrombosis
- Giant cell arteritis (GCA) (May produce CRAO or an ischemic optic neuropathy. See the previous discussion for concomitant symptoms.)
- Collagen-vascular disease other than giant cell arteritis (e.g., systemic lupus erythematosus, polyarteritis nodosa)
- Hypercoagulation disorders (e.g., oral contraceptives, polycythemia, antiphospholipid syndrome)
- Rare causes (e.g., migraine, Behçet's disease, syphilis, sickle-cell disease)
- Trauma

Treatment

To be instituted immediately after the diagnosis is made, before the work-up, *if* the CRAO has been present <24 hours.

1. Immediate ocular massage (fundus contact lens or digital massage).
2. Anterior-chamber paracentesis (Fig. 12.1): Place a drop of topical anesthetic (e.g., cocaine 2–4%) in the eye and anesthetize the base of the medial rectus muscle by holding a cotton-tipped applicator dipped in the topical anesthetic against the muscle for 1 minute. Retract the eyelid with an eyelid speculum, and using an operating microscope or slit-lamp (a microscope is easier), grasp the base of the medial rectus muscle with fixation forceps at the anesthetized site. With a 30-gauge short needle on a tuberculin syringe, enter the eye temporally at the limbus with the bevel of the needle pointing up and away from the eye. Make sure to keep the tip of the needle over the iris (not the lens) when entering the anterior chamber. Withdraw fluid until the chamber shallows slightly (usually 0.1–0.2 cc). Withdraw the needle and place a drop of antibiotic on the eye (e.g., gentamicin).
3. Acetazolamide 500 mg IV or two 250-mg tablets po and/or a topical beta-blocker (e.g., timolol 0.5% bid or levobunolol 0.5% bid) is used to lower the intraocular pressure.
4. Consider admission to the hospital for Carbogen (95% oxygen, 5% carbon dioxide) therapy, 10 minutes every 2 hours around the clock for 48 hours. The patient's blood pressure, pulse, and mental status must be monitored.

Work-up

1. Immediate ESR to rule out GCA if the patient is ≥55 years of age. (This is obtained immediately after the paracentesis. If the patient's history and/ or ESR are consistent with GCA, high-dose systemic steroids are started.

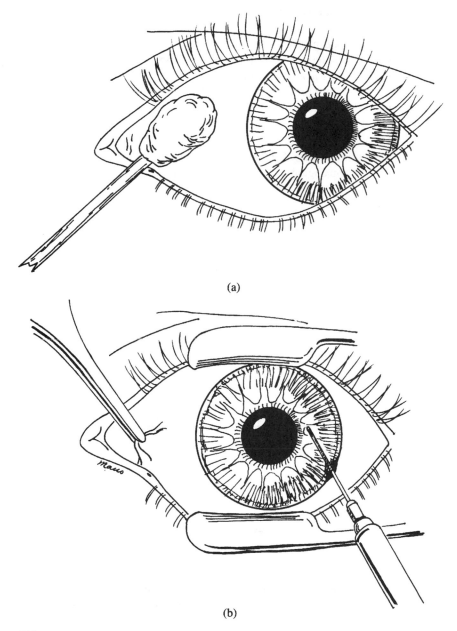

(a)

(b)

Figure 12.1
Anterior-chamber paracentesis. (a) The base of the medial rectus muscle is anesthetized with a cotton-tipped applicator dipped in cocaine 2–4%. (b) While fixating the globe with forceps, a 30-gauge needle is passed through the cornea into the anterior chamber. The needle should stay over the iris.

See "Arteritic Ischemic Optic Neuropathy," Section 11.16, for additional details.)

2. Check blood pressure.

3. Other blood tests: Fasting blood sugar (FBS), 3-hour glucose tolerance test if the FBS is negative, complete blood count (CBC) with differential and platelets, lipid profile, PT, PTT, ANA, rheumatoid factor, and FTA-ABS. Consider serum protein electrophoresis, hemoglobin electrophoresis, and antiphospholipid antibodies.

4. Carotid artery evaluation (Doppler and ultrasound of the carotid arteries).

5. Cardiac evaluation (echocardiogram and Holter monitor).

6. Fluorescein angiogram, electroretinogram, or both to confirm the diagnosis.

Follow up

The patient is discharged from the hospital after 2–3 days and is seen by an internist to complete the medical work-up above. A repeat eye examination is performed in 1–2 weeks, checking for neovascularization of the iris/disc, which develops in up to 20% of patients, at a mean of 4 weeks after onset. If neovascularization develops, panretinal photocoagulation should be performed.

12.2 BRANCH RETINAL ARTERY OCCLUSION (BRAO)

Symptoms

Unilateral painless abrupt loss of partial visual field; a history of transient visual loss (amaurosis fugax) may be elicited.

Critical Sign

Superficial opacification or whitening along the distribution of a branch retinal artery. The affected retina becomes edematous.

Other Signs

Narrowed branch retinal artery; boxcarring, segmentation of the blood column, or emboli are sometimes seen in the branch retinal artery. Cotton-wool spots may appear in the involved area.

Etiology
See "Central Retinal Artery Occlusion," Section 12.1.

Work-up
See "Central Retinal Artery Occlusion," Section 12.1. An electroretinogram, however, is not obtained.

Treatment
1. No ocular therapy of proven value is available. Ocular massage (and rarely, anterior-chamber paracentesis) may dislodge a cholesterol embolus (cholesterol emboli appear as bright, reflective crystals, generally at a vessel bifurcation).
2. Treat any underlying medical problem.

Follow-up
Patients need to be evaluated emergently to treat any underlying disorders (especially giant cell arteritis). Reevaluate every 3–6 months after concluding the work-up.

12.3 CENTRAL RETINAL VEIN OCCLUSION (CRVO)

Symptoms
Painless loss of vision, usually unilateral.

Critical Signs
Diffuse retinal hemorrhages in all quadrants of the retina; dilated, tortuous retinal veins.

Other Signs
Cotton-wool spots; disc edema and hemorrhages; retinal edema; optociliary shunt vessels on the disc; neovascularization of the optic disc, retina, or iris.

Types
Ischemic   Multiple cotton-wool spots (usually >10), extensive retinal hemorrhage, and widespread capillary nonperfusion on fluorescein angiogram. Often, a relative afferent pupillary defect is present and acuity is 20/200 or worse.

Nonischemic   Mild fundus changes. No afferent pupillary defect is present, and often, acuity is better than 20/200.

Etiology

- Atherosclerosis of the adjacent central retinal artery   (The artery compresses the central retinal vein in the region of the lamina cribrosa, secondarily inducing thrombosis in the lumen of the vein.)
- Hypertension
- Optic-disc edema
- Glaucoma (open- or narrow-angle; most commonly associated ocular disease)
- Optic-disc drusen
- Hypercoagulable state (e.g., polycythemia, lymphoma, leukemia, sickle-cell disease, multiple myeloma, cryoglobulinemia, Waldenström's macroglobulinemia, antiphospholipid syndrome)
- Vasculitis (e.g., sarcoid, syphilis, systemic lupus erythematosus)
- Drugs (e.g., oral contraceptives, diuretics)
- Abnormal platelet function (e.g., mitral valve prolapse)
- Retrobulbar external compression (e.g., thyroid disease, orbital tumor)
- Migraine   (Rare.)

Differential Diagnosis

- Ocular ischemic syndrome (carotid occlusive disease)   (Veins are usually dilated and irregular in caliber, but are not usually tortuous; disc edema does not usually occur; hemorrhages are not usually present on the disc, although neovascularization of the disc is present in one third of cases; hemorrhages tend to be in the midperiphery; patients may have a history of amaurosis fugax, transient ischemic attacks, or orbital pain. Intraocular pressure [IOP] is often low. Central retinal artery perfusion pressure is low in this entity. See Section 12.7.)
- Diabetic retinopathy   (Hemorrhages and microaneurysms are usually concentrated in the posterior pole, exudate is more prominent, and the condition is typically bilateral. Fluorescein angiography may be required to distinguish this condition from CRVO. See Section 14.6.)
- Papilledema   (Bilateral disc swelling with flame-shaped hemorrhages surrounding the disc but not extending to the peripheral retina; secondary to increased intracranial pressure. See Section 11.13.)
- Radiation retinopathy   (History of prior irradiation is critical in diagnosis. Disc swelling with radiation papillopathy, and retinal neovascularization may be present. Generally, cotton-wool spots are a more prominent feature than hemorrhages.)

Work-up

1. History: Medical problems, medications, eye diseases?
2. Complete ocular examination, including an IOP measurement and slit-lamp and gonioscopic examinations to rule out iris and angle neovascularization or the presence of a narrow angle, and a dilated fundus examination.
3. Fluorescein angiogram.
4. Check blood pressure.
5. Blood tests: fasting blood sugar, CBC with differential, platelets, serum protein electrophoresis, lipid profile, FTA-ABS, and ANA. (Other tests that may be considered include hemoglobin electrophoresis, PTT, PT, ESR, VDRL, cryoglobulins, and antiphospholipid antibodies.)
6. Chest x-ray (when an underlying medical problem is to be ruled out).
7. Complete medical evaluation, especially to rule out cardiovascular disease.
8. If the diagnosis is uncertain, oculopneumoplethysmography (OPG) or ophthalmodynamometry may help to distinguish CRVO from carotid disease (ophthalmic artery pressure is low in carotid disease but is normal to elevated in CRVO).
9. Consider electroretinogram to determine amount of ischemia.

Treatment

1. Discontinue oral contraceptives; change diuretics to other antihypertensive medications if possible.
2. Lower IOP if elevated (e.g., >20 mm Hg) in either eye (see "Primary Open-Angle Glaucoma," Section 10.1).
3. Treat underlying medical disorders.
4. If neovascularization of the iris, retina, or optic nerve is present, or if the CRVO is ischemic, laser therapy [panretinal photocoagulation (PRP)] is performed.
5. Aspirin 60–360 mg po daily.
6. Photocoagulation for persistent macular edema may lead to resolution of fluid but has not been proven to be visually beneficial.

Follow-up

Nonischemic Every 4 weeks for the first 6 months; if the fundus picture worsens and can be categorized as ischemic, treat as ischemic.

Ischemic Every 2–3 weeks after treatment for the first 6 months; watch for neovascularization of the iris.

12.4 BRANCH RETINAL VEIN OCCLUSION (BRVO)

Symptoms

Blind spot in the visual field or loss of vision, generally unilateral.

Critical Signs

Superficial hemorrhages in a sector of the retina along a retinal vein. The hemorrhages almost never cross the horizontal raphé (midline).

Other Signs

Cotton-wool spots, retinal edema, a dilated and tortuous retinal vein, narrowing and sheathing of the adjacent artery, retinal neovascularization, vitreous hemorrhage.

Etiology

Disease of the adjacent arterial wall (usually the result of hypertension, arteriosclerosis, or diabetes) compresses the venous wall at a crossing point.

Differential Diagnosis

- Diabetic retinopathy   (Dot and blot hemorrhages and microaneurysms extend across the horizontal raphé. Nearly always bilateral. See Section 14.6.)
- Hypertensive retinopathy   (Narrowed retinal arterioles. Hemorrhages are not confined to a sector of the retina and usually cross the horizontal raphé. Bilateral in most. See Section 12.15.)

Work-up

1. History: Systemic disease, particularly hypertension or diabetes?
2. Complete ocular examination, including dilated retinal examination with indirect ophthalmoscopy to look for retinal neovascularization and a macular examination using a slit-lamp and a Hruby, 60- or 90-diopter, or fundus contact lens to detect macular edema.
3. Check blood pressure.
4. Consider obtaining fasting blood sugar, CBC with differential and platelets, PT, PTT, ESR, ANA, rheumatoid factor, and chest x-ray.
5. Medical examination (usually performed by an internist to check for cardiovascular disease).
6. A fluorescein angiogram is obtained after the hemorrhages have cleared or sooner if neovascularization is suspected.

Treatment

1. Retinal laser photocoagulation is indicated for:

    a. Chronic macular edema (3–6 months duration) reducing vision below 20/40 in the absence of macular capillary nonperfusion. Grid treatment to the area of macular edema is employed.

    b. Retinal neovascularization. Sector panretinal photocoagulation to the ischemic area, as delineated by fluorescein angiographic evidence of capillary nonperfusion, is performed.

2. Underlying medical problems are treated.

Follow-up

Every 1–2 months at first, then every 3–12 months, checking for neovascularization, macular edema, or both.

12.5 HYPERTENSIVE RETINOPATHY

Symptoms

Usually asymptomatic, although may have decreased vision.

Critical Sign

Generalized or localized retinal arteriolar narrowing, almost always bilateral.

Other Signs

Arteriovenous crossing changes, retinal arteriolar sclerosis ("copper" or "silver" wiring), cotton-wool spots, hard exudates often in a "macular star" configuration, flame-shaped hemorrhages, retinal edema, arterial macroaneurysms, chorioretinal atrophy (Elschnig spots of choroidal nonperfusion). Rarely, retinal detachment, vitreous hemorrhage, central or branch occlusion of an artery or vein, or neovascular complications can develop.

Signs of "malignant hypertension" Swelling of the optic-nerve head (disc edema) in addition to the signs listed previously.

❖ **Note** *When hypertensive changes are only found in one eye, suspect carotid artery obstruction on the side of the normal-appearing eye, sparing the retina from the effects of the hypertension.*

Etiology

- Essential hypertension   (No known underlying cause.)
- Secondary hypertension   (Typically the result of preeclampsia/eclampsia, pheochromocytoma, kidney disease, adrenal disease, or coarctation of the aorta.)

Differential Diagnosis
- Diabetic retinopathy   (Hemorrhages are generally dot and blot, micro-aneurysms are common, vessel attenuation is less common. See Section 14.6.)
- Collagen vascular disease   (May show multiple cotton-wool spots, but few-to-no other fundus findings characteristic of hypertension.)
- Anemia   (Hemorrhage predominates without marked arterial changes.)
- Radiation retinopathy   (Can appear similar to hypertension. A history of irradiation to the eye or an adnexal structure such as the brain, sinus, or nasopharynx can usually be elicited. It may develop anytime after the radiation therapy, but it most commonly occurs within a few years.)
- Central or branch retinal vein occlusion   (Unilateral, multiple hemor-rhages, venous dilatation and tortuosity, no arteriolar narrowing. May be secondary to hypertension. See Sections 12.3 or 12.4.)

Work-up
1. History: Known hypertension, diabetes, or adnexal radiation?
2. Complete ocular examination, particularly dilated retinal examination.
3. Check blood pressure.
4. Refer patient to a medical internist or the emergency room of a hospital. (The urgency generally depends on the blood pressure reading and whether the patient is symptomatic. As a general rule, a diastolic blood pressure of 110–120 mm Hg or the presence of chest pain, difficulty breathing, headache, or blurred vision with optic disc swelling require immediate medical attention.)

Treatment
Control the hypertension (as per the internist).

Follow-up
Every 2–3 months at first, then every 6–12 months.

12.6 AMAUROSIS FUGAX

Symptoms
Monocular visual loss that usually last seconds to minutes, but may last up to 1–2 hours. Vision returns to normal.

Critical Signs
May see an embolus within an arteriole or the ocular examination may be normal.

Other Signs

Signs of the ocular ischemic syndrome (dilated veins; midperipheral dot and blot hemorrhages; neovascularization of the iris, disc, or retina), an old branch retinal artery occlusion (BRAO) (sheathed arteriole), or neurologic signs caused by ischemia of a cerebral hemisphere (e.g., contralateral arm or leg weakness).

Etiology

Embolus from the carotid artery (most common), heart, or aorta; talc emboli from IV drug abuse; vascular insufficiency as a result of arteriosclerotic disease of vessels anywhere along the path from the aorta to the globe precipitated by a postural change or cardiac arrhythmia; hypercoagulable/hyperviscosity state. Rarely, an intraorbital tumor may compress the optic nerve or a nourishing vessel in certain gaze positions, causing transient visual loss.

Differential Diagnosis

All of the following conditions may produce transient visual loss:

- Papilledema   (Optic-disc swelling is evident. Visual loss is usually bilateral and is often associated with postural change or Valsalva's maneuver. See Section 11.13.)
- Giant cell arteritis (GCA)   (Patients are typically ≥55 years of age and have an elevated ESR, temporal headache, scalp tenderness, jaw claudication, or muscle pains. Transient visual loss may precede an ischemic optic neuropathy or central retinal artery occlusion. See Section 11.16.)
- Impending central retinal vein occlusion (CRVO)   (Dilated, tortuous retinal veins are observed on funduscopic examination. See Section 12.3.)
- Glaucoma   (Characteristic optic-nerve changes. See Section 10.1.)
- Retinal migraine   (Usually a diagnosis of exclusion. Typically occurs in patients <40 years of age. May have recurrent episodes. See Section 15.4.)
- Intermittent intraocular hemorrhage (e.g., vitreous hemorrhage)
- Others (e.g., optic nerve drusen)

Work-up

1. History: Monocular visual loss or homonymous hemianopsia? (Did the patient cover one eye to test vision?) Duration of visual loss? Previous episodes of amaurosis fugax or transient cerebral ischemia? Atherosclerotic risk factors? Use of oral contraceptives? Heart disease or operations? IV drug abuse?
2. Ocular examination, including a confrontational visual field examination and a dilated retinal evaluation. Look for an embolus or signs of other disorders mentioned previously.
3. Medical examination (cardiac and carotid auscultation).
4. Consider a fluorescein angiogram (focal arterial staining at the site of the embolus may be seen).

5. Immediate ESR when GCA is suspected.
6. CBC with differential and platelet count, fasting blood sugar with or without glucose tolerance test, and lipid profile (to rule out polycythemia, thrombocytosis, diabetes, and hyperlipidemia).
7. Noninvasive carotid artery evaluation (e.g., Doppler, ultrasound).
8. Cardiac evaluation (including an echocardiogram).
9. Check the arms of patients for signs of IV drug abuse.

Treatment
A. Carotid disease
   1. Consider aspirin 325 mg po daily.
   2. Consider carotid endarterectomy in the presence of a surgically accessible, high-grade carotid stenosis or occlusion *if* the potential benefit of the procedure outweighs the risks.
   3. Control hypertension and diabetes (follow-up with a medical internist).
   4. Stop smoking.
B. Cardiac disease
   1. Consider aspirin 325 mg po daily for mitral valve prolapse.
   2. Consider hospitalization and anticoagulation (e.g., heparin therapy) in the presence of a mural thrombus.
   3. Consider cardiac surgery as needed.
   4. Control arteriosclerotic risk factors as described previously.
C. If carotid and cardiac disease are ruled out, a vasospastic etiology can be considered. Treatment with a calcium channel blocker can be beneficial.

Follow-up
Patients with recurrent episodes of amaurosis fugax (especially if accompanied by signs of cerebral transient ischemic attacks) require immediate diagnostic and sometimes therapeutic attention.

12.7 OCULAR ISCHEMIC SYNDROME
(CAROTID OCCLUSIVE DISEASE)

Symptoms
Decreased vision, ocular or periorbital pain, after-images or prolonged recovery of vision following exposure to bright light, may have a history of transient monocular visual loss (amaurosis fugax). Usually unilateral. Typically occurs in patients who are 50–80 years of age.

Critical Signs
Dilated but nontortuous retinal veins that are irregular in caliber, narrowed retinal arterioles, midperipheral retinal hemorrhages; often neovascularization of the iris, disc, and/or retina.

Other Signs

Episcleral injection, corneal edema, mild anterior uveitis, neovascular glaucoma, iris atrophy, cataract, retinal microaneurysms, cotton-wool spots, spontaneous pulsations of the central retinal artery, and cherry-red spot. Central retinal artery occlusion may occur.

Etiology

Carotid disease (usually >90% stenosis). Rarely, ophthalmic artery disease.

Differential Diagnosis

- Central retinal vein occlusion (CRVO)   (Similar signs, but may have optociliary shunt vessels or edema of the disc and dilated retinal veins that are tortuous and regular in caliber. Decreased vision after exposure to light and orbital pain are not typically found. Ophthalmodynamometry may distinguish this condition from ocular ischemic syndrome. See Section 12.3.)
- Diabetes   (Bilateral, usually symmetric. Retinal hemorrhages usually concentrate in the posterior pole, and hard exudates are often present. See Section 14.6.)
- Aortic arch disease (caused by atherosclerosis, syphilis, or Takayasu's disease)   (Ocular ischemia producing an identical picture, usually bilaterally. Examination reveals absent arm and neck pulses, cold hands, and spasm of the arm muscles with exercise.)

Work-up

1. History: Previous episodes of transient monocular visual loss? Cold hands or spasm of arm muscles with exercise?
2. Complete ocular examination: Search carefully for neovascularization of the iris, disc, or retina.
3. Medical examination (arm pulses, cardiac and carotid auscultation). Evaluate for hypertension, diabetes, and atherosclerotic disease.
4. Consider fluorescein angiography for diagnostic or therapeutic purposes.
5. Noninvasive carotid artery evaluation (e.g., ultrasound, Doppler, oculoplethysmography).
6. Consider ophthalmodynamometry if the diagnosis of CRVO cannot be excluded (ophthalmic artery pressure is low in carotid disease but is normal to elevated in CRVO).
7. Carotid arteriography is reserved for patients in whom surgery is to be performed.
8. Consider a cardiology consultation, because there is a high association with cardiac disease.

Treatment

Often unsuccessful.

1. Consider carotid surgery, if indicated.
2. Consider panretinal photocoagulation in the presence of neovascularization.

3. Manage glaucoma if present (see "Neovascular Glaucoma," Section 10.13).
4. Control hypertension and diabetes and reduce cholesterol level (follow-up with internist).
5. Stop smoking.

Follow-up

Depends upon the age and general health of the patient and the symptoms and signs of disease. Surgical candidates should be evaluated urgently.

12.8 CENTRAL SEROUS CHORIORETINOPATHY

Symptoms

Blurred or dim vision, objects appear distorted and miniature in size, colors appear washed-out, central scotoma. Usually unilateral, sometimes asymptomatic. Generally occurs in men age 25–50 years (has been reported in women, particularly during pregnancy, and in patients >60 years of age).

Critical Signs

Localized detachment of the sensory retina from the underlying pigment epithelium by clear, serous fluid in the macular area. The margins of the detachment are sloping and merge gradually into the attached retina. It is best seen with a fundus contact lens (e.g., Goldmann contact lens) using a slit-lamp. No blood is present.

Other Signs

Visual acuity generally ranges from 20/20–20/80, Amsler's grid testing reveals distortion of straight lines often with scotoma; a small afferent pupillary defect or a concomitant retinal pigment epithelial detachment may be present.

Differential Diagnosis

The entities below may produce a serous detachment of the sensory retina in the macular area.

- Age-related macular degeneration (ARMD)   [Patient generally >50 years of age, drusen, pigment epithelial alterations, may have a choroidal (subretinal) neovascular membrane, often bilateral. See Section 12.10.]
- Optic pit   (The optic disc has a small defect, a pit, in the nerve tissue. A serous retinal detachment may be present contiguous with the optic disc. See Section 12.9.)
- Macular detachment as a result of a rhegmatogenous retinal detachment   (A hole in the retina can be found. See Section 12.19.)
- Choroidal tumor   (A mass is visible by indirect ophthalmoscopy. See Section 8.3.)

- Pigment epithelial detachment (The margins of a pigment epithelial detachment are more distinct than those of central serous chorioretinopathy. It may accompany central serous choroidopathy or ARMD.)
- Others (Idiopathic choroidal effusion, inflammatory choroidal disorders.)

Work-up

1. Amsler's grid test to document the area of field involved (see Appendix 3).
2. Slit-lamp examination of the macula with a fundus contact, Hruby, or 60- or 90-diopter lens to rule out a concomitant choroidal neovascular membrane. Additionally, search for an optic pit of the disc.
3. Dilated retinal examination using indirect ophthalmoscopy to rule out a choroidal tumor and rhegmatogenous retinal detachment.
4. Obtain an intravenous fluorescein angiogram if the diagnosis is uncertain, a choroidal neovascular membrane is suspected, or laser treatment is to be instituted.

Treatment/Follow-up

The prognosis for spontaneous recovery of visual acuity to $\geq 20/30$ is excellent. The prognosis is worse for patients with recurrent disease, multiple areas of detachment, or prolonged course. Final degree of visual outcome has not been shown to be improved or worsened by laser therapy, but vision is restored more rapidly. Because of the small but significant risks of laser photocoagulation, however, the following recommendations have been made:

1. Examine most patients every 6–8 weeks until the condition spontaneously resolves or, if no resolution occurs, for 4–6 months.
2. Laser photocoagulation may be considered under the following circumstances:
   a. Persistence of a serous detachment beyond 4–6 months.
   b. Recurrence of the condition in an eye that sustained a permanent visual deficit from a previous episode.
   c. Occurrence in the contralateral eye after a permanent visual deficit resulted from a previous episode.
   d. Patient requires prompt restoration of vision (e.g., occupational requirement).

12.9 OPTIC PIT

Symptoms

Asymptomatic if isolated. May notice distortion of straight lines or edges, blurred vision, a blind spot, or micropsia if a serous macular detachment develops.

Critical Sign

Small defect (usually hypopigmented or gray in appearance) in the nerve tissue of the optic disc. The majority are temporal, but some are central.

Other Signs

May develop a localized detachment of the sensory retina extending from the disc to the macula, usually unilateral.

Differential Diagnosis

- Pseudopit   (See in patients with low-tension glaucoma or primary open-angle glaucoma, occasionally accompanied by flame hemorrhages.)
- Other causes of a serous macular detachment (see "Central Serous Chorioretinopathy," Section 12.8).

Work-up

1. Optic-disc evaluation to detect the pit.
2. Slit-lamp examination of the macula with a fundus contact lens or 60- or 90-diopter lens to evaluate for a serous macular detachment and to rule out a choroidal (subretinal) neovascular membrane.
3. Measure intraocular pressure.
4. Consider a fluorescein angiogram to help detect a pit and rule out a choroidal neovascular membrane in patients with a serous macular detachment.

Treatment

Isolated optic pit   No treatment required.

Optic pit with a serous macular detachment   Laser photocoagulation to the temporal margin of the optic disc is used in most cases. Surgery (vitrectomy) may be used in refractory cases.

Follow-up

Isolated optic pits   Yearly examination; sooner if symptomatic.

Optic pits with serous macular detachment   Reexamine every few weeks after treatment to check for resorption of subretinal fluid. Watch for amblyopia in children.

12.10 AGE-RELATED MACULAR DEGENERATION (ARMD)

Two types: Nonexudative (dry form) and exudative (wet form). Both forms almost always occur in patients older than 50 years of age.

A. Nonexudative

Symptoms

Gradual loss of central vision; may be asymptomatic.

Critical Sign

Drusen, almost always in the macular area of both eyes.

Other Signs

Clumps of pigment in the outer retina, retinal pigment epithelial atrophy (e.g., geographic atrophy), dystrophic calcification, Amsler's grid defects.

Differential Diagnosis

- Peripheral drusen   (Drusen are located outside of the macular area, not within it.)
- Myopic degeneration   (Typically, high myopia with characteristic peripapillary changes in addition to the macular degeneration. Drusen are not seen.)

Work-up

1. Amsler's grid to document or detect a central or paracentral scotoma (see Appendix 3).
2. Macular examination with a 60- or 90-diopter or a fundus contact lens: Look for signs of the exudative form.

Treatment

No proven treatment is available. Some physicians advocate the use of oral zinc preparations with or without antioxidant vitamins (e.g., vitamins C, E), but this has not been scientifically confirmed to be beneficial. Low-vision aids may benefit patients with bilateral loss of macular function.

Follow-up

Every 6 months. Patients are given an Amsler's grid to take home and use on a daily basis. They are instructed to return immediately if a change is noted on Amsler's grid.

B. Exudative

1. Choroidal (Subretinal) Neovascular Membrane Without a Pigment Epithelial Detachment

Symptoms

Distortion of straight lines or edges, rapid onset of visual loss, blind spot in the central or paracentral visual field.

Critical Signs

Drusen accompanied by a choroidal neovascular membrane (CNVM; dirty grayish green membrane beneath the retina).

Other Signs

Subretinal hemorrhages, subretinal exudates, subretinal pigment ring, subretinal fibrosis (disciform scar), retinal or vitreous hemorrhage. Nonexudative signs may be present.

Risk Factors for Loss of Vision

Advanced age, hyperopia, family history, soft drusen, focal pigment clumping, retinal pigment epithelial (RPE) detachments.

❖ **Note** *The risk of a CNVM in the contralateral eye is 10–12% per year. Eyes at highest risk are those with multiple or confluent soft drusen or RPE clumping.*

Differential Diagnosis

All of the following are associated with a choroidal neovascular membrane:

- Ocular histoplasmosis syndrome   (Small white-yellow chorioretinal scars are seen in the midperiphery and posterior pole along with chorioretinal scarring adjacent to the optic disc. See Section 12.11.)
- Angioid streaks   (Bilateral subretinal red-brown or gray bands of irregular contour which radiate from the optic disc. See Section 12.13.)
- High myopia   (Significant myopic refractive error, lacquer cracks in the posterior pole, myopic disc changes. See Section 12.12.)
- Traumatic choroidal rupture   (History of trauma, usually unilateral; a choroidal tear concentric to the optic disc is often noted. See Section 3.10.)
- Others   (Drusen of the optic nerve, choroidal tumors, photocoagulation scars, inflammatory chorioretinal lesions, and idiopathic.)

Work-up

1. Amsler's grid testing to detect and document the degree of central field involved (see Appendix 3).
2. Macular slit-lamp examination with a 60- or 90-diopter or fundus contact lens to detect a choroidal neovascular membrane. Must examine *both* eyes.
3. Blood pressure measurement. The presence of systemic hypertension in patients with a CNVM appears to have a negative effect on the response to laser therapy.
4. Fluorescein angiography (FA) is performed as soon as possible if a CNVM is suspected on clinical examination. FA classically shows an area of lacy, fine capillaries at the outer retinal level or beneath the RPE in early transit phase, with leakage obscuring the boundaries of these vessels in the middle and late phases.

5. Indocyanine green (ICG) angiograms may be a helpful adjuvant test in delineating the borders of some CNVM, especially in the presence of subretinal blood or exudate.

❖ **Note** *Neither FA nor ICGA are indicated when there is no hope of preserving central vision, such as in advanced stages of macular scarring (despite the presence of choroidal neovascularization).*

Treatment

Laser photocoagulation should be applied within 72 hours of the FA to reduce the risk of severe visual loss in patients with treatable macular CNVM as outlined by the Macular Photocoagulation Study (MPS) Group. Argon blue-green or green is used to treat CNVM located greater than 200 microns from the center of the foveal avascular zone (FAZ).[1] Krypton red should be considered for juxtafoveal CNVM (i.e., membrane or associated blood or pigment extending within 200 microns from the FAZ center). The treatment of subfoveal CNVM is controversial, although the macular photocoagulation study showed the degree of scarring to be less with laser treatment when compared with no treatment.

Follow-up

PATIENTS TREATED FOR CNVM WITH LASER PHOTOCOAGULATION

Because of the high rate of neovascular activity following treatment (persistent and new CNVM), patients need to be followed closely, especially during the first posttreatment year:

1. Amsler's grid to be used at home daily. The patient is instructed to return immediately if a change is noted.
2. Scheduled examinations at 2 weeks, 6 weeks, 3 months, and 6 months posttreatment, and then every 6 months. Careful macular examination is performed as described previously.
3. FA is repeated 2 weeks following treatment and again when renewed neovascular activity is suspected.
4. Retreatment with laser photocoagulation should be considered when renewed neovascular activity is identified.

Risk Factors

1. Persistance: Incomplete treatment of CNVM.
2. Recurrence: Hypertension, cigarette smoking, contralateral eye with

---

[1]The FAZ is an avascular area about 500 microns in diameter in the center of the fovea. It is easily observed with FA.

CNVM or disciform scar and or high-risk fundus features (soft drusen and pigment clumping).

RPE Detachment

May have any of the symptoms or signs described previously, but RPE detachment always has a well-defined elevated area of retina and retinal pigment epithelium with sharp borders. The work-up is the same as described previously.

Treatment

Laser therapy is typically applied to a CNVM when it is located adjacent to the pigment epithelial detachment, but there is a risk of an RPE tear. If no CNVM is present, patients are usually observed.

Follow-up

Follow closely for the development of a treatable CNVM. Some pigment epithelial detachments may flatten or tear spontaneously. Amsler's grid should be used as described in Appendix 3.

References

Macular Photocoagulation Study Group. Argon laser photocoagulation for neovascular maculopathy: Five year results from randomized clinical trials. *Arch Ophthalmol* 109:1109, 1991.
Macular Photocoagulation Study Group. Krypton laser photocoagulation for neovascular lesions of age-related macular degeneration: Results of a randomized clinical trial. *Arch Ophthalmol* 108:816, 1990.
Macular Photocoagulation Study Group. Subfoveal neovascular lesions in age-related macular degeneration: Guidelines for evaluation and treatment in the macular photocoagulation study. *Arch Ophthalmol* 109:1242, 1991.

12.11 OCULAR HISTOPLASMOSIS SYNDROME

Symptoms

May be asymptomatic or have decreased or distorted vision. Patients often have lived in or visited the Ohio-Mississippi River Valley area and are usually in the 20- to 50-year age range.

Critical Signs

Classic triad.

1. Yellow-white punched-out round spots usually <1 mm in diameter, deep to the retina in any fundus location ("histo-spots").
2. A macular choroidal neovascular membrane (CNVM) appearing as a gray-

green patch beneath the retina, associated with detachment of the sensory retina, subretinal blood or exudate, or a pigment ring evolving into a disciform scar.
3. Atrophy or scarring adjacent to the optic disc, sometimes with nodules or hemorrhage. There may be a rim of pigment separating the disc from the area of atrophy or scarring.

Other Signs

Linear streaks of chorioretinal atrophy in the peripheral fundus. The eye is uninflamed with minimal to no vitreous cells and no aqueous cells or flare.

Differential Diagnosis

- High myopia [May have atrophic spots in the posterior pole and a myopic crescent on the temporal side of the disc. A choroidal neovascular membrane may develop. The atrophic spots are whiter than histo-spots and are not seen beyond the posterior pole. The myopic crescent has a rim of pigment on the outer (not inner) edge, separating the crescent from the retina. May have lacquer cracks. The disc is often tilted. See Section 12.12.]
- Age-related macular degeneration (ARMD) (The macular changes may appear similar, but typically, there are macular drusen and patients are older than 50 years of age. There are no atrophic round spots similar to histoplasmosis and no scarring or atrophy around the disc. See Section 12.8.)
- Toxoplasmosis (White chorioretinal lesion associated with vitreous and sometimes aqueous cells. See Section 13.3.)
- Angioid streaks (Histo-like spots may be seen in the midperiphery, and macular degeneration may occur. Jagged red, brown, or gray lines appearing deep to the retinal vessels and radiating from the optic disc are typically seen. Often associated with pseudoxanthoma elasticum, sickle-cell anemia, Paget's disease, and other rarer systemic diseases. See Section 12.13.)
- Multifocal choroiditis with panuveitis (Similar clinical findings, except anterior and/or vitreous inflammatory cells are also present. See Section 13.2.)

Work-up

1. History: Time spent in the Ohio-Mississippi River Valley area? Prior exposure to fowl?
2. Amsler's grid test (see Appendix 3) to evaluate the central visual field of each eye.
3. Slit-lamp examination: Anterior-chamber cells and flare should not be present.
4. Dilated fundus examination: Concentrate on the macular area with a slit-lamp and fundus contact, Hruby, or 60- or 90-diopter lens. Look for signs of CNVM and vitreous cells.
5. Fluorescein angiography (to help detect or treat a CNVM).

Treatment

Laser photocoagulation is used to treat CNVM in the macula. Guidelines established by the Macular Photocoagulation Study (MPS) trials should be followed (see "Age-Related Macular Degeneration," Section 12.10). Knowledge of the patient's blood pressure status may be important in considering treatment. (In the MPS trials, patients with hypertension had a reduction in treatment benefit for both extrafoveal and juxtafoveal CNVM.) Prophylactic laser photocoagulation (i.e., in the absence of CNVM) is usually not recommended. Antifungal treatment is not helpful.

Follow-up

Treatment should be instituted within 72 hours of confirming the presence of CNVM by FA. All patients (whether they will be, will not be, or have been treated) are to use an Amsler's grid daily. Patients are instructed to return immediately if any sudden visual change is noted. Treated patients are seen at 2–3 weeks, 4–6 weeks, 3 months, and 6 months post-treatment and then every 6 months. A careful macular examination is performed at each visit. FA is repeated at the 2- to 3-week post-treatment visit and whenever renewed neovascular activity is suspected. Patients without CNVM are seen every 6 months when macular changes are present in one or both eyes and yearly when no macular pathology is present in either eye.

12.12 HIGH MYOPIA

Symptoms

Decreased vision. (Patients are usually beyond the fifth decade of life before progressive decrease in visual acuity occurs.)

Critical Signs

Myopic crescent (a crescent-shaped area of white sclera or choroidal vessels adjacent to the disc, separated from the normal-appearing fundus by a hyperpigmented line; this crescent may enlarge with time); an oblique (tilted) insertion of the optic disc; macular pigmentary abnormalities, a hyperpigmented spot in the macula (Fuchs' spot); typically, but not always, a refractive correction of more than -6.00 to -8.00 diopters.

Other Signs

Temporal optic-disc pallor, posterior staphyloma, entrance of the retinal vessels into the nasal part of the cup, the retina and choroid may be seen to extend over the nasal border of the disc, well-circumscribed areas of atrophy, spots of subretinal hemorrhage, choroidal sclerosis, yellow subretinal streaks (lacquer cracks), peripheral retinal thinning, lattice degeneration. A choroidal neovascular membrane (CNVM) or retinal detachment may develop. Visual field defects may be present. Increased intraocular pressure (IOP) with other evidence for primary open-angle glaucoma may be seen.

Differential Diagnosis
- Age-related macular degeneration (May develop CNVM and a similar macular appearance, but typically, drusen are present, and the myopic features of the optic disc described previously are absent. See Section 12.10.)
- Ocular histoplasmosis [May develop CNVM and exhibit a peripapillary scar. A pigmented ring may separate the disc from the peripapillary atrophy, as opposed to pigmented ring separating the atrophic area from the adjacent retina. Round choroidal scars (punched-out lesions) are often seen scattered throughout the fundus. See Section 12.11.]
- Tilted discs [Anomalous discs with a scleral crescent, most often inferonasally, an irregular vascular pattern as the vessels emerge from the disc (situs inversus), and an area of fundus ectasia in the direction of the tilt (inferonasally). Many patients have myopia and astigmatism. They do not have chorioretinal degeneration or lacquer cracks. Visual field defects corresponding to the areas of fundus ectasia are often seen. Most cases are bilateral.]
- Gyrate atrophy (Rare. Multiple, sharply defined areas of chorioretinal atrophy beginning in the midperiphery in childhood and then coalescing to involve a large portion of the fundus. Body fluid levels of ornithine are markedly elevated. Patients are often highly myopic. Autosomal recessive. See Section 12.26.)

Work-up
1. Manifest and/or cycloplegic refraction.
2. IOP measurement by applanation tonometry (Schiötz's tonometry may underestimate IOP in highly myopic eyes.)
3. Dilated retinal examination, using indirect ophthalmoscopy to search for retinal breaks or detachment. Scleral depression helps to reveal the far peripheral retina, but should not be performed over a staphyloma.
4. Slit-lamp and fundus contact. Hruby, or 60- or 90-diopter lens examination of the macula, searching for CNVM (dirty-gray or green lesion beneath the retina, subretinal blood or exudate, or subretinal fluid).
5. Fluorescein angiography when a CNVM is suspected.
6. Formal visual field examinations (e.g., Humphrey, Octopus) to document field stability or change when glaucoma is suspected.

Treatment
1. Symptomatic retinal breaks are treated with laser photocoagulation, cryotherapy, or scleral-buckling surgery. Treatment of asymptomatic retinal

breaks should be considered when there is no surrounding pigmentation or demarcation line.

2. Extrafoveal or juxtafoveal CNVM may be considered for laser photocoagulation therapy within several days of obtaining an FA (see "Age-Related Macular Degeneration," Section 12.10).

3. For glaucoma suspects, a single visual field often cannot distinguish myopic visual field loss from early glaucoma. Progression of visual field loss in the absence of progressive myopia, however, suggests the presence of glaucoma and the need for therapy (see "Primary Open-Angle Glaucoma," Section 10.1).

Follow-up

In the absence of complications, reexamine every 6–12 months, watching for the related disorders discussed above. See "Primary Open-Angle Glaucoma," Section 10.1; "Age-Related Macular Degeneration," Section 12.10 (for treatment of choroidal neovascularization); "Retinal Break," Section 12.18; and "Retinal Detachment," Section 12.19 for further information on these conditions.

12.13 ANGIOID STREAKS

Symptoms

Usually asymptomatic; decreased vision may result from choroidal (subretinal) neovascularization.

Critical Signs

Bilateral reddish brown or gray bands located deep to the retina, radiating in an irregular or spokelike pattern from the optic disc. Choroidal neovascular membranes leading to macular degeneration may occur.

Other Signs

Mottled-background fundus appearance ("peau d'orange"); subretinal hemorrhages (after mild blunt trauma); reticular pigmentary changes in the macula; small, white, pinpoint chorioretinal scars ("histo-like spots") in the midperiphery; drusen of the optic disc (especially with pseudoxanthoma elasticum).

Etiology

(Fifty percent of cases are associated with systemic diseases, the remainder are idiopathic.)

- Pseudoxanthoma elasticum (Most common. Loose skin folds in the neck and on flexor aspects of joints, cardiovascular complications, increased risk of GI bleeds.)
- Paget's disease (Enlarged skull, bone pain, history of bone fractures, hearing loss, possible cardiovascular complications. May be asymptomatic. Increased serum alkaline phosphatase and urine calcium.)
- Sickle-cell disease [May be asymptomatic; may have decreased vision from fundus abnormalities (see "Sickle-Cell Disease," Section 12.23), or may have a history of recurrent infections or painless or painful crises. Positive sickle-cell preparation and abnormal hemoglobin [Hgb] electrophoresis.)
- Ehlers-Danlos syndrome (Hyperelasticity of skin, loose-joints.)
- Less common (Acromegaly, senile elastosis, lead poisoning, Marfan's syndrome.)

Differential Diagnosis
- Myopic chorioretinal degeneration (lacquer cracks) (High myopia, often with a tilted disc and peripapillary atrophy; may have macular degeneration.)
- Choroidal rupture (Subretinal streaks are usually concentric to the optic disc, yellow-white in color, and result from ocular trauma.)

Work-up
1. History: Any known systemic disorders? Previous ocular trauma?
2. Complete ocular examination: Look carefully at the macula with a slit lamp and a Hruby, 60- or 90-diopter, or a fundus contact lens to detect choroidal neovascularization.
3. Fluorescein angiogram if uncertain of the diagnosis or if choroidal neovascularization is suspected.
4. Physical examination: Look for clinical signs of etiologic diseases.
5. Serum alkaline phosphatase and urine calcium levels if Paget's disease is suspected.
6. Sickle-cell preparation and Hgb electrophoresis in African-American patients.
7. Skin biopsy if pseudoxanthoma elasticum is suspected.

Treatment
1. Focal laser photocoagulation for treatable choroidal neovascularization (see "Age-Related Macular Degeneration," Section 12.10).
2. Management of any underlying systemic disease, if present, by a medical internist.

Follow-up

Fundus examination every 6 months, observing for choroidal neovascularization. Amsler's grid (see Appendix 3) is to be used at home on a daily basis. Patients are instructed to return immediately if a change is noted on Amsler's grid.

See "Age-Related Macular Degeneration," Section 12.10, for management of choroidal neovascularization.

12.14 CYSTOID MACULAR EDEMA (CME)

Symptoms

Decreased vision.

Critical Signs

Irregularity and blurring of the foveal light reflex, thickening with or without small intraretinal cysts in the foveal region.

Other Signs

Loss of the choroidal vascular pattern underlying the macula. Vitreous cells and optic-nerve swelling can appear in severe cases. A lamellar macular hole causing permanent visual loss can develop.

Etiology

- After any type of ocular surgery (including laser photocoagulation and cryotherapy)   (The peak incidence after cataract surgery is about 6–10 weeks; the incidence increases with surgical complications including vitreous to the wound, iris prolapse, and vitreous loss.)
- Diabetic retinopathy
- Central and branch retinal vein occlusions
- Uveitis (particularly pars planitis; see Section 13.5)
- Retinitis pigmentosa
- Topical epinephrine (or dipivefrin) drops, especially in postoperative cataract patients   (Often reversed by discontinuing the drops.)
- Retinal vasculitis (e.g., Eales' disease, Behçet's syndrome, sarcoidosis, necrotizing angiitis, multiple sclerosis, cytomegalovirus retinitis)
- Retinal telangiectasias (e.g., Coats' disease)
- Nicotinic acid maculopathy (Relatively high doses of nicotinic acid are used to treat hypercholesterolemia.)

- Others (Intraocular tumors, systemic hypertension, collagen-vascular disease, surface-wrinkling retinopathy, others.)

Work-up
1. History: Recent intraocular surgery? Diabetes? Previous uveitis or eye inflammation? Night blindness or family history of eye disease? Medications, including topical epinephrine or dipivefrin?
2. Complete ocular examination, including a peripheral fundus evaluation (scleral depression inferiorly may be required to detect pars planitis). A macular examination is best performed with a slit-lamp and a fundus contact lens, a Hruby lens, or a 60- or 90-diopter lens.
3. Fluorescein angiography often shows early leakage of dye out of perifoveal capillaries and late macular staining, classically in a flower-petal or spoke-wheel pattern. Optic-nerve head leakage is sometimes observed. Fluorescein leakage does not occur in nicotinic acid maculopathy.)
4. Other diagnostic tests when indicated (e.g., fasting blood sugar or glucose tolerance test, electroretinogram)

❖ **Note** *Subclinical CME commonly develops after cataract extraction and is noted on FA. These cases are not treated.*

Treatment
Not well established for macular edema developing after ocular surgery. Most of these cases resolve spontaneously within 6 months.

1. Treat the underlying disorder if possible.
2. Discontinue topical epinephrine or dipivefrin drops and medications containing nicotinic acid.
3. Consider acetazolamide 500 mg po daily, especially for postoperative patients, but also for those with retinitis pigmentosa and uveitis.
4. Other forms of therapy that have unproven efficacy, but are occasionally used:
   a. Systemic nonsteroidal antiinflammatory drugs (e.g., indomethacin 25 mg po tid for 6 weeks).
   b. Topical nonsteroidal antiinflammatory drugs (e.g., flurbiprofen or ketorolac qid).
   c. Topical steroids (e.g., prednisolone acetate 1% qid for 3 weeks, then taper over 3 weeks).
   d. Systemic steroids (e.g., prednisone 40 mg po daily for 5 days, then taper over 2 weeks).
   e. SubTenon's steroid (e.g., methylprednisolone 80 mg/mL, 0.5 mL).

- Diabetic macular edema may benefit from focal laser treatment (see "Diabetes Mellitus," Section 14.6).

- Macular edema persisting for 3–6 months after a BRVO and reducing vision below 20/40 may improve with laser photocoagulation (see "Branch Retinal Vein Occlusion," Section 12.4).
- Macular edema in the presence of vitreous incarceration in a surgical wound may be improved by anterior vitrectomy or YAG-laser lysis of the vitreous strand.
- Macular edema from pars planitis is often treated with steroids when vision is reduced below 20/40 (see "Pars Planitis," Section 13.5).

Follow-up

Postsurgical CME is not an emergent condition. Other forms of macular edema may require an etiologic work-up and may benefit from early treatment (e.g., elimination of nicotinic acid-containing medications).

REFERENCES

Cox SN, Hay E, Bird AC. Treatment of chronic macular edema with acetazolamide. *Arch Ophthalmol* 106:1190, 1988.

12.15 MACULAR HOLE

Symptoms

Decreased vision, typically around the 20/200 level for a full-thickness hole, better for a partial-thickness hole; sometimes distortion of vision. More commonly, middle-aged to elderly women are affected.

Critical Signs

A round, red spot in the center of the macula, usually from one third to two thirds of a disc diameter in size, surrounded by a gray halo (marginal retinal detachment). An impending idiopathic macular hole demonstrates loss of the normal foveolar depression and often a yellow spot or ring in the center of the macula.

Other Signs

Small, yellow deposits within the hole, deep to the retina; retinal cysts at the margin of the hole and/or a small operculum above the hole, anterior to the retina.

❖ **Note** *A partial-thickness (lamellar) hole is not as red in color, and the surrounding gray halo is usually not present.*

Etiology

May be caused by vitreous or epiretinal membrane traction on the macula, trauma, or cystoid macular edema.

Differential Diagnosis

- Macular pucker with a pseudohole   (A condensation of a membrane on the surface of the retina may stimulate a macular hole.)
- Solar retinopathy   (Small, round, red or yellow lesion at the center of the fovea, with surrounding fine gray pigment in a sun-gazer or eclipse-watcher.)

Work-up

1. History: Previous trauma? Previous eye surgery? Sun-gazer?
2. Complete ocular examination, including a macular examination with a slit lamp and 60- or 90-diopter, Hruby, or fundus contact lens.

Treatment

In selected cases of macular hole or impending macular hole, vitrectomy may be beneficial. The risk of retinal detachment is very small. However, symptoms of a retinal detachment (e.g., sudden increase in flashes and floaters, abundant "cobwebs" in the vision, or a curtain coming across the field of vision) are explained to patients, particularly those with high myopia. It is in this latter group that the macular hole sometimes leads to a retinal detachment. Retinal detachment requires repair.

Follow-up

Patients with high myopia are seen every 6 months, other patients may be seen yearly. All patients are seen sooner if retinal detachment symptoms develop. Because there is a small risk that the condition may develop in the contralateral eye, patients are given an Amsler's grid for periodic home monitoring.

12.16 MACULAR PUCKER
(SURFACE-WRINKLING RETINOPATHY)

Symptoms

Decreased and/or distorted vision. Occasionally bilateral. Typically occurs in middle-aged or elderly patients.

Critical Signs

Spectrum ranges from a fine, glistening membrane (cellophane retinopathy) to a thick, gray-white membrane (macular pucker) present on the surface of the retina in the macular area.

❖ **Note** *When the preretinal membrane is thin, it is often best appreciated with an indirect ophthalmoscope by moving the lens up and down in the examiner's hand. A glistening sparkle, much like cellophane, may be observed in the macular area.*

Other Signs

Retinal folds radiating out from the membrane, displacement or straightening of the macular retinal vessels, macular edema or detachment, signs of other ocular disease. A round, dark condensation of the epiretinal membrane in the macula may simulate a macular hole.

Etiology

Idiopathic, retinal break, rhegmatogenous retinal detachment, following retinal cryotherapy or photocoagulation, following intraocular surgery, trauma, uveitis, retinal vascular disease, others.

Differential Diagnosis

- Diabetic retinopathy   (May produce preretinal fibrovascular tissue, which may displace retinal vessels or detach the macula. Macular edema may be present. Hemorrhages and microaneurysms are usually found in addition, and the changes are commonly bilateral.)

Work-up

1. History: Previous eye surgery or eye disease? Diabetes?
2. Complete ocular examination, particularly a thorough dilated fundus evaluation. The macula is often best seen with a slit lamp and a 60- or 90-diopter, Hruby, or fundus contact lens.

Treatment

Treat the underlying disorder. Surgical peeling of the membrane can be performed when it reduces the vision to 20/80–20/100 or worse.

Follow-up

This is not an emergent condition, and treatment may be instituted at any time. Some membranes separate from the retina, and vision may improve spontaneously. A small percentage of preretinal membranes recur after surgical removal.

12.17 POSTERIOR VITREOUS DETACHMENT (PVD)

Symptoms

Floaters ("cobwebs" or "flies" that move with eye movement), blurred vision, flashes of light which are more common in dim illumination and are temporally located.

Critical Signs

One or more discrete pigmented vitreous opacities, often in the shape of a ring, suspended over the optic disc. The opacities float within the vitreous as the eye moves from side to side.

Other Signs

Vitreous hemorrhage, peripheral retinal and disc-margin hemorrhages, pigmented cells in the anterior vitreous, retinal break or detachment.

❖ **Note** *The presence of pigmented cells in the anterior vitreous or vitreous hemorrhage in association with acute PVD indicates a high probability of a coexisting retinal break (see Section 12.18).*

Differential Diagnosis

- Vitritis   (It may be difficult to distinguish PVD with pigmented anterior vitreous cells from vitreous inflammatory cells. In vitritis, the vitreous cells may be found in both the posterior and anterior vitreous, the condition may be bilateral, and the cells are not typically pigmented. A history of uveitis may be elicited. See Section 13.2.)
- Migraine   (Patients complain of flashing lights in a fortified pattern that last approximately 20 minutes. A headache may or may not follow. No vitreous or retinal abnormalities are found on examination. See Section 15.3.)

The following may occur with or without PVD, producing similar symptoms:

- Retinal break
- Vitreous hemorrhage
- Retinal detachment

Work-up

1. History: Distinguish between the flashing lights of migraine, which typically occur in a "zig-zag" pattern, obstruct vision, and last approximately

20 minutes, from the light sparks of PVD, which are commonly accompanied by floaters. Determine the duration of the symptoms.

2. Complete ocular examination, particularly a dilated retinal examination using indirect ophthalmoscopy and scleral depression to rule out a retinal break and detachment. A slit-lamp examination of the anterior vitreous, looking for pigmented cells, is often performed (see Appendix 8).

3. PVD may be visualized by focusing in the vitreous, above the disc, using:
   a. Indirect ophthalmoscopy.
   b. Direct ophthalmoscopy. (The ophthalmoscope is initially focused on the cornea, the lens wheel is moved from a higher black number toward a lower black number, and the patient is asked to move his or her eye from left to right. The PVD is seen to float by.)
   c. A slit lamp and a 60- or 90-diopter or Hruby lens examination. (Pull the slip lamp back once focus on the disc is obtained. A black strand may be seen in the vitreous.)

Treatment

No treatment is indicated for PVD. If a retinal break is found, the patient should receive laser or cryotherapy within 24–72 hours to avoid the development of a retinal detachment (see Section 12.18).

❖ **Note** *A retinal break surrounded by pigment is old and usually does not require treatment.*

Follow-up

The patient should be given a list of retinal detachment symptoms (an increase in floaters or flashing lights, or the appearance of a curtain or shadow anywhere in the field of vision), and told to return immediately if these symptoms develop.

- If no retinal break or hemorrhage is found, the patient should be scheduled for repeat examination with scleral depression in 2–4 weeks, 2–3 months, and 6 months after the symptoms first developed.
- If no retinal break is found, but mild vitreous hemorrhage or peripheral punctate retinal hemorrhages are present, repeat examinations are performed 1–2 weeks, 4 weeks, 3 months, and 6 months after the event.
- If a vitreous hemorrhage dense enough to obscure the entire retina is found, ultrasonography is indicated to rule out a retinal detachment or tumor. Bed rest, with the head of the bed elevated, often with bilateral patches, is employed for 24–48 hours to hasten settling of the blood (see Section 12.22).

12.18 RETINAL BREAK

Symptoms

Acute retinal break   Blurred vision, flashes of light, floaters ("cobwebs" or "flies" that move with eye movement).

Chronic retinal break or an atrophic retinal fold   Usually asymptomatic.

Critical Sign

A full-thickness retinal defect.

Other Signs

Acute retinal break   Pigmented cells in the anterior vitreous, vitreous hemorrhage, posterior vitreous detachment, retinal flap, an operculum (a free-floating piece of retina) suspended in the vitreous cavity above the retinal hole.

Chronic retinal break   A ring of pigmentation surrounding the break, demarcation line between attached and detached retina, signs (but not symptoms) of an acute retinal break.

Predisposing Lesions

Lattice degeneration, high myopia, aphakia, senile retinoschisis, vitreoretinal tufts, meridional folds, history of previous retinal break or detachment in the fellow eye.

Work-up

Complete ocular examination, particularly a dilated fundus examination of both eyes using indirect ophthalmoscopy and scleral depression. Scleral depression is generally *not* performed until 3–4 weeks following a traumatic hyphema or microhyphema. A slit-lamp examination with a fundus contact lens is often quite helpful in evaluating retinal breaks.

Treatment

In general, laser therapy, cryotherapy, or scleral-buckling surgery is required within 24–72 hours for acute retinal breaks, and only rarely for chronic breaks. Each case must be individualized; however, we follow these general guidelines:

A. Treatment recommended
   1. Acute symptomatic break (e.g., a horseshoe or operculated tear).
   2. Acute traumatic break (including a dialysis).
B. Treatment to be considered
   1. Asymptomatic retinal break that is large (e.g., >1.5 mm) and/or above

the horizontal meridian, particularly if there is no posterior vitreous detachment.

2. Asymptomatic retinal break in an aphakic or pseudophakic eye, an eye in which the involved or the contralateral eye has had a retinal detachment, or in a highly myopic eye.

Follow-up

Patients with predisposing lesions or retinal breaks that do not require treatment are followed every 6–12 months. Patients treated for a retinal break are reexamined in 1 week, 1 month, 3 months, and then every 6–12 months. Retinal detachment symptoms (an increase in floaters or flashing lights or the appearance of a curtain or shadow anywhere in the field of vision) are explained to all patients, and patients are told to return immediately if these symptoms develop.

12.19 RETINAL DETACHMENT

There are three distinct types of retinal detachment (RD). All three forms show an elevation of the retina.

A. Rhegmatogenous (RRD)

Symptoms

Flashes of light, floaters, a curtain or shadow moving over the field of vision, peripheral and/or central visual loss.

Critical Sign

Elevation of the retina and a flap tear or break in the retina.

Other Signs

Pigmented cells in the anterior vitreous, vitreous hemorrhage, posterior vitreous detachment, usually lower intraocular pressure in the affected eye than the contralateral eye, clear subretinal fluid that does not shift with body position, sometimes fixed retinal folds. The detached retina moves with eye motion and is corrugated in appearance. An afferent pupillary defect (APD) may be present.

❖ **Note** *A chronic RRD often shows a pigmented demarcation line at the posterior extent of the RD, intraretinal cysts, fixed folds, or white dots underneath the* *retina (subretinal precipitates). It should be differentiated from retinoschisis, which produces an absolute visual field defect.*

B. Exudative (ERD)

Symptoms

Minimal-to-severe visual loss or a visual field defect.

Critical Sign

Serous elevation of the retina with shifting subretinal fluid (SRF). (The area of detached retina changes when the patient changes position: while sitting, the SRF accumulates inferiorly, detaching the retina inferiorly; while in the supine position, the fluid accumulates in the posterior pole, detaching the macula.)

Other Signs

The detached retina is smooth and may become so elevated that it reaches the lens. A mild APD may be present.

Etiology

- Neoplastic (e.g., choroidal malignant melanoma, multiple myeloma, metastasis, choroidal hemangioma, capillary retinal hemangioma)   (Fluorescein angiography and ultrasound may be helpful in making a differential diagnosis.)
- Inflammatory disease (e.g., Vogt-Koyanagi-Harada syndrome, posterior scleritis, other chronic inflammatory processes)
- Congenital abnormalities (e.g., optic pit, morning-glory syndrome, choroidal coloboma, Coats' disease)
- Nanophthalmos   (Small eyes with a small cornea and a shallow anterior chamber but a large lens and a thick sclera.)
- Idiopathic central serous chorioretinopathy   (May present with bullous retinal detachment from multiple, large retinal pigment epithelial detachment.)
- Uveal effusion syndrome   (Bilateral detachments of the peripheral choroid, ciliary body, and retina; leopard-spot retinal pigment epithelial changes; cells in the vitreous; dilated episcleral vessels.)

C. Tractional (TRD)

Symptoms

Visual loss or visual field defect; may be asymptomatic.

Critical Signs

The detached retina appears concave with a smooth surface; vitreous membranes pulling the retina are present. (Detachment may become a convex RRD if traction tears the retina.)

Other Signs
The retina is immobile, and the detachment rarely extends to the ora serrata. A mild APD may be present.

Etiology
Fibrous bands in the vitreous (e.g., resulting from proliferative diabetic retinopathy, sickle-cell retinopathy, retinopathy of prematurity, toxocariasis, trauma, previous giant retinal tear) contract and pull the retina off of the RPE.

Differential Diagnosis for All Three Types of RD
- Senile retinoschisis (Commonly bilateral, usually temporal, no pigmented cells or hemorrhage is present in the vitreous, the retinal vessels over the schisis are often sheathed, white "snowflakes" are often seen on the inner layer of the schisis near the ora serrata, the patient is asymptomatic. An absolute scotoma, as opposed to a relative scotoma as seen with a RRD, is found on visual field testing. A demarcation line is generally not present unless an RD develops from the schisis.)
- Juvenile retinoschisis (Cystoid foveal changes are present, X-linked recessive, bilateral, the retinoschisis does not extend to the ora serrata.)
- Choroidal detachment (Orange-brown in color, more solid in appearance than an RD, the ora serrata can usually be seen without scleral depression, the detachment often extends 360 degrees around the globe. Hypotony is generally present.)

Treatment/Follow-up
1. Patients with acute RRD that involves or threatens the macula or those with TRD that involves the macula should be placed at bed rest with bilateral patching until surgical repair can be performed.
2. All other RRDs that do not threaten the macula are repaired at the earliest convenience, preferably within 1–2 days.
3. Chronic retinal detachments are treated within 1 week.
4. For ERD, successful treatment of the underlying condition often leads to resolution of the detachment.

REFERENCE

Michels RG, Wilkinson CP, Rice TA. Retinal Detachment. CV Mosby, Philadelphia: 1990.

12.20 RETINOSCHISIS

Retinoschisis, a splitting of the retina, occurs in juvenile (X-linked) and senile forms.

A. Juvenile (X-Linked) Retinoschisis

Symptoms

Decreased vision (often due to vitreous hemorrhage) or asymptomatic. The condition is congenital, but may not be detected until years later. A positive family history may or may not be elicited.

Critical Signs

Cystoid foveal changes with retinal folds that radiate from the center of the foveal configuration (petaloid pattern). Unlike the cysts of cystoid macular edema, they do not stain on fluorescein angiography.

Other Signs

Separation of the nerve fiber layer from the outer retinal layers in the retinal periphery with the development of nerve fiber–layer breaks; this peripheral retinoschisis occurs most commonly in the inferotemporal quadrant of the fundus and is bilateral. The retinoschisis does not extend to the ora serrata. Retinal detachment, vitreous hemorrhage, and a pigmentary degeneration similar to retinitis pigmentosa may also occur.

Inheritance

X-linked recessive.

Differential Diagnosis

- Senile retinoschisis (see the following)
- Rhegmatogenous retinal detachment   (Usually unilateral and acquired. It extends to the ora serrata and lacks the foveal changes described previously. Anterior-chamber cells and flare and pigment in the vitreous are often seen. See Section 12.19.)

Work-up

1. Family history.
2. Dilated retinal examination with scleral depression to rule out an outer-layer retinal break or detachment.

Treatment

Surgical repair of a retinal detachment should be performed if present. Superimposed amblyopia should always be considered in children younger than 9–11 years of age when one eye is more severely affected, and a trial of patching should be considered (see Section 9.6).

Follow-up

Every 6 months; sooner if treating amblyopia.

B. Senile Retinoschisis

Symptoms
Usually none, may have decreased vision.

Critical Signs
The retinal split is usually bilateral and may show sheathing of retinal vessels and "snowflakes," or "frosting" on the elevated inner wall of the schisis cavity. (In contrast to juvenile retinoschisis, splitting usually occurs at the level of the outer plexiform layer.) The schisis cavity is dome-shaped with a smooth surface and is usually located temporally, especially inferotemporally.

Other Signs
Prominent cystoid degeneration near the ora serrata, an absolute scotoma is found on visual field testing, hyperopia is common, and there are no pigment cells nor hemorrhage in the vitreous. A rhegmatogenous retinal detachment may occasionally develop.

Differential Diagnosis
- Rhegmatogenous retinal detachment   (The surface is not smooth, but corrugated in appearance and can be seen to move more with eye movements than schisis does; retinal vessels are not sheathed, and no "snowflakes" or "frosting" can be seen on the retinal elevation; one or more full-thickness holes are present, and pigmented cells or hemorrhage may be present in the vitreous. A long-standing retinal detachment may resemble retinoschisis, but intraretinal cysts, demarcation lines between attached and detached retina, and white retroretinal dots may be seen. A relative scotoma is found on visual field testing. See Section 12.19.)
- Juvenile (X-linked) retinoschisis (see previous)

Work-up
1. Slit-lamp evaluation to rule out the presence of anterior-chamber inflammation or pigmented anterior-vitreous cells, both of which should not be present in isolated retinoschisis.
2. Dilated retinal examination with scleral depression to rule out a concomitant retinal detachment or an outer-layer retinal hole, which may lead to a retinal detachment.
3. A fundus contact lens evaluation of the retina as needed to aid in recognizing outer-layer retinal breaks.

Treatment
Surgery is indicated when a clinically significant retinal detachment develops. A small retinal detachment walled off by a demarcation line is generally not treated.

Follow-up

Every 6 months. Retinal detachment symptoms (an increase in floaters or flashing lights or the appearance of a curtain or shadow anywhere in the field of vision) are explained to all patients, and patients are told to return immediately if these symptoms develop.

12.21 CHOROIDAL DETACHMENT

Symptoms

Decreased vision or asymptomatic in a serous choroidal detachment. Severe pain, decreased vision, and red eye in a hemorrhagic choroidal detachment.

Critical Signs

Smooth, bullous, orange-brown elevation of the retina and choroid, usually extending 360 degrees around the periphery in a lobular configuration. The ora serrata can be seen without scleral depression.

Other Signs

Serous choroidal detachment Low intraocular pressure (IOP) (often <6 mm Hg), shallow anterior chamber with mild cell and flare, positive transillumination.

Hemorrhagic choroidal detachment High IOP, shallow anterior chamber with mild cell and flare, no transillumination.

Etiology

SEROUS

- Postsurgical (Wound leak, perforation of the sclera from a superior rectus bridle suture, iritis, cyclodialysis cleft, leakage or excess filtration from a filtering bleb, or following laser photocoagulation or cryotherapy. May occur days to weeks after the surgery.)
- Traumatic (Often associated with a ruptured globe.)
- Inflammatory [e.g., scleritis, Vogt-Koyanagi-Harada (VKH) syndrome]
- Tumor (Primary or metastasis.)
- Rhegmatogenous retinal detachment or after scleral buckling repair of a detachment
- Others (Nanophthalmos, uveal effusion syndrome, carotid-cavernous fistula.)

HEMORRHAGIC

- Postsurgical (From anterior displacement of the ocular contents and rupture of the short posterior ciliary arteries.)

- Spontaneous (e.g., after perforation of a corneal ulcer)
- Rupture of a choroidal neovascular membrane in a patient on anticoagulants

Differential Diagnosis
- Melanoma of the ciliary body   (Not typically multilobular or symmetrical in each quadrant of the globe. Pigmented melanomas do not transilluminate. B-scan ultrasound may help to differentiate between the two. See Section 8.3.)
- Rhegmatogenous retinal detachment   (Appears white and undulates with eye movements. A break usually seen in the retina, and pigment cells are present in the vitreous. See Section 12.19.)

Work-up
1. History: Recent ocular surgery or trauma? Known eye or medical problem?
2. Slit-lamp examination: Check for the presence of a filtering bleb and perform Seidel's test to rule out a wound leak (see Appendix 4).
3. Gonioscopy of the anterior-chamber angle: Look for a cyclodialysis cleft.
4. Dilated retinal examination: Determine whether there is subretinal fluid, indicating a concomitant retinal detachment, and whether an underlying choroidal disease or tumor is present. Examination of the contralateral eye may be helpful in diagnosis.
5. In cases suspicious for melanoma, B-scan ultrasonography and transillumination of the globe are helpful in making a diagnosis.
6. Check the skin for vitiligo and the head for alopecia (VKH).

Treatment
A. General treatment
    1. Cycloplegic (e.g., atropine 1% tid).
    2. Topical steroid (e.g., prednisolone acetate 1% 4–6 times per day).
    3. Surgical drainage of the suprachoroidal fluid may be indicated for a flat or progressively shallow anterior chamber, particularly in the presence of inflammation (because of the risk of peripheral anterior synechiae), corneal decompensation secondary to lens-cornea touch, or "kissing" choroidals (apposition of two lobules of detached choroid).
B. Specific treatment: Repair the underlying problem.

SEROUS

- Wound leak or leaky filtering bleb: Patch for 24 hours, suture the site, use cyanoacrylate glue, and/or place a bandage contact lens on the eye.
- Cyclodialysis cleft: Laser therapy, diathermy, cryotherapy, or suture the cleft to close it.
- Uveitis: Topical cycloplegic and steroid as discussed previously.
- Inflammatory disease: See the specific entity.
- Retinal detachment: Surgical repair.

HEMORRHAGIC

An anterior vitrectomy and drainage of the choroidal detachment is performed for severe cases with vitreous to the wound. Otherwise use general treatment above.

Follow-up
In accordance with the underlying problem.

12.22 VITREOUS HEMORRHAGE

Symptoms
Sudden painless loss of vision or sudden appearance of black spots with flashing lights.

Critical Signs
In a severe vitreous hemorrhage, the red fundus reflex may be absent, and there may be no fundus view on ophthalmoscopy. Red blood cells can sometimes be appreciated when a slit lamp is focused posterior to the lens. In a mild vitreous hemorrhage, blood may be seen to obscure part of the retina and retinal vessels. Chronic vitreous hemorrhage has a yellow ochre appearance secondary to the breakdown of hemoglobin.

Other Signs
A mild afferent pupillary defect. Depending on the etiology, there may be other fundus abnormalities.

Etiology
- Diabetic retinopathy   (Almost always have a known history of diabetes and usually one of diabetic retinopathy. Diabetic retinopathy is usually evident in the contralateral eye. See Section 14.6.)
- Retinal break   (Commonly superior in cases of dense vitreous hemorrhage. This may be demonstrated by ultrasonography and scleral depression. See Section 12.18.)
- Retinal detachment   (May be diagnosed by ultrasound if the retina cannot be viewed on clinical examination. See Section 12.19.)
- Retinal vein occlusion (usually a branch retinal vein occlusion)   (Commonly occurs in older patients with a history of high blood pressure. May have a history of a vein occlusion or sudden visual loss in the eye months to years previously. See Section 12.4.)
- Posterior vitreous detachment   (Common in middle-aged or elderly patients. Usually, patients note floaters and flashing lights. See Section 12.17.)
- Age-related macular degeneration (ARMD)   (Patients often acknowledge poor vision prior to the vitreous hemorrhage as a result of their underlying

disease. Macular drusen and/or other findings of ARMD are found in the contralateral eye. See Section 12.10.)
- Sickle-cell disease (particularly SC disease)   African-American patients. May have peripheral retinal neovascularization in the contralateral eye, typically in a "sea-fan" configuration. See Section 12.23.)
- Trauma (by history)
- Intraocular tumor   (May be visible on ophthalmoscopy or B-scan ultrasonography. See Sections 12.2 and 12.3.)
- Subarachnoid or subdural hemorrhage (Terson's syndrome)   (Frequently bilateral preretinal or vitreous hemorrhages may occur. A severe headache usually precedes the fundus findings. Coma may occur.)
- Eales' disease   (Usually occurs in men 20–30 years of age with peripheral retinal ischemia and neovascularization of unknown etiology. Decreased vision as a result of vitreous hemorrhage is frequently the presenting sign. The disease is often bilateral and is a diagnosis of exclusion.)
- Others   (Coats' disease, retinopathy of prematurity, retinal capillary angiomas of von Hippel-Lindau syndrome, congenital prepapillary vascular loop, hypertension, radiation retinopathy, anterior-segment hemorrhage because of an intraocular lens, bleeding diathesis, others.)

❖ **Note** *In infancy and childhood consider birth trauma, shaken baby syndrome, traumatic child abuse, juvenile X-linked retinoschisis.*

Differential Diagnosis
- Vitritis (*white* blood cells in the vitreous)   (The onset is rarely as sudden as in vitreous hemorrhage; anterior or posterior uveitis may also be present. No red blood cells and no hemorrhage in the vitreous are present. See Section 13.2.)
- Retinal detachment   (May occur without a vitreous hemorrhage, yet the symptoms may be identical. The fundus view may be difficult in a highly elevated detachment; however, the retina can usually be viewed with an indirect ophthalmoscope. In cases of highly elevated detachments, slit-lamp examination may show the retina behind the lens. See Section 12.19.)

Work-up
1. History: Any ocular or systemic diseases, specifically the ones mentioned previously? Trauma?
2. Complete ocular examination, including a slit-lamp examination to check for iris neovascularization, intraocular pressure measurement, and a dilated fundus examination of *both eyes* using direct ophthalmoscopy. In cases of spontaneous vitreous hemorrhage, scleral depression is performed if a retinal view can be obtained (we do not generally depress eyes until 3–4 weeks after traumatic hemorrhages.)
3. When no retinal view can be obtained, a B-scan ultrasound is performed to detect an associated retinal detachment or intraocular tumor. Flap retinal tears may be detected with scleral depression.

4. A fluorescein angiogram may aid in defining the etiology, although the quality of the angiogram may depend on the density of the hemorrhage.

Treatment

1. If the etiology of the vitreous hemorrhage is not known and a retinal break and/or a retinal detachment cannot be ruled out (e.g., there is no known history of one of the diseases mentioned previously, there are no changes in the contralateral eye, and the fundus is obscured by a total vitreous hemorrhage), the patient is admitted to the hospital or followed closely as an outpatient.
2. Bed rest with the head of the bed elevated (and sometimes bilateral patching) for 2–3 days (this reduces the chance of recurrent bleeding and allows the blood to settle inferiorly, permitting a view of the superior peripheral fundus, a common site for responsible retinal breaks).
3. Eliminate aspirin, nonsteroidal antiinflammatory drugs, and other anticlotting agents unless they are medically necessary.
4. The underlying etiology is treated as soon as possible (e.g., retinal breaks are sealed with cryotherapy or laser photocoagulation, detached retinas are repaired, and proliferative retinal vascular diseases are treated with laser photocoagulation or cryotherapy when there is no retinal view).
5. Surgical removal of the blood (vitrectomy) is usually performed for:
   a. Vitreous hemorrhage accompanied by retinal detachment.
   b. Chronic vitreous hemorrhage (>6 months in duration).
   c. Vitreous hemorrhage with neovascularization of the iris.
   d. Hemolytic or ghost cell glaucoma.

❖ **Note** *Vitrectomy for isolated vitreous hemorrhage (e.g., without retinal detachment) may be considered earlier than 6 months for diabetics or patients with bilateral vitreous hemorrhage.*

Follow-up

The patient is evaluated daily for the first 2–3 days. If a total vitreous hemorrhage persists, and the etiology remains unknown, the patient is followed with a B-scan ultrasound every 1–3 weeks to rule out a retinal detachment.

12.23 SICKLE-CELL DISEASE
(SICKLE-CELL HEMOGLOBIN C DISEASE, SICKLE-CELL THALASSEMIA, SICKLE-CELL ANEMIA, AND SICKLE-CELL TRAIT)

Symptoms

Usually without ocular symptoms. May have floaters, flashing lights, or loss of vision with advanced disease. Systemically, patients with sickle-cell anemia often have painful crises with severe abdominal or musculoskeletal discomfort. Patients are of African or Mediterranean extraction in most cases.

Critical Signs

Peripheral retinal neovacularization in the shape of a fan ("sea-fan" sign), sclerosed peripheral retinal vessels, or an abnormal dull gray peripheral fundus background color (as a result of peripheral arteriolar occlusions and ischemia).

Other Signs

Tortuosity of retinal veins, black midperipheral fundus lesions with spiculated borders (black sunbursts), intraretinal and subretinal hemorrhages (salmon patch), refractile (iridescent) deposits, angioid streaks, comma-shaped capillaries of the conjunctiva (especially along the inferior fornix). Vitreous hemorrhage and traction bands, retinal detachment, central retinal artery occlusion, and macular arteriolar occlusions may develop.

❖ **Note** *Proliferative sickle-cell retinopathy is thought to progress from peripheral arteriolar occlusions (stage 1) to peripheral arteriovenous anastomoses (stage 2) to retinal neovascularization (stage 3). The retinal neovascularization may spontaneously regress or may produce vitreous hemorrhage (stage 4) or traction retinal detachment (stage 5).*

Differential Diagnosis

(Other causes of peripheral retinal neovascularization.)

- Sarcoidosis   (May also produce peripheral sea-fan neovascularization in young black individuals. However, granulomatous uveitis, vitritis with vitreous opacities, and sheathing of retinal veins are often present. See Section 13.4.)
- Diabetes   (Tends to have a more posterior retinal location, dot/blot hemorrhages, and elevated blood sugar. See Section 14.6.)
- Branch retinal vein occlusion   [Flame-shaped hemorrhages involving a sector or one half of the retina (the inferior or superior half); the hemorrhages do not cross the horizontal raphé. May only see a sclerosed arteriole in late stages. See Section 12.4.]
- Embolic (e.g., talc) retinopathy   (History of IV drug abuse. May see refractile talc particles in the macular arterioles.)
- Eales' disease   (Peripheral retinal vascular occlusion of unknown etiology; a diagnosis of exclusion.)
- Others   (Retinopathy of prematurity, familial exudative vitreoretinopathy, chronic myelogenous leukemia, radiation retinopathy, pars planitis, carotid-cavernous fistula, ocular ischemic syndrome, collagen-vascular disease.)

Work-up

1. Past medical history and family history: Sickle-cell disease, diabetes, or known medical problems? IV drug abuse?

2. Dilated fundus examination using indirect ophthalmoscopy.
3. Sickle-cell preparation and hemoglobin electrophoresis (patients with sickle-cell trait, as well as hemoglobin C disease, may have a negative sickle-cell preparation).
4. Consider fluorescein angiography to aid in diagnostic and therapeutic considerations.

Treatment

There are no well-established indications or guidelines for treatment. The presence of vitreous hemorrhage or retinal detachment, however, typically warrants treatment. Laser photocoagulation or retinal surgery is typically performed.

Follow-up

- No retinal pathology present: Repeat dilated fundus examination yearly.
- Retinal pathology present: Repeat dilated fundus examination every 1–6 months, depending upon the degree of pathology.

12.24 RETINITIS PIGMENTOSA (RP)

Symptoms

Difficulty with night vision (often night blindness) and loss of peripheral vision are most common. Poor central vision or difficulty with color vision may ensue. Often, relatives have the same problem.

Critical Signs

Classically, clumps of pigment dispersed throughout the peripheral retina in a perivascular pattern, often assuming a "bone spicule" arrangement, areas of depigmentation or atrophy of the retinal pigment epithelium (RPE), narrowing of arterioles, vitreous cells, and later, optic-disc pallor. The diagnosis is confirmed by finding an abnormal or nonrecordable electroretinogram (ERG) and progressive visual field loss (initially, the visual field defect is in the form of a ring scotoma), which may precede fundus findings.

Other Signs

Chicken-track or bone corpuscular retinal pigmentation, focal or sectorial pigment clumping, visual deterioration, cystoid macular edema, epiretinal membrane, posterior subcapsular cataract.

Inheritance

May be autosomal recessive, autosomal dominant, X-linked recessive, or simplex (only one affected member in the pedigree).

Systemic Diseases Associated with Hereditary Retinal Degeneration

There are many systemic diseases and syndromes associated with RP. The following is a short list of conditions that should be considered when evaluating an RP patient, as treatment may be beneficial.

- Refsum's disease   (Autosomal recessive RP with increased serum phytanic acid level. May have ataxia, progressive weakness of distal extremities, deafness, dry skin, anosmia, or progressive restriction of ocular motility.)
- Hereditary abetalipoproteinemia (Bassen-Kornzweig syndrome)   (RP with fat intolerance, diarrhea, crenated erythrocytes [acanthocytes], ataxia, progressive restriction of ocular motility, and other neurologic symptoms as a result of deficiency in lipoproteins and malabsorption of the fat-soluble vitamins A, D, E, and K.)
- Kearns-Sayre syndrome   (Pigmentary degeneration of the retina, often salt-and-pepper in appearance, with normal arterioles, progressive limitation of ocular movement, ptosis, and later, heart block. Ocular signs generally appear before age 20 years. See Section 11.11.)

Differential Diagnosis

DISORDERS THAT PRODUCE A FUNDUS PICTURE SIMILAR TO RP (PSEUDORETINITIS PIGMENTOSA)

- Phenothiazine toxicity   (Especially in patients with taking >800 mg/day of thioridazine.)
- Syphilis   (Positive FTA-ABS, asymmetric visual fields, abnormal fundus appearance, may have a history of recurrent uveitis, no family history of RP; the ERG is generally preserved to some degree.)
- Congenital rubella   (A salt-and-pepper fundus appearance may be accompanied by microphthalmos, cataract, deafness, a congenital heart abnormality, or another systemic abnormality. The ERG is usually normal.)
- Following resolution of an exudative retinal detachment, often from toxemia of pregnancy or Harada's disease   (The history is diagnostic.)
- Pigmented paravenous retinochoroidal atrophy   (Paravenous localization of RPE degeneration and pigment deposition. No definite hereditary pattern. Variable visual fields and ERG. May be nonprogressive, but long-term follow-up is not available.)

DISORDERS THAT PRODUCE NIGHT BLINDNESS

- Gyrate atrophy [The fundus shows well-demarcated, scalloped areas of full-thickness atrophy white-yellow in appearance with thin margins of pigment outlining the areas of atrophy; the changes extend from the periphery toward the macula. Patients have high levels of ornithine in their blood (often 10 times normal levels), urine, aqueous humor, and cerebrospinal fluid. Abnormal or nonrecordable ERG, visual field defects, high myopia, and cataracts are common. Autosomal recessive. See Section 12.26.]
- Choroideremia (Choroidal atrophy accompanies scattered, small pigment granules, sparing the macula. Bone spicules are not seen. X-linked recessive. See Section 12.25.)
- Vitamin A deficiency [Usually acquired from malnutrition or surgical resection of the bowel, but may be inherited (familial carotinemia). Marked night blindness; numerous small, yellow-white, well-demarcated spots deep in the retina seen peripherally; dry eye and/or Bitot's spots (white lesions) on the conjunctiva. See Section 14.10.]
- Congenital stationary night blindness (Night blindness from birth, normal visual fields, may have a normal or abnormal fundus, not progressive. Paradoxical pupillary response.)

Work-up
1. Medical and ocular history pertaining to the diseases discussed previously.
2. Drug history.
3. Family history (for diagnostic and counseling purposes).
4. Ophthalmoscopic examination.
5. Formal visual field testing (e.g., Goldmann's).
6. ERG (may help distinguish stationary rod-cone dysfunction from RP, a progressive disease) and dark adaptation studies.
7. Fundus photographs.
8. FTA-ABS if the diagnosis is uncertain.
9. If the patient is male and the type of inheritance is unknown, examine his mother and perform an ERG on her (women carriers of X-linked disease often have abnormal pigmentation in the midperiphery and have abnormal dark-adapted ERGs.)
10. If neurological abnormalities such as ataxia, polyneuropathy, deafness, or anosmia are present, obtain a fasting (at least 14 hours) serum phytanic acid level to rule out Refsum's disease.
11. If hereditary abetalipoproteinemia is suspected, obtain a serum cholesterol and triglyceride level (levels are low), a serum protein and lipoprotein electrophoresis (lipoprotein deficiency is detected), and peripheral blood smears (acanthocytosis is seen).
12. If Kearns-Sayre syndrome is suspected, the patient must be examined by

a cardiologist with sequential electrocardiograms, checking for a cardiac conduction abnormality.

Treatment/Follow-up

See "Choroideremia," Section 12.25; "Gyrate Atrophy," Section 12.26; "Acquired Syphilis," Section 14.2; and "Vitamin A Deficiency," Section 14.10 if these conditions are suspected. No effective treatment for RP is currently known. However, there may be an effective treatment for some of the systemic conditions mentioned previously. All patients will benefit from genetic counseling and instruction on how to deal with their visual handicap. In advanced cases, low-vision aids and vocational rehabilitation are helpful.

REFSUM'S DISEASE

1. Place on a low–phytanic acid, low-phytol diet (minimize the amount of milk products, animal fats, and green leafy vegetables in the patient's diet).
2. Examine serum phytanic acid levels every 6 months.

HEREDITARY ABETALIPOPROTEINEMIA

1. Water-miscible vitamin A 10,000–15,000 IU po daily.
2. Vitamin E 200–300 IU/kg po daily.
3. Vitamin K 5 mg po weekly.
4. Restrict dietary fat to 15% of caloric intake.
5. Biannual serum levels of vitamin A and E; yearly ERG, dark adaptometry, and prothrombin time; periodic nerve conduction studies.
6. Consider supplementing the patient's diet with zinc.

KEARNS-SAYRE SYNDROME

Refer the patient to a cardiologist for yearly electrocardiograms. Patients may need a pacemaker.

12.25 CHOROIDEREMIA

Symptoms

Night blindness in male patients 4–30 years of age, followed by insidious loss of peripheral vision. Decreased central vision occurs late in the disease. Women are asymptomatic carriers.

Critical Signs

Males Dispersed pigment granules throughout the fundus accompanied by atrophy of the choroid, sparing the macula. The choroidal vasculature is not well seen despite a light fundus background.

Females Small, scattered, square intraretinal pigment granules overlying choroidal atrophy, most marked in the midperiphery.

Other Signs

Retinal arteriolar narrowing and optic atrophy can occur late in the process; constriction of visual fields, normal color vision, abnormal electroretinogram (ERG).

Inheritance

X-linked recessive.

Differential Diagnosis

- Retinitis pigmentosa (No choroidal atrophy, may see bone spicules of pigment. See Section 12.24.)
- Gyrate atrophy (Scalloped RPE and choriocapillaris atrophy, posterior subcapsular cataract, high myopia with astigmatism, hyperornithinemia. Autosomal recessive. See Section 12.26.)
- Albinism (Blond fundus without RPE clumping; the choroidal vasculature is easily seen. Iris transillumination defects are present, and the foveal reflex is absent. See Section 14.7.)
- Thioridazine (e.g., Mellaril) retinopathy (Patients taking >800 mg/day of thioridazine. See Section 12.29.)

Work-up

1. History: Family history? Medications?
2. Dilated fundus examination of the patient's mother and other family members if possible.
3. Formal visual fields (e.g., Octopus, Humphrey).
4. ERG with or without dark-adaptation studies.
5. Fluorescein angiography may be diagnostic.

Treatment

No effective treatment for this condition is currently available. The following may be helpful in management.

1. Darkly tinted sunglasses may ameliorate symptoms.
2. Genetic counseling.

12.26 GYRATE ATROPHY

Symptoms
Decreased vision, night blindness.

Critical Signs
Multiple sharply defined areas of chorioretinal atrophy separated from each other by thin margins of pigment. The lesions begin in the midperiphery in childhood and then coalesce to involve the entire fundus, sparing the fovea until late in the disease, usually in midlife. Ornithine levels are markedly elevated in all body fluids.

Other Signs
Posterior subcapsular cataract, high myopia, and astigmatism; optic-disc pallor and narrowing of the retinal vessels appear later in the disease. Constriction of visual fields and abnormal-to-nonrecordable electroretinogram (ERG), electro-oculogram, and dark-adaptation studies occur. Color vision typically remains relatively intact until late in the course of the disease. Carriers have normal fundi, but may have mild elevation of ornithine levels.

Inheritance
Autosomal recessive.

Differential Diagnosis
All of the following can be distinguished by the presence of normal ornithine levels.

- Paving stone degeneration   (Patches of chorioretinal atrophy limited to the retinal periphery, usually inferiorly.)
- Choroideremia   (Diffuse retinal pigment epithelial and choroidal atrophy spread throughout the fundus. X-linked recessive. See Section 12.25.)
- High myopia   (Chorioretinal atrophy, most marked in the posterior pole, often with a staphyloma. See Section 12.12.)
- Thioridazine retinopathy   (Patient taking >800 mg/day of thioridazine. See Section 12.29.)

Work-up
1. Family history: Check for night blindness or severely decreased vision.
2. Dilated fundus examination.
3. Plasma ornithine and amino acid levels (expect ornithine to be 6–10 times normal).
4. Consider ERG and fluorescein angiography if the ornithine level is not markedly elevated.

Treatment

1. Supplemental vitamin B$_6$ (pyridoxine). The dose is not currently established—can try 20 mg/day po initially and increase up to 500 mg/day po if there is no response.

❖ **Note** *Only a small percentage of patients are vitamin B$_6$ responders.*

2. Reduce dietary protein consumption and substitute artificially flavored solutions of essential amino acids without arginine.

Follow-up

- Frequent serum ornithine levels are obtained initially to determine the amount of supplemental vitamin B$_6$ and the degree to which dietary protein needs to be restricted. Serum ornithine levels between 0.15–0.20 mM are optimal. The frequency of blood tests may be reduced after the ornithine levels stabilize in this range.
- Serum ammonia levels are followed in patients restricting dietary arginine.

12.27 CONE DYSTROPHIES

Symptoms

Slowly progressive bilateral visual loss, photophobia, and poor color vision. Vision is worse during the day than at night.

Critical Signs

Early Essentially, a normal fundus examination, even with poor visual acuity. Abnormal cone function on the electroretinogram (ERG) (i.e., a reduced single-flash photopic response and a reduced flicker response).
Late Bull's-eye macular appearance or central geographic atrophy of the retinal pigment epithelium (RPE) and choriocapillaris.

Other Signs

Nystagmus, temporal pallor of the optic disc, spotty pigment clumping in the macular area, tapetal-like retinal sheen. Rarely, rod degeneration may ensue, leading to a retinitis pigmentosa–like picture (i.e., a cone-rod degeneration, which may have an autosomal dominant inheritance pattern).

Inheritance

Usually sporadic. Hereditary forms are usually autosomal dominant, but autosomal recessive and X-linked also occur.

Differential Diagnosis

- Stargardt's disease or fundus flavimaculatus   (Bilateral visual loss in the first or second decades of life often precedes the fundus findings, normal night vision and peripheral visual fields, macular atrophy with accompanying yellow flecks may develop. A normal ERG is usually present in the early stage. Primarily autosomal recessive. See Section 12.28.)
- Chloroquine retinopathy   (May produce a bull's-eye macular appearance and poor color vision. History of chloroquine or hydroxychloroquine use, no family history of cone degeneration, no nystagmus. See Section 12.30.)
- Central areolar choroidal dystrophy   (Geographic atrophy of the RPE with normal photopic ERG.)
- Age-related macular degeneration   (Can have geographic atrophy of the RPE, but with normal color vision and photopic ERG. See Section 12.10.)
- Congenital color blindness   (Normal visual acuity, onset at birth, not progressive.)
- Retinitis pigmentosa   (Night blindness and peripheral visual field loss are the first symptoms. Often peripheral retinal bone spicules are seen. Can be distinguished by dark-adaptation testing and ERG. See Section 12.24.)
- Optic neuropathy or atrophy (Decreased acuity, impaired color vision, temporal and/or diffuse optic-disc pallor. May have a positive family history. See Sections 11.16, 11.17 and 11.18.)
- Nonphysiologic visual loss   [Normal ophthalmoscopic examination, fluorescein angiogram (FA), ERG, and electro-oculogram. Patients can often be tricked into seeing better by special testing. See Section 11.22.]

Work-up

1. Family history.
2. Complete ophthalmic examination, including color plates and formal color testing (e.g., Farnsworth-Munsell 100-hue test, red test object for chloroquine).
3. Formal visual field test (e.g., Humphrey, Octopus).
4. ERG.
5. FA to help detect the bull's-eye macular pattern.

Treatment

There is no proven cure for this disease. The following measures may be palliative:

1. Heavily tinted glasses or contact lenses may help maximize vision.
2. Miotic drops (e.g., pilocarpine 0.5–1% qid during the day) are occasionally tried to improve vision and reduce photophobia.
3. Genetic counseling.
4. Low-vision aids as needed.

Follow-up

Yearly.

12.28 STARGARDT'S DISEASE
(FUNDUS FLAVIMACULATUS)

Symptoms

Usually bilateral decreased vision in childhood or young adulthood. In the early stages, the decrease in vision is often out of proportion to the clinical ophthalmoscopic appearance.

Critical Signs

Any of the following may be present.

A. A relatively normal-appearing fundus except for a heavily pigmented retinal pigment epithelium (RPE).
B. Yellow or yellow-white flecklike deposits at the level of the RPE, usually in a pisciform (fish-tail) configuration.
C. Atrophic macular degeneration: May have a bull's-eye appearance as a result of atrophy of the RPE around a normal central core of RPE, a "beaten-metal" appearance, pigment clumping, or marked geographic atrophy.

Other Signs

Atrophy of the RPE just outside of the macula or in the midperipheral fundus, normal peripheral visual fields in most cases, and rarely an accompanying cone or rod dystrophy. The electroretinogram (ERG) is typically normal in the early stages, but may become abnormal late in the disease. The electrooculogram (EOG) is usually normal.

Inheritance

Usually autosomal recessive, rarely autosomal dominant.

Differential Diagnosis

- Fundus albipunctatus   (Diffuse, small, white, discrete dots, most prominent in the midperipheral fundus and rarely present in the fovea; nonprogressive congenital night blindness; no atrophic macular degeneration or pigmentary changes. Visual acuity and visual fields remain normal.)
- Retinitis punctata albescens   (Similar clinical appearance to fundus albipunctatus, but visual acuity, visual field, and night blindness progressively worsen. A markedly abnormal ERG develops.)
- Drusen   (Small, yellow-white spots deep to the retina, sometimes calcified, usually developing later in life. Fluorescein angiography (FA) helps distinguish: All drusen hyperfluoresce, whereas some lesions of fundus flavimaculatus do and some lesions do not hyperfluoresce, and some areas without flecks show hyperfluorescence.)

- Cone or cone-rod dystrophy   (May have a bull's-eye macula, but have a significant color vision deficit and a characteristic ERG. See Section 12.27.)
- Chloroquine/hydroxychloroquine maculopathy   (History of use of this medication. Dose-related. See Section 12.30.)
- Nonphysiologic visual loss   (Normal ophthalmoscopic examination, FA, ERG, and EOG. Patients can often be tricked into seeing better by special testing. See Section 11.22.)

Work-up
Indicated when the diagnosis is uncertain or needs to be confirmed.

1. History: Age at onset, medications, family history?
2. Dilated retinal examination.
3. FA often shows blockage of choroidal fluorescence producing a "silent choroid" or "midnight fundus" as a result of increased lipofuscin in the RPE cells.
4. ERG and EOG.
5. Formal visual field examination (e.g., Octopus, Humphrey).

Treatment
No known medical or surgical therapy is beneficial. The patient may benefit from low-vision aids, services dedicated to helping the visually handicapped, and genetic counseling.

12.29 PHENOTHIAZINE TOXICITY

A. Thioridazine (e.g., Mellaril)

Symptoms
Blurred vision, brownish vision, difficulty with night vision.

Signs
Pigment clumps between the posterior pole and the equator, areas of retinal depigmentation, retinal edema, visual field abnormalities (central scotoma and general constriction), depressed or extinguished electroretinogram (ERG).

❖ **Note** *Symptoms and signs may occur within weeks of starting phenothiazine therapy, particularly if very large doses (>2000 mg/day) are taken.*

Dosage Generally Required to Produce Toxicity
800 mg/day chronically.

Differential Diagnosis
(Pigment clumps in the retina.)

- Retinitis pigmentosa   (Positive family history, pale optic disc, narrowed arterioles. See Section 12.24.)
- Old syphilitic chorioretinopathy   (Positive FTA-ABS, may have a history of an acute visual problem.)
- Viral chorioretinitis   (Often associated with an anterior-chamber reaction, vitreous cells, and other ocular signs.)
- Trauma   (Usually unilateral, history of trauma.)

Treatment
Discontinue the medication.

Baseline Work-up
(For patients in whom long-term treatment is anticipated.)

1. Visual acuity.
2. Complete ophthalmoscopic examination.
3. Fundus photographs.
4. Visual field, preferably automated (e.g., Humphrey, Octopus, with or without a red test object).
5. Consider ERG.
6. Color vision testing, preferably with a Farnsworth-Munsell 100-hue test.

Follow-up
Every 6 months.

B. Chlorpromazine (e.g., Thorazine)

Symptoms
Blurred vision or none.

Signs
Abnormal pigmentation of the eyelids, cornea, conjunctiva (especially within the palpebral fissure), and anterior-lens capsule; anterior and posterior subcapsular cataract; rarely, a pigmentary retinopathy with the visual field and ERG changes described for thioridazine.

Dosage Generally Required to Produce Toxicity
1200–2400 mg/day for longer than 12 months.

Treatment
Discontinue the medication if vision is affected.

Baseline Work-up
Same as for thioridazine.

Follow-up
Every 6 months.

12.30 CHLOROQUINE/HYDROXYCHLOROQUINE TOXICITY

Symptoms
Decreased vision, abnormal color vision, difficulty adjusting to darkness.

Critical Signs
Bull's-eye macula (a ring of depigmentation surrounded by a ring of increased pigmentation), loss of the foveal reflex.

Other Signs
Increased pigmentation in the macula, arteriolar narrowing, vascular sheathing, peripheral pigmentation, decreased color vision, visual field abnormalities (central, paracentral, or peripheral scotoma), abnormal ERG and EOG, and normal dark adaptation. Whorl-like corneal changes may also be observed.

Dosage Generally Required to Produce Toxicity
Chloroquine: >300 g total cumulative dose.
Hydroxychloroquine: >750 mg/day taken over months to years.

(Some feel that retinopathy will not develop if the daily dose is kept <4.4 mg/kg/day of chloroquine and 7.7 mg/kg/day of hydroxychloroquine.)

Differential Diagnosis
The following can produce a bull's-eye macula.

- Cone dystrophy   (Positive family history, generally <30 years old, severe

photophobia, abnormal to nonrecordable photopic ERG. See Section 12.27.)
- Stargardt's disease/fundus flavimaculatus   (Positive family history, generally <25 years old, may have white-yellow flecks in the posterior pole and midperiphery. See Section 12.28.)
- Age-related macular degeneration   (Drusen; pigment clumping and atrophy and detachment of the retinal pigment epithelium or sensory retina may or may not occur. See Section 12.10.)
- Spielmeyer-Vogt syndrome   (Retinitis pigmentosa, seizures, ataxia, and progressive dementia.)

Treatment
Discontinue the medication if signs of toxicity develop.

Baseline Work-up
(For patients in whom long-term treatment is anticipated.)

1. Visual acuity.
2. Ophthalmoscopic examination.
3. Posterior-pole fundus photographs.
4. Visual field, preferably automated (e.g., Humphrey, Octopus, with or without red test object).
5. Color vision testing, preferably Farnsworth-Munsell 100-hue test.

Follow-up
Every 6 months.

❖ **Note** *Once ocular toxicity develops, it usually does not regress even if the drug is withdrawn. In fact, new toxic effects may develop, and old ones may progress even after the chloroquine/hydroxychloroquine has been discontinued.*

12.31 BEST'S DISEASE
(VITELLIFORM MACULAR DYSTROPHY)

Symptoms
Decreased vision or asymptomatic. Onset at birth, but may not be detected until years later.

Critical Signs
Yellow, round, subretinal lesion(s) likened to an egg yolk or in some cases to a pseudohypopyon. Typically bilateral and located in the fovea, measuring

approximately one to two disc areas in size. Ten percent of lesions are multiple and extrafoveal. Normal electroretinogram (ERG), abnormal electro-oculogram (EOG).

Other Signs

The lesions may degenerate, and macular choroidal neovascularization, hemorrhage, and scarring may develop. In the scar stage, it may be indistinguishable from age-related macular degeneration (ARMD).

Inheritance

Autosomal dominant with variable penetrance and expression. Carriers may have normal fundi but an abnormal EOG.

Work-up

1. Family history (often helpful to examine family members).
2. Complete ocular examination, including a dilated retinal examination, carefully inspecting the macula with a slit lamp and a fundus contact, Hruby, or 60- or 90-diopter lens.
3. EOG to confirm the diagnosis or to detect the carrier state of the disease.
4. Consider fluorescein angiography to confirm the presence of or delineate a choroidal neovascular membrane.

Treatment

There is no effective treatment for the underlying disease. Choroidal neovascularization may need to be treated by laser photocoagulation, but is not as devastating as in ARMD.

Follow-up

Patients with treatable CNVM should be attended to promptly. Otherwise, there is no urgency in seeing patients with this disease. Patients are given an Amsler's grid (see Appendix 3), instructed on its use, and told to return immediately if a change is noted.

❖ **Note** *An adult form of vitelliform macular dystrophy (a "pattern dystrophy") has been described. The egg-yolk lesions usually appear from age 30–50 years, the disease is dominantly inherited, and the EOG may or may not be abnormal. There is also no effective treatment for this entity.*

UVEITIS

13.1 ANTERIOR UVEITIS
(IRITIS/IRIDOCYCLITIS)

Symptoms
    Acute   Pain, red eye, photophobia, mild decreased vision, tearing.
    Chronic   Recurrent episodes, fewer or none of the acute symptoms.

Critical Signs
    Cells and flare in the anterior chamber.

Differentiating Signs
    Nongranulomatous   Fine keratic precipitates (KP) (white cells on the corneal
       endothelium).
    Granulomatous   Large "mutton-fat" KP, Koeppe's nodules (clusters of cells
       on the pupillary border), Busacca's nodules (clusters of cells on the anterior
       iris surface).

Other Signs
    Cells in the anterior vitreous (spillover), posterior synechiae (adhesions of the
iris to the lens), miosis, low intraocular pressure (IOP) but occasionally elevated, injection of the perilimbal blood vessels, hypopyon (layering of white
cells in the anterior chamber) if severe, cystoid macular edema if chronic,
occasionally a cataract.

❖ **Note** *Patients will often complain of increased pain in the involved eye when
light is shined in the uninvolved eye.*

The Wills Eye Manual: Office and Emergency Room Diagnosis and Treatment of Eye Diseases,
Second Edition, edited by R. Douglas Cullom, Jr., M.D., and Benjamin Chang, M.D. © 1994 J. B.
Lippincott Company.

Etiology

ACUTE, NONGRANULOMATOUS

- Trauma (see "Traumatic Iritis," Section 3.7)
- Ankylosing spondylitis (Young adult men, often with low back pain, abnormal sacroiliac spine x-rays, elevated ESR, positive HLA B27.)
- Inflammatory bowel disease (Chronic intermittent diarrhea, often alternating with constipation.)
- Reiter's syndrome (Young adult men, conjunctivitis, urethritis, polyarthritis, occasionally keratitis, elevated ESR, positive HLA B27, may have recurrent episodes.)
- Psoriatic arthritis (Iritis is not associated with psoriasis without arthritis.)
- Glaucomatocyclitic crisis (Recurrent episodes of acute IOP rise, open angle on gonioscopy, corneal edema, fine KP, fixed mid-dilated pupil, and mild iritis. See Section 10.12.)
- Lens-induced uveitis (Often after incomplete extracapsular cataract extraction or trauma damaging the lens capsule; may also be secondary to a hypermature cataract.)
- Herpes simplex/herpes zoster/varicella (Usually with a dendritic keratitis, occasionally skin vesicles, glaucoma, iris atrophy.)
- Postoperative iritis (An anterior-chamber reaction is expected after intraocular surgery. Severe reactions with excessive pain, however, must make the examiner consider endophthalmitis. See "Postoperative Uveitis," Section 13.9.)
- UGH syndrome (uveitis-glaucoma-hyphema) (Usually secondary to irritation from an intraocular lens.)
- Behçet's disease (Young adults, acute hypopyon, iritis, aphthous mouth ulcers, genital ulcerations, erythema nodosum, positive Behçet's skin-puncture test if active systemic disease is present, often retinal vasculitis and hemorrhages, may have recurrent episodes.)
- Lyme disease (Often a history of a tick bite. May have a skin rash and/or arthritis. See Section 14.4.)
- Mumps, influenza, adenovirus, measles, chlamydia (Rare causes of transient anterior uveitis.)
- Other rare causes of anterior uveitis (Tight contact lens, leptospirosis, Kawasaki's disease, rickettsial disease.)

CHRONIC, USUALLY NONGRANULOMATOUS

- Juvenile rheumatoid arthritis (JRA) [Usually young girls, eye may be white and without pain, often bilateral, iritis can occur before the arthritis, pauciarticular arthritis (fewer than 5 joints involved), positive ANA, negative rheumatoid factor, elevated ESR, occasionally fever and lymphadenopathy.]

- Chronic iridocyclitis of children (Usually young girls, same as JRA except no arthritis.)
- Fuchs' heterochromic iridocyclitis (Usually unilateral, few symptoms, diffuse iris stromal atrophy often causing a lighter colored iris, iris transillumination defects, blunting of the iris architecture, fine KP over the *entire* corneal endothelium, mild anterior-chamber reaction, few if any posterior synechiae. Vitreous opacities, glaucoma, and cataracts are common.)

CHRONIC, USUALLY GRANULOMATOUS

- Sarcoidosis [Usually African-American, usually bilateral; may have dense posterior synechiae, conjunctival nodules, or signs of posterior uveitis (see Section 13.2). Mild-to-moderate anergy, an abnormal chest x-ray, positive gallium scan, and elevated serum angiotensin converting enzyme (ACE) are common. See Section 13.4.]
- Syphilis [May have a maculopapular rash (often on the palms and soles), iris roseola (vascular papules on the iris), and interstitial keratitis with ghost vessels in late stages. A positive VDRL or RPR and positive FTA-ABS are usually present. See Section 14.2.]
- Tuberculosis [Positive PPD, typical chest x-ray, occasionally phlyctenular keratitis, sometimes signs of posterior uveitis (see Section 13.2).]
- Others [Rare (e.g., leprosy, brucellosis).]

Differential Diagnosis
The following may be associated with an anterior-chamber reaction.

- Rhegmatogenous retinal detachment (Elevated retina with a retinal break, pigment cells in the vitreous or anterior chamber. See Section 12.19.)
- Posterior segment tumor (e.g., retinoblastoma or leukemia in children, malignant melanoma in adults. See Section 8.3.)
- Juvenile xanthogranuloma (Age <15 years, often with a spontaneous hyphema, yellow-gray poorly demarcated iris nodule or nodules, and slightly raised orange skin lesions.)
- Intraocular foreign body
- Sclerouveitis (Uveitis secondary to scleritis.)

Work-up
1. Obtain a history, attempting to define the etiology.
2. Complete ocular examination, including an IOP check and a dilated fundus examination. The vitreous should be evaluated for cells (see Appendix 8).

If a unilateral, nongranulomatous uveitis develops for the first time *and* the history and examination are unremarkable, then no further work-up is pursued.

If the uveitis is bilateral, granulomatous, *or* recurrent and the history and examination are unremarkable, then a nonspecific initial work-up is conducted:

3. Complete blood count (CBC).
4. ESR.
5. ANA.
6. RPR or VDRL.
7. FTA-ABS or MHA-TP.
8. PPD and anergy panel.
9. Chest x-ray, especially to rule out sarcoidosis and tuberculosis.
10. In endemic areas, a Lyme titer is recommended (see the following).
11. Consider HLA-B27.

If the history, symptoms, and/or signs point strongly to a certain etiology, then the work-up should be tailored accordingly:

- Ankylosing spondylitis: Sacroiliac spine x-rays show sclerosis and narrowing of the joint spaces, ESR, consider an HLA B27.
- Inflammatory bowel disease: Medical or gastrointestinal consult, consider an HLA B27.
- Reiter's syndrome: Conjunctival, urethral, and prostatic cultures if indicated; joint x-rays if arthritis is present; a medical or rheumatology consult; consider an HLA B27.
- Psoriatic arthritis: A rheumatology or dermatology consult, consider an HLA B27.
- Glaucomatocyclitic crisis: Diagnosed clinically.
- Lens-induced uveitis: Diagnosed clinically. See "Phacolytic Glaucoma," Section 10.8; "Lens-Particle Glaucoma," Section 10.9; and "Phacoanaphylactic Endophthalmitis," Section 13.14.
- Herpes: Diagnosed clinically.
- UGH: Diagnosed clinically.
- Behçet's disease: Behçet's skin-puncture test (if a blister develops minutes to hours after puncturing the skin intradermally with a sterile 25- to 30-gauge needle, a positive test is noted), a medical or rheumatology consult, consider an HLA B27 or HLA B5.
- Lyme disease: Lyme immunofluorescent assay or enzyme-linked immunosorbent assay.
- JRA: ANA, rheumatoid factor, x-rays of arthritic joints (if no arthritic symptoms are present, then x-rays of the knees are obtained), and a pediatric or rheumatology consult.
- Chronic iridocyclitis of children: Same as JRA.
- Fuchs' heterochromic iridocyclitis: Diagnosed clinically.
- Sarcoidosis: Chest x-ray, ACE, serum lysozyme and a PPD and anergy panel, gallium scan of the head and neck; consider a biopsy of any skin or

conjunctival nodule for pathological diagnosis (see "Sarcoidosis," Section 13.4).

❖ **Note** *ACE and gallium scans may give false-negative results if the patient is taking systemic steroids.*

- Syphilis: RPR or VDRL, FTA-ABS or MHA-TP.
- Tuberculosis: PPD and anergy panel, chest x-ray, referral to a medical specialist.

Treatment

1. Cycloplegic (e.g., cyclopentolate 1–2% tid for mild-to-moderate inflammation; scopolamine 0.25% or atropine 1% tid for moderate-to-severe inflammation).
2. Topical steroid (e.g., prednisolone acetate 1% q 1–6 h depending on the severity).

   If the anterior uveitis is severe and is not responding well to frequent topical steroids, then consider periocular repository steroids (e.g., methylprednisolone 40–80 mg subtenons). Before injecting depot steroids periocularly, it is wise to use topical steroids at full strength for 6 weeks to make certain that the patient is not a steroid responder (i.e., develops a significant IOP rise secondary to steroids). See Appendix 7, which describes the technique of a subtenons injection.

   If there is no improvement on maximal topical and repository steroids, then consider systemic steroids or lastly, systemic immunosuppressive agents. A medical or rheumatology consult is often advisable when systemic therapy is to be instituted. See medical glossary for a systemic steroid work-up.

3. Treat secondary glaucoma. Glaucoma may result from:
   a. A severe inflammatory reaction with cellular blockage of the trabecular meshwork. See "Inflammatory Open-Angle Glaucoma," Section 10.4.
   b. Synechiae formation giving rise to secondary angle-closure. See "Acute Angle-Closure Glaucoma," Section 10.10.
   c. Neovascularization of the iris producing blockage of the trabecular meshwork or closure of the angle. See "Neovascular Glaucoma," Section 10.13.
   d. A response to steroids. See "Steroid-Response Glaucoma," Section 10.5.
4. If an exact etiology for the anterior uveitis is determined, then the specific management outlined below should be added to the above treatment.
   Ankylosing spondylitis Often requires systemic antiinflammatory agents (e.g., aspirin, indomethacin). Consider cardiology consult (there is a high incidence of heart block and aortic insufficiency), rheumatology consult, and physical therapy consult.

Inflammatory bowel disease   Often benefits from systemic steroids and/
or sulfadiazine and supplemental vitamin A. Consider a medical or
gastrointestinal consult.

Reiter's syndrome   If urethritis is present, then the patient and sexual
partners are treated (e.g., tetracycline 250–500 mg qid, doxycycline 100
mg bid, or erythromycin 250–500 mg qid for 3–4 weeks). Obtain medical,
rheumatology, and/or physical therapy consult.

Psoriatic arthritis   Consider a rheumatology consult.

Glaucomatocyclitic crisis   See Section 10.12.

Lens-induced uveitis   Usually requires removal of lens material, see "Phacolytic Glaucoma" Section 10.8; "Lens-Particle Glaucoma," Section
10.9; and "Phacoanaphylactic Endophthalmitis," Section 13.14.

Herpes uveitis   See "Herpes Simplex Virus," Section 4.15; or "Herpes
Zoster Virus," Section 4.16.

UGH   See "Postoperative Glaucoma," Section 10.15.

Behçet's disease   Often needs systemic steroids or immunosuppressive
agents (responds well to chlorambucil); consider a medical or rheumatology consult.

Lyme disease   See Section 14.4.

JRA   The steroid dosage is adjusted according to the degree of cells, not
flare, present in the anterior chamber; chronic cycloplegic therapy (e.g.,
tropicamide 0.5% qhs) may be required. A rheumatology or pediatric
consult for possible aspirin or systemic steroid therapy is usually obtained.

❖ **Note** *There is a high complication rate with cataract surgery.*

Chronic iridocyclitis of children   Same as JRA.

Fuchs' heterochromic iridocyclitis   Usually does not respond to nor require steroids (a trial of steroids may be attempted, but they should be
tapered quickly if there is no response); cycloplegics are rarely necessary.

❖ **Note** *Patients usually do well with cataract surgery.*

Sarcoidosis   Often needs periocular and systemic steroids; a medicine or
pulmonary consult is advisable for systemic evaluation (see Section
13.4).

Syphilis   See "Acquired Syphilis," Section 14.2; or "Congenital Syphilis," Section 14.3.

Tuberculosis   Refer the patient to an internist for consideration of systemic
antituberculous treatment.

Follow-up

Every 1–7 days in the acute phase, depending on the severity; every 1–6
months chronically when stable. At each visit, the anterior-chamber reaction
and IOP should be evaluated. A vitreous and fundus examination should be

performed for all flare-ups, when vision is affected, or every 3–6 months. If the anterior-chamber reaction is improving, then the steroid drops can be slowly tapered [usually 1 drop per day every 3–7 days (e.g., qid for 1 week, then tid for 1 week, then bid for 1 week]. Steroids are usually discontinued once all cells have disappeared from the anterior chamber (flare is often still present). Rarely, chronic low-dose steroids every day or every other day are required to keep the inflammation from recurring. The cycloplegic agents can also be tapered as the anterior-chamber reaction improves. Slow tapering is advised for granulomatous reactions because of a higher tendency to form posterior synechiae. Cycloplegics should be used at least qhs until the anterior chamber is free of cells.

❖ **Note** *As with most ocular and systemic diseases requiring steroid therapy, the steroid (be it topical or systemic) should never be discontinued abruptly. Sudden discontinuation of steroids can lead to severe rebound inflammation.*

13.2 POSTERIOR UVEITIS

Symptoms
Blurred vision, floaters; occasionally redness, pain, and photophobia.

Critical Signs
White blood cells and opacities in the vitreous (vitritis), retinal or choroidal infiltrates, edema, vascular sheathing.

Other Signs
Disc swelling, retinal hemorrhages or exudates, or signs of anterior-segment inflammation (e.g., aqueous cells and flare, posterior synechiae) may be present. Glaucoma, cataract, choroidal neovascularization, or retinal detachment may develop.

Etiology
A. More common
   • Toxoplasmosis   [A yellow-white, fuzzy retinal lesion, commonly in the posterior pole. It may be difficult to see the lesion because of a severe accompanying vitritis. A chorioretinal scar is frequently seen adjacent to the acute, active lesion. May be associated with retinal vascular occlusive disease. A negative anti-toxoplasma antibody titer (undiluted) in an immunocompetent host usually rules out toxoplasmosis. See Section 13.3.]

- Sarcoidosis [White-yellow exudates or sheathing around retinal veins, retinal or vitreous white nodules, and other retinal or choroidal abnormalities may be present. Vitritis and granulomatous uveitis are common. Patients are typically African-American and often have pulmonary, skin, central nervous system (CNS), or other systemic involvement. An elevated angiotensin converting enzyme (ACE) level is often present. See Section 13.4.]
- Syphilis (Produces an acute chorioretinitis and vitritis that may mimic almost any other condition. A concomitant skin rash on the palms, soles, or both may be present. Retinal pigment clumping, sometimes similar to retinitis pigmentosa, may later occur. May be associated with retinal vascular occlusive disease. Congenital syphilis typically produces a salt-and-pepper fundus. Positive FTA-ABS. See Sections 14.2 and 14.3.)
- Pars planitis [Considered an intermediate uveitis. Usually a bilateral vitritis in patients age 15–40 years with white exudative material covering the inferior ora serrata and pars plana. Cellular clumps in the vitreous (appearing as "snowballs") and peripheral vascular sheathing may be present. See Section 13.5.]
- Ocular histoplasmosis (Common in the Ohio-Mississippi River Valley area. Yellow-white choroidal spots, usually <1 mm in diameter, macular degenerative changes, sometimes with choroidal neovascularization, and peripapillary atrophy or scarring is seen. Minimal-to-no vitreous nor aqueous cells are seen. See Section 12.11.)

B. Following surgery or trauma: See "Postoperative Uveitis," Section 13.9; "Postoperative Endophthalmitis," Section 13.10; "Traumatic Endophthalmitis," Section 13.11; and "Sympathetic Ophthalmia," Section 13.15.

C. Immunocompromised host (e.g., AIDS, patients being treated with chemotherapy)
- Cytomegalovirus (CMV) (Yellow-white patches of necrotic retina are mixed with retinal hemorrhage. Also seen in neonates. See "Acquired Immunodeficiency Syndrome," Section 14.1.)
- Candida (Seen also in hospitalized patients being treated with prolonged antibiotic therapy, IV drug abusers, and patients with long-standing catheters. Yellow-white, fluffy, retinal or preretinal lesions are found initially. Later, associated "cotton balls" develop in the vitreous. Candida may be cultured from the blood, urine, or an IV site.)
- Herpetic retinitis (Clinically similar to acute retinal necrosis, but may not have vitreous cells and may spare retinal vessels. May involve deep retina. Rapidly progressive. Treat like acute retinal necrosis.
- Endogenous endophthalmitis (Patients are typically septic, and many have an anterior-chamber reaction or hypopyon in addition to the vitritis. See Section 13.12.)

- Others (Herpes simplex, varicella-zoster, fungi, mycobacteria, others.)

D. Less common

- Acute posterior multifocal placoid pigment epitheliopathy (AMP-PE) (Acute visual loss, typically in young adults, sometimes following a viral illness. Multiple creamy-white subretinal lesions with indistinct margins approximately one half of the disc diameter in size are usually found in the posterior poles of both eyes. Vitreous cells, disc edema, serous retinal detachment, and rarely CNS signs may be present. Vision usually returns to normal in 2–6 weeks.)
- Acute retinal necrosis (Unilateral or bilateral multiple opaque white patches of thickened retina with vascular sheathing, usually in the retinal periphery. The patches of necrotic retina gradually enlarge and coalesce. Vitreous cells are abundant. May have a retinal detachment. See Section 13.6.)
- Acute retinal pigment epitheliitis (Krill's disease) (Young adults with sudden visual loss. Gray spots are seen at the level of the retinal pigment epithelium in the macula, each of which is surrounded by a lighter-colored halo. The spots occur in 2–4 distinct clusters. The condition may be unilateral or bilateral. It resolves in 6–12 weeks without treatment.)
- Behçet's disease (Usually a bilateral ocular disease of young adult men. Retinal and optic-disc edema, vascular sheathing, and occasionally hemorrhages or exudate may accompany a vitritis and anterior uveitis, sometimes with a hypopyon. The eye is typically not red. Recurrent oral and/or genital ulcers, erythema nodosum, or arthritis may be noted. See "Anterior Uveitis," Section 13.1.)
- Birdshot (vitiliginous) retinochoroidopathy (Usually middle-aged adults with bilateral multiple creamy-yellow spots deep to the retina, approximately 1 mm in diameter, scattered around the equator of the fundus. With time, the spots coalesce and spread to the macula. Vitreous cells are more abundant than aqueous cells. Retinal and/or optic-nerve edema may be present. Positive HLA A29 in most patients. Visual loss appears to be irreversible.)
- Diffuse unilateral subacute neuroretinitis (Unilateral visual loss in children and young adults, thought to be caused by a nematode. Optic-nerve swelling, vitreous cells, and deep gray-white retinal lesion are present initially. Later, optic atrophy, narrowing of retinal vessels, and atrophic pigment epithelial changes develop. Vision and visual fields deteriorate with time.)
- Embolic retinitis [Sudden onset of decreased vision in a systemically ill patient. Retinal edema, vascular sheathing, and hemorrhages with

white centers (Roth's spots) may be accompanied by vitreous cells. Diseased heart valves are common sources.]

- Lyme disease (Produces varied forms of posterior uveitis. More common in New England and Middle Atlantic states, particularly in patients who camp outdoors. A history of a tick bite, skin rash, Bell's palsy, or arthritis may be elicited. See Section 14.4.)

- Multiple evanescent white-dot syndrome (Acute unilateral visual loss, often following a viral illness, usually in young women. May be bilateral or sequential. Multiple creamy-white lesions at the level of the retinal pigment epithelium are accompanied by a granularity of the fovea. There are few vitreous cells and occasional sheathing of retinal vessels. There is often an enlarged blind spot on formal visual field testing. Vision typically returns to normal within weeks without treatment.)

- Recurrent multifocal choroiditis (multifocal choroiditis with panuveitis) [Unilateral visual loss in young women, who often have bilateral fundus involvement. Multiple, small, round, pale inflammatory lesions at the level of the pigment epithelium and choriocapillaris are found (similar to "histo-spots"), sometimes associated with choroidal neovascularization. Vitreous cells, mild disc edema, and less commonly, anterior-chamber cells and flare may be present. The lesions are predominantly in the macular area and frequently respond to oral or periocular steroids, but typically recur. Chronic cases may exhibit nominal or extensive subretinal fibrosis. Myopia is common. Laser photocoagulation may be considered in the presence of a choroidal neovascular membrane.]

- Rubella (Usually seen in infants whose mother developed rubella during the pregnancy. Salt-and-pepper pigmentation of the retina is typical. A small eye, cataract, or iris transillumination defects may be present. The optic nerve may be pale. An elevated anti-rubella antibody titer can usually be demonstrated.)

- Serpiginous choroidopathy [Typically bilateral, recurrent chorioretinitis characterized by acute lesions (yellow-white subretinal patches with indistinct margins) bordering old atrophic scars. The chorioretinal changes usually extend from the optic disc outward. Patients are typically 30–60 years of age. A choroidal neovascular membrane may develop, requiring laser photocoagulation to prevent visual loss.]

- Toxocariasis (Usually occurs in children, affecting only one eye. An elevated, white retinal lesion may be seen in the posterior pole or peripheral fundus. The peripheral lesion may be associated with a fibrous band extending to the optic disc, sometimes dragging the macular vessels away from their normal course. A severe vitritis and anterior uveitis may be present. A negative undiluted toxocara titer in an immunocompetent host usually rules out this disease. See Section 9.1.)

- Tuberculosis   [Produces varied clinical manifestations. The diagnosis is usually made by ancillary laboratory tests. Miliary tuberculosis may produce multifocal, small, yellow-white choroidal lesions. Most patients have concomitant anterior granulomatous or nongranulomatous uveitis. A 2-week therapeutic trial of isoniazid 300 mg po daily and pyridoxine (vitamin B_6) 10 mg/day may be given. If the uveitis is the result of tuberculosis, it should improve significantly in patients on this regimen.]

- Vogt-Koyanagi-Harada syndrome   (Exudative retinal detachment with vitreous cells, a swollen optic disc, or atrophic patches at the level of the retinal pigment epithelium may accompany an anterior-chamber reaction. Patients are darkly pigmented, typically of Asian or Native American ancestry, and have or develop systemic signs including meningeal signs, vitiligo, alopecia, and poliosis. See Section 13.7.)

- Whipple's disease   (Rare. Small white vitreous opacities, retinal hemorrhages and exudates, or exudative material over the pars plana in a patient with diarrhea, arthralgia, and weight loss. The diagnosis is made by intestinal biopsy or, less commonly, by pars plana vitrectomy.)

- Others   [Nocardia, *Coccidioides* species, *Aspergillus* species, *Cryptococcus* species, meningococcus, ophthalmomyiasis, onchocerciasis and cystericercosis (seen in Africa and Central and South America), measles, Eales' disease, Crohn's disease, multiple sclerosis, subacute sclerosing panencephalitis, and age-related vitritis.)

Differential Diagnosis
(Masquerade syndromes.)

- Reticulum cell sarcoma (large cell lymphoma)   (Persistent vitreous cells in patients older than 50 years of age, that usually do not respond completely to systemic steroids. Yellow-white subretinal infiltrates, retinal edema and hemorrhage, anterior-chamber inflammation, or neurologic signs may be present. See Section 13.8.)

- Malignant melanoma   (A retinal detachment and associated vitritis may obscure the underlying tumor. B-scan ultrasound will usually detect the tumor in cases not detectable by indirect ophthalmoscopy. See Section 8.3.)

- Retinitis pigmentosa   (Vitreous cells and macular edema may accompany "bone-spicule" pigmentary changes and attenuated retinal vessels. Drusen of the optic disc may be mistaken for disc swelling. Electroretinography aids in diagnosis. See Section 12.24.)

- Rhegmatogenous retinal detachment   (A small number of pigmented anterior vitreous cells and a mild anterior uveitis frequently accompany a rhegmatogenous retinal detachment. See Section 12.19.)
- Retained intraocular foreign body   (Persistent inflammation following a penetrating ocular injury. May have iris heterochromia. Diagnosed by indirect ophthalmoscopy, B-scan ultrasound, or CT scan of the globe. See Section 3.16.)
- Posterior scleritis   (May or may not have an accompanying anterior scleritis. Vitritis is accompanied by a subretinal mass and often an exudative retinal detachment. Chorioretinal folds may be seen. Fluorescein angiography and B-scan ultrasonography are helpful in diagnosis.)
- Retinoblastoma   (Almost always occurs in young children. May present with a pseudohypopyon and vitreous cells. One or more elevated white retinal lesions is usually, but not always, present. A retinal detachment, iris neovascularization, or both may be found. Fluorescein angiography, CT scan, and B-scan ultrasonography may aid in diagnosis. See Section 9.1.)
- Leukemia   (Unilateral retinitis and vitritis may occur in patients already known to have leukemia.)
- Amyloidosis   (Rare. Vitreous globules or membranes without any signs of anterior-segment inflammation. A serum protein electrophoresis and diagnostic vitrectomy confirm the diagnosis.)
- Asteroid hyalosis [Small, white refractile particles (calcium soaps) adherent to collagen fibers and floating in the vitreous)   (Usually asymptomatic and of no clinical significance.]

Work-up

1. History: Systemic disease or infection, skin rash, IV drug abuse, indwelling catheter, risk factors for AIDS? Recent eye trauma or surgery? Travel to the Ohio-Mississippi River Valley, New England, or Middle Atlantic area? Tick bite?
2. Complete ocular examination, including IOP measurement and careful ophthalmoscopic examination. Indirect ophthalmoscopy with scleral depression of the inferior ora seratta is essential.
3. Consider fluorescein angiography to help in diagnosis or plan for therapy.
4. Blood tests (any of the following are obtained, depending on the suspected diagnosis): Toxoplasma titer, ACE level, FTA-ABS, RPR, ESR, ANA, HLA B5 (Behçet's), HLA A29 (birdshot), *Toxocara* titer, Lyme immunofluorescent assay or enzyme-linked immunosorbent assay (ELISA), and in neonates or immunocompromised patients, titers for CMV, herpes simplex, varicella-zoster, or rubella virus. Cultures of blood and IV sites may be helpful when infectious etiologies are suspected.

5. PPD with anergy panel.
6. Chest x-ray.
7. Urine for CMV in immunocompromised patients.
8. CT scan of the brain and lumbar puncture when reticulum cell sarcoma is suspected and when HIV-associated opportunistic infections indicate a potential for systemic, and in particular, CNS involvement.
9. Diagnostic vitrectomy when appropriate (see individual sections).

See the individual sections for more specific guidelines for work-up and treatment.

13.3 TOXOPLASMOSIS

Symptoms
Blurred vision, floaters, may have pain.

Critical Signs
Unilateral white-yellow retinal lesion associated with a hazy vitreous as a result of the presence of vitreous cells. An old chorioretinal scar can often be seen adjacent to the new white-yellow lesion but is not always present.

Other Signs
Vitreous precipitates on the posterior surface of the detached vitreous, vitreous debris, optic-disc swelling, neuroretinitis, mild granulomatous iritis, localized vasculitis, retinal artery or vein occlusion in the area of the inflammation. Chorioretinal scars are occasionally found in the uninvolved eye. Large visual field loss may result from peripapillary toxoplasmosis. Cystoid macular edema may be present. A choroidal (subretinal) neovascular membrane develops on rare occasions as a late sequela.

❖ **Note** *Toxoplasmosis can also develop in the deep retina, in which case few to no vitreous cells may be present.*

Differential Diagnosis
See "Posterior Uveitis," Section 13.2, for a complete list. The following may closely simulate toxoplasmosis.

- Syphilis   (Positive FTA-ABS. See Section 14.2.)
- Tuberculosis   (Positive PPD with possible abnormal chest x-ray. Rare.)
- Toxocariasis   (Usually affects children. A fibrous band may be seen radiating from a white retinal mass. Old chorioretinal scars are not typically

seen. May have a history of exposure to puppies or eating dirt. Positive *Toxocara* ELISA.)

Work-up

See "Posterior Uveitis," Section 13.2, for a nonspecific work-up when the diagnosis is in doubt.

1. History: Does the patient eat raw meat or has he or she been exposed to cats (sources of acquired infection)? Inquire about risk factors for AIDS in atypical cases (e.g., several active lesions without old chorioretinal scars).
2. Complete ocular examination, including a dilated fundus evaluation.
3. Serum anti-toxoplasma antibody titer. Should have a positive titer from current or previous infection (the dilution is unimportant).

❖ **Note** *Ask the lab to do a 1:1 dilution, as only a positive result is necessary.*

4. FTA-ABS, PPD with anergy panel, chest x-ray, and a *Toxocara* ELISA when the diagnosis is uncertain.
5. Fluorescein angiogram if a choroidal neovascular membrane is suspected.
6. Consider an HIV test in atypical cases or when the patient is a high-risk candidate for AIDS.

Treatment

A. Small peripheral retinochoroiditis (not affecting or threatening vision): If an anterior-chamber reaction is present, a topical cycloplegic (e.g., cyclopentolate 2% tid) with or without a topical steroid (e.g., prednisolone acetate 1%) qid is given. No additional treatment is indicated. The drops are tapered as the anterior-chamber reaction resolves.

B. Active lesions that are within 2–3 millimeters of the disc or fovea and threaten or are affecting vision, or extramacular lesions accompanied by severe vitritis:

1. Usual first-line therapy (for 3–6 weeks):
   a. Pyrimethamine 75 mg po load (or two 50-mg doses po 12 hours apart), then 25 mg po bid.
   b. Folinic acid 3–5 mg po twice weekly (to minimize bone marrow toxicity of pyrimethamine).
   c. Sulfadiazine 2 g po load then 1 g po qid.
2. Prednisone may be added, after initiation of antibiotic therapy, at a dose of 20–80 mg po daily. Periocular steroids should never be given.
3. Clindamycin 300 mg po qid may be used with sulfadiazine as alternative therapy or as an adjunct to previously discussed therapy.
4. Other alternative therapies are used with success. One alternative treatment is trimethoprim/sulfamethoxazole (160 mg/800 mg) one tablet orally bid, with or without clindamycin and prednisone.
5. Anterior-segment inflammation is treated with cyclopegia (e.g., cyclo-

pentolate 1–2% tid) and topical steroid (e.g., prednisolone acetate 1% qid).

❖ **Note** *Systemic steroids should never be used without antimicrobial treatment and rarely used in immunocompromised patients.*

If a patient is placed on pyrimethamine, a platelet count and CBC are obtained once or twice per week to check for a low platelet count and a low red or white blood cell count (pyrimethamine can depress the bone marrow). If the platelet count falls below 100,000 then reduce the dosage of pyrimethamine and increase the folinic acid.

Patients on pyrimethamine should not take vitamins that contain folic acid. The medication should be given with meals to reduce anorexia. A small amount of pyrimethamine pills should be given at each visit to ensure compliance.

Patients on clindamycin should be warned about pseudomembranous colitis and the medication should be stopped if diarrhea develops.

C. Laser photocoagulation, cryotherapy, and vitrectomy have been employed as adjunctive treatment modalities.

Follow-up

In 3–7 days for blood tests and/or ocular assessment, then every 1–2 weeks on therapy.

❖ **Notes**

1. *If a patient cannot use or must discontinue clindamycin, tetracycline 2 g load po followed by 250 mg po qid is used alternatively. Do not give tetracycline to children or pregnant or breast-feeding women.*
2. *Pyrimethamine should not be given to pregnant or breast-feeding women.*
3. *Only women who develop toxoplasmosis* during *pregnancy can transmit it to their fetus. A woman cannot transmit congenital toxoplasmosis.*

See "AIDS" for additional information.

REFERENCES

Engstrom RE, et al. Current practices in the management of ocular toxoplasmosis. *Am J Ophthalmol* 111:601, 1991.
Opremcak EM, et al. Trimethoprim-sulfamethoxazole therapy for ocular toxoplasmosis. *Ophthalmology* 99:920, 1992.

13.4 SARCOIDOSIS

Symptoms

Pain, photophobia, decreased vision. Typically affects African-Americans in the 20- to 50-year age group.

Critical Ocular Signs

Granulomatous iritis with large "mutton-fat" keratic precipitates on the corneal endothelium (or less commonly, a nongranulomatous iritis), vitritis with white, fluffy opacities in the inferior vitreous or yellow-white nodules or exudates ("candle-wax drippings") and sheathing along peripheral retinal veins.

Other Ocular Signs

Iris and/or choroidal nodules, retinal hemorrhage, conjunctival granuloma, band keratopathy, posterior synechiae, glaucoma, cataract, lacrimal-gland enlargement, dry eye, optic-disc swelling, optic-nerve granuloma, optic neuritis, extraocular muscle palsy, and proptosis. Retinal neovascularization and cystoid macular edema may occur.

Systemic Signs

Facial-nerve palsy, salivary-gland enlargement, bilateral hilar adenopathy on chest x-ray, erythema nodosum (erythematous, tender nodules beneath the skin, often in the anterior tibial area), arthritis, lymphadenopathy, hepatosplenomegaly, and other skin, CNS, and bone changes may be found.

Differential Diagnosis

- Sickle-cell disease   (May also produce peripheral retinal neovascularization in young African-American individuals, but it is more commonly "sea-fan" in appearance. The aqueous and vitreous have few-to-no cells, and a hemoglobin electrophoresis is abnormal in sickle-cell disease. See Section 12.23.)
- Tuberculosis (TB)   (Rare. May appear identical to sarcoidosis. Positive PPD may have abnormal chest x-ray.)
- Idiopathic pars planitis   (White, fluffy vitreous opacities and cells and white exudative material accumulating along the ora serrata and pars plana, typically inferiorly. See Section 13.5.)
- Others   (See "Anterior Uveitis," Section 13.1, and "Posterior Uveitis," Section 13.2.)

Work-up

The following are the tests that are obtained when sarcoidosis is suspected clinically. See "Anterior Uveitis," Section 13.1, and "Posterior Uveitis," Section 13.2, for nonspecific uveitis work-ups.

1. Chest x-ray.
2. Serum angiotensin converting enzyme (ACE): Usually, but not always elevated in active systemic sarcoidosis. May also be elevated in TB, diabetes, leprosy, histoplasmosis, and other conditions that do *not* produce uveitis. Normal ACE values vary with age, requiring comparison with age-matched

controls. Steroids usually suppress the ACE level soon after starting treatment.

3. PPD with anergy panel: Used to distinguish TB (induration of 10 mm or more in most cases) from sarcoidosis (anergy in 50% of cases).
4. Biopsy of any conjunctival granuloma or the palpebral lobe of the lacrimal gland when it is enlarged. (An acid-fast stain and a methenamine-silver stain should be performed at the time of biopsy to rule out TB and fungal infection.) A "blind conjunctival" biopsy has an extremely low yield and generally is not recommended.

If the above work-up is inconclusive, yet sarcoidosis is still suspected, the following tests may be obtained:

5. Gallium scan of the head, neck, and mediastinum (often shows increased uptake in patients with active systemic sarcoidosis).
6. Serum lysozyme (may be elevated) and serum protein electrophoresis (may show hypergammaglobulinemia).
7. Skin, lymph node, or lung biopsy by the appropriate physician.
8. Kveim's skin test (rarely available).
9. Pulmonary function tests may be indicated.

Serum calcium levels are sometimes obtained in patients diagnosed with sarcoidosis to ascertain that the blood calcium is not dangerously high.

Treatment

All patients are referred to an internist for medical management.

A. Uveitis
   1. Cycloplegic (e.g., cyclopentolate 2% or scopolamine 0.25% tid).
   2. Topical steroid (e.g., prednisolone acetate 1% q 1–6 h, depending on the degree of inflammation).
   3. Periocular steroids (e.g., triamcinolone 40 mg subtenons every 3–4 weeks) may be required when the uveitis does not respond to q 1 h topical steroids. See Appendix 7 for the technique.
   4. Systemic steroids (e.g., prednisone 60–100 mg po daily) and a histamine H_2 blocker (e.g., ranitidine 150 mg po bid) are often required in the presence of posterior uveitis (including optic neuritis). See Drug Glossary when considering systemic steroids.
   5. Cyclosporin A has been used effectively in patients who are intolerant of or refractory to systemic steroids.
B. Cystoid macular edema: See Section 12.14.
C. Glaucoma: See "Inflammatory Open-Angle Glaucoma," Section 10.4; "Steroid-Response Glaucoma," Section 10.5; "Acute Angle-Closure Glaucoma," Section 10.10; or "Neovascular Glaucoma," Section 10.13, depending on the etiology of the glaucoma.
D. Retinal neovascularization: May require panretinal photocoagulation.

E. Orbital disease is managed with systemic steroids as described previously.

F. Seventh-nerve palsy, CNS disease, pulmonary disease, and renal disease require systemic steroids and management by an internist. Hypercalcemia may also require medical treatment.

Follow-up

Patients are reexamined in 3–7 days. The steroid dosages are adjusted in accordance with the patient's response to treatment. As the inflammation subsides, the steroids and cycloplegic agent are tapered slowly. Intraocular pressure is monitored, and fundus reevaluation is performed periodically. Asymptomatic patients with quiet eyes are seen every 6 months. Patients being treated with steroids need to be followed more closely (e.g., every 1–3 months). Children with sarcoidosis are reexamined every 3 months because of the frequent occurrence of asymptomatic but damaging uveitis.

13.5 PARS PLANITIS

Symptoms

Floaters and cloudy vision, rarely red eye, pain, or photophobia. Usually age 15–40 years and bilateral.

Critical Signs

"Snowbanking" (white exudative material over the inferior ora serrata and pars plana), vitreous cells.

❖ **Note** *Snowbanking can often only be seen with indirect ophthalmoscopy and scleral depression.*

Other Signs

Cellular aggregates in the vitreous, especially inferiorly ("snowball" opacities), peripheral retinal vascular sheathing, anterior-chamber inflammation, cystoid macular edema (CME), posterior subcapsular cataract, secondary glaucoma, posterior vitreous detachment, vitreous hemorrhage, retinal detachment, retinal tears, or peripapillary edema may develop.

Differential Diagnosis

See "Posterior Uveitis," Section 13.2.

Work-up

See "Posterior Uveitis," Section 13.2.

Treatment

No treatment is necessary for patients who have a visual acuity of 20/40 or better. For patients with a visual acuity worse than 20/40 as a result of CME, any or all of the following may be tried (although (2) and (3) are not generally given simultaneously).

1. Topical prednisolone acetate 1% (e.g., Pred-Forte) q 1–2 h may serve a dual purpose, relieving discomfort from an anterior-chamber reaction, and sometimes improving the CME.
2. Periocular repository steroids (e.g., methylprednisolone 40 mg subTenons). Repeat the injections every 1–2 months until the vision and CME are no longer improving, then slowly taper the frequency of injections. See Appendix 7 for the technique.
3. If there is no improvement after the first three subTenons injections, then consider systemic steroids (e.g., prednisone 60 mg po daily for 4–6 weeks, tapering gradually according to the patient's response.

❖ **Note** *In bilateral cases, systemic steroid therapy is often preferred over bilateral periocular injections.*

4. In patients who fail to respond to either oral or subTenon's corticosteroids, transcleral cryotherapy to the area of snowbanking may be tried. If cryotherapy fails, pars plana vitrectomy can be considered.
5. As a last resort, some physicians advocate the use of systemic immunosuppressive agents (e.g., cyclophosphamide, cyclosporin A).

❖ **Notes**
  1. *Some physicians delay periocular repository steroid therapy for several weeks in order to observe whether the patient is a steroid responder (i.e., develops a significant IOP rise secondary to the topical steroids). If a steroid response is found, then the periocular steroid may need to be withheld.*
  2. *Acetazolamide 500 mg po daily may be tried in refractory patients.*

Follow-up
In the acute phase, patients are reevaluated every 1–4 weeks, depending on the severity of the condition. In the chronic phase, rexamination is performed every 3–6 months.

13.6 ACUTE RETINAL NECROSIS (ARN)

Symptoms
Blurred vision (often with floaters), ocular pain, photophobia. Most patients are in good systemic health, but underlying AIDS should be considered.

Critical Signs

Multiple white opaque patches of thickened retina, usually in the periphery, which gradually enlarge and coalesce. There is a sharp demarcation line between the involved and normal retina. Vitreous cells are often abundant. Bilateral (simultaneously or sequentially) in one third of patients.

Other Signs

Anterior-chamber reaction (sometimes granulomatous); increased intraocular pressure (IOP); sheathed retinal arterioles and sometimes venules, especially in the periphery; retinal hemorrhages (minor finding); optic-disc edema; rheg-matogenous retinal detachments (RRD). (The RRD typically has multiple, large, irregular posterior breaks and is usually a late finding.) An optic neuropathy (disc edema or pallor with an afferent pupillary defect, decreased color vision, and a central scotoma) sometimes develops.

Etiology

Herpesvirus family (varicella-zoster or herpes simplex; CMV less likely).

Differential Diagnosis

See "Posterior Uveitis," Section 13.2.

Work-up

See "Posterior Uveitis," Section 13.2, for a nonspecific uveitis work-up.

1. History: Risk factors for AIDS? Immunocompromised? If yes, CMV retinitis may be more likely.
2. Complete ocular examination: Evaluate the anterior chamber and the vitreous for cells, measure the IOP, and perform a dilated retinal examination using indirect ophthalmoscopy and scleral depression.
3. Consider a CBC with differential, FTA-ABS, RPR, ESR, toxoplasmosis titers, PPD with anergy panel, and chest x-ray to rule out other etiologies and before instituting medical treatment.
4. Consider testing for HIV.
5. Acute and convalescent serum titers for herpes simplex, varicella-zoster, and CMV (limited utility).
6. Consider a fluorescein angiogram.
7. An orbital CT scan or B-scan ultrasound to look for an enlarged optic nerve in cases of suspected optic-nerve dysfunction.
8. CT scan or MRI of the brain and lumbar puncture if large cell lymphoma, tertiary syphilis, or encephalitis is suspected.
9. Consider vitreous or retinal biopsy for viral cultures and to rule out other possible infectious causes (selected cases).

Treatment
1. Admit to the hospital.
2. Acyclovir[1] 1500 mg/m² of body surface area/day IV in 3 divided doses for 7–10 days. Then oral acyclovir (400–600 mg 5 times daily) for up to 6 weeks from the onset of infection.[2] Regression of the retinitis is usually seen within 4 days. (The lesions may progress during the first 48 hours of treatment.)
3. Topical cycloplegic (e.g., atropine 1% tid) and topical steroid (e.g., prednisolone acetate 1% q 2–6 h) in the presence of anterior-segment inflammation.
4. Consider anticoagulation (e.g., heparin or warfarin for a total of 2–3 weeks) or antiplatelet therapy (aspirin 125–650 mg daily).
5. Systemic steroids (controversial): Some physicians administer steroids aggressively at the time of diagnosis (e.g., methylprednisolone 250 mg IV qid for 3 days followed by prednisone 60 mg po bid for 1–2 weeks), particularly when the optic nerve is thought to be involved. Others delay steroid therapy for one or more weeks until the retinitis begins to clear. A typical oral corticosteroid regimen (initial or delayed therapy) is prednisone 60–80 mg/day for 1–2 weeks followed by a taper over 2–6 weeks.
6. See "Inflammatory Open-Angle Glaucoma," Section 10.4, for treatment of elevated IOP.
7. Consider prophylactic laser photocoagulation (confluent laser spots posterior to active retinitis) to wall-off or prevent subsequent RRD.
8. Consider pars plana vitrectomy with internal tamponade (long-acting gas or silicone oil) for the associated complex RRD. (Proliferative vitreoretinopathy is common.)
9. Consider optic-nerve-sheath decompression surgery for ARN optic neuropathy when the optic nerve is enlarged and the patient's condition worsens or does not improve with medical therapy.

Follow-up
Patients are seen daily in the hospital and are then examined every few weeks to months for the following year. A careful fundus evaluation with scleral depression is performed at each visit to rule out retinal holes that may lead to a detachment. If the retinitis crosses the margin of prior laser treatment, consider applying additional laser therapy. A pupillary examination should always be performed, and an optic neuropathy should be considered if the retinopathy does not explain the amount of visual loss.

---

[1]The dosage of acyclovir needs to be reduced in patients with renal insufficiency. Blood urea nitrogen and creatinine levels are followed closely.

[2]Six weeks of treatment is based on the observation that occurrences in the second eye most often begin within 6 weeks of the onset in the first eye.

REFERENCE

Duker JS, Blumenkranz MS. Diagnosis and management of the acute retinal necrosis syndrome. *Surv Ophthalmol* 35:327, 1991.

13.7 VOGT-KOYANAGI-HARADA (VKH) SYNDROME

Symptoms

Bilaterally decreased vision, photophobia, pain, and red eyes, accompanied by or preceded by a headache, stiff neck, nausea, vomiting, fever, and malaise. Hearing loss, dysacusis, and tinnitus frequently occur.

Critical Signs

Bilateral serous retinal detachments with underlying choroidal infiltrates, posterior vitreous cells and opacities, retinal hemorrhages, optic-disc edema, anterior-chamber flare and cells, and keratic precipitates. Perilimbal vitiligo is common. Alopecia, vitiligo, and poliosis may develop later.

Other Signs

May see mottling and atrophy of the retinal pigment epithelium after the serous retinal detachment resolves (sunset fundus), hyphema, iris nodules, peripheral anterior and posterior synechiae, scleritis, hypotony, venous engorgement, retinal vasculitis, or choroidal neovascularization. Neurologic signs, including loss of consciousness, paralysis, and seizures, may occur. Typically, patients are 20–50 years of age and are of a darkly pigmented heritage such as Asian or Native American.

Differential Diagnosis

See "Posterior Uveitis," Section 13.2, for a complete list. In particular, consider the following:

- Sympathetic ophthalmia   (Prior history of trauma or surgery to the uninvolved eye. Generally no CNS, skin, or hair manifestations. See Section 13.15.)
- Acute posterior multifocal placoid pigment epitheliopathy (AMPPE) (Ophthalmoscopic and fluorescein angiographic features may be very similar, but there is less vitreous inflammation and no anterior-segment involvement.)
- Other granulomatous panuveitides (e.g., syphilis, sarcoidosis, TB)

Work-up

See "Posterior Uveitis," Section 13.2, for a nonspecific uveitis work-up.

1. History: Neurologic symptoms, hearing loss, or hair loss? Previous eye surgery or trauma?

2. Complete ocular examination, including a dilated retinal evaluation.
3. CBC, RPR, FTA-ABS, angiotensin converting enzyme (ACE), and PPD with anergy panel and possibly chest x-ray to rule out similar-appearing disorders.
4. Consider a CT scan with and without contrast or MRI of the brain during attacks with neurologic signs to rule out a CNS disorder.
5. Lumbar puncture during attacks with meningeal symptoms for cell count and differential, protein, glucose, VDRL, Gram's and methenamine-silver stains, and culture. (Lymphocytosis is often seen in VKH and AMPPE.)
6. Fluorescein angiogram may help in diagnosis.

Treatment

Inflammation is controlled with steroids; the dose depends on the severity of the inflammation. In moderate-to-severe cases, the following regimen can be used initially. Steroids are tapered slowly as the condition improves.

1. Topical steroids (e.g., prednisolone acetate 1% q 1 h).
2. Systemic steroids (e.g., prednisone 60–80 mg po daily) and a histamine H_2 blocker (e.g., ranitidine 150 mg po bid). See Drug Glossary for a systemic steroid work-up.
3. Topical cycloplegic (e.g., scopolamine 0.25% tid).
4. Treatment of any specific neurologic disorders (e.g., seizures or coma).
5. Immunosuppressive agents (e.g., methotrexate, azathioprine, chlorambucil, cyclosporine) can be used under the supervision of a medical consultant in patients who cannot tolerate or are unresponsive to systemic steroids.

Follow-up

Initial management may require hospitalization. Weekly, then monthly reexamination is performed, watching for recurrent inflammation and increased IOP. The steroids are tapered slowly. Inflammation may recur up to 9 months after the steroids have been discontinued. If this occurs, the previously described treatment regimen should be reinstituted.

13.8 RETICULUM CELL SARCOMA
(LARGE CELL LYMPHOMA)

Symptoms

Painless decrease in vision, floaters. Usually no history of prior uveitis

Critical Signs

Large amount of vitreous cells and debris in a patient older than 40 years of age (typically >50 years) that do not respond well to systemic steroids. Usually bilateral.

Other Signs

May see patches of yellow-white chorioretinal or subretinal pigment epithelial infiltrates, retinal edema and hemorrhages, or a mild anterior-chamber reaction with fine keratic precipitates. Neurologic manifestations may be present.

Differential Diagnosis

See "Posterior Uveitis," Section 13.2.

Work-up

See "Posterior Uveitis," Section 13.2, for a nonspecific uveitis work-up. Evaluate for CNS disorders and visceral lymphoma.

1. History: Previous uveitis? Recent intraocular surgery? Immunocompromised or risk group for AIDS? Concomitant systemic symptoms or signs (e.g., skin rash, difficulty breathing, diarrhea)? If yes, see "Posterior Uveitis," Section 13.2.
2. Complete ocular examination.
3. CT scan (axial and coronal views) with and without contrast or MRI of the orbit and head (and a body CT scan, if indicated).
4. Lumbar puncture for cell count, cytology, VDRL, protein, glucose, culture, and Gram's and methenamine-silver stains.
5. Consider a diagnostic vitrectomy with cytologic and immunohistologic studies.
6. Biopsy suspicious lymph nodes as needed.
7. Bone marrow biopsy, if indicated.

Treatment

In cooperation with an oncologist and radiation therapist.

1. Ocular and brain radiation therapy.
2. Intravenous chemotherapy.
3. Systemic radiation therapy (if there is visceral involvement).
4. Intrathecal chemotherapy, if indicated.

Follow-up

In conjunction with the oncologist and radiation therapist.

13.9 POSTOPERATIVE UVEITIS

Postoperative inflammation is typically mild-to-moderate, usually resolving within 6 weeks. This section presents several etiologies of postoperative uveitis and a work-up that may be considered when postoperative inflammation is atypical.

Etiology

A. Severe intraocular inflammation in the early postoperative course

- Infectious endophthalmitis [Progressive and often severe ocular pain (but not always), deteriorating vision, corneal edema, eyelid swelling, chemosis, sometimes a hypopyon, and commonly vitreous inflammation and blunting of the red reflex. See Section 13.10.)
- Phacoanaphylactic endophthalmitis (A severe granulomatous inflammation with mutton-fat keratic precipitates, resulting from an autoimmune reaction to lens protein exposed during surgery. See Section 13.14.)
- Aseptic endophthalmitis (A severe sterile postoperative uveitis caused by excess tissue manipulation, especially vitreous manipulation, during surgery. A hypopyon and a mild vitreous cellular reaction may develop. Generally *not* characterized by profound or progressive pain or visual loss. Eyelid swelling and chemosis are atypical. Usually resolves with topical steroid therapy.)

B. Persistent postoperative inflammation (e.g., beyond 6 weeks)
- Patient noncompliance with steroid drops (e.g., not taking the drops or not shaking them properly)
- Steroid drops tapered too abruptly
- Iris or vitreous incarceration in the wound
- Uveitis-glaucoma-hyphema (UGH) syndrome (Irritation of the iris or ciliary body by an intraocular lens. Increased intraocular pressure (IOP) and red blood cells in the anterior chamber accompany the anterior-segment inflammation.)
- Retinal detachment (Often produces a low-grade anterior-chamber reaction. See Section 12.19.)
- Low-grade endophthalmitis (e.g., *Proprionibacterium acnes,* fungal, or partially treated bacterial endophthalmitis)
- Inflammatory reaction to contaminants on the intraocular lens (e.g., polishing substances or substances used to sterilize the lens) or to the viscoelastic substance
- Epithelial downgrowth or fibrous ingrowth (Corneal or conjunctival epithelium or fibrous tissue grows into the eye through a corneal wound and may be seen on the posterior corneal surface. The iris may appear flattened because of the spread of the membrane over the anterior-chamber angle onto the iris. Large cells may be seen in the anterior chamber, and glaucoma may be present. The diagnosis of epithelial downgrowth can be confirmed by observing the immediate appearance of white spots after medium-power argon laser treatment to the areas of iris covered by the membrane.)
- Preexisting uveitis (see "Anterior Uveitis," Section 13.1)

C. Sympathetic ophthalmia (Diffuse granulomatous inflammation in *both* eyes, following trauma or surgery to one eye. See Section 13.15.)

Work-up
1. History: Is the patient taking and shaking the steroid drops properly? Did the patient stop the steroid drops abruptly? Was there a postoperative wound

leak allowing for epithelial downgrowth or fibrous ingrowth? Previous history of uveitis?

2. Complete ocular examination of both eyes, including a slit-lamp assessment of the anterior-chamber reaction, a determination of whether vitreous or residual lens material is present in the anterior chamber, and an inspection of the posterior lens capsule looking for posterior capsular opacities (as is seen in some cases of *P. acnes*). Gonioscopy (checking for iris or vitreous to the wound), an IOP measurement, a dilated indirect ophthalmoscopic examination (to rule out a retinal detachment or signs of chorioretinitis), and a posterior vitreous evaluation with a slit-lamp and a 60-diopter, Hruby, or Goldmann's contact lens looking for inflammatory cells should be performed.

3. Obtain a B-scan ultrasound when the fundus view is obscured.

4. A diagnostic surgical vitrectomy is usually performed for smears and cultures when infectious endophthalmitis is suspected. Anaerobic cultures, using both solid media and broth, should be obtained to isolate *P. acnes* (routine cultures are also obtained, see "Postoperative Endophthalmitis," Section 13.10). The anaerobic cultures should be incubated in an anaerobic environment as rapidly as possible and allowed to grow for at least 2 weeks.

5. Consider an anterior-chamber paracentesis for diagnostic smears and cultures.

6. Consider diagnostic medium-power argon laser treatment to the areas of iris thought to be covered by epithelial downgrowth.

If the above work-up is negative, no underlying etiology can be elicited, and a trial of steroids only transiently reduces the inflammation, surgical removal of the capsular bag and intraocular lens should be considered in an effort to isolate *P. acnes*.

See "Anterior Uveitis," Section 13.1; "Posterior Uveitis," Section 13.2; "Postoperative Endophthalmitis," Section 13.10; "Phacoanaphylactic Endophthalmitis," Section 13.14; and "Sympathetic Ophthalmia," Section 13.15 for more specific information on diagnosis and treatment.

13.10 POSTOPERATIVE ENDOPHTHALMITIS

Acute (One to Several Days after Surgery)

Symptoms
Sudden onset of progressively decreasing vision, redness, and increasing eye pain.

Critical Signs

More ocular inflammation than would be expected after the ocular procedure performed. Intense flare and cell in the anterior chamber and vitreous, with or without hypopyon, eyelid edema, chemosis, and a reduced red reflex.

❖ **Note** *Pain and a hypopyon may not be present.*

Other Signs

Corneal edema, iris hyperemia, purulent discharge.

Organisms

Most common *Staphylococcus epidermidis.*
Common *Staphylococcus aureus,* streptococcal species (except pneumococcus, which is not a common cause).
Less common Gram-negative bacteria (*Pseudomonas* species, *Aerobacter* species, *Proteus* species, *Haemophilus influenzae, Klebsiella,* species, *Escherichia coli* species, *Bacillus* species, *Enterobacter* species) and anaerobes.

Differential Diagnosis

See "Postoperative Uveitis," Section 13.9.

Work-up

1. Complete ocular history and examination.
2. Consider a B-scan ultrasound (may confirm the clinical suspicion by revealing marked vitreous cells, and establishes a baseline against which the success of therapy can be measured.)
3. A diagnostic (and therapeutic) vitrectomy is often performed. Cultures (blood, chocolate, Sabouraud's, thioglycolate) and smears (Gram's and Giemsa stains) are obtained, and intravitreal antibiotics are given as described in the following section. An anterior-chamber paracentesis should be considered.
4. CBC with differential and serum electrolytes.

Treatment

1. Hospitalization.
2. Topical fortified antibiotics (e.g., fortified cefazolin or fortified vancomycin q 1 h and fortified gentamicin or tobramycin q 1 h alternating every one-half hour). See Appendix 9, which describes fortified drop preparation.
3. Subconjunctival antibiotics (e.g., gentamicin 40 mg and vancomycin 25-50 mg or clindamycin 40 mg); can be repeated daily if bacteria are isolated. See Appendix 7 for the technique.
4. Systemic antibiotics (e.g., cefazolin 500-1000 mg IV q 6 h or vancomycin 500 mg IV q 6 h and gentamicin 2.0 mg/kg IV load followed by 1 mg/kg

q 8 h, add clindamycin 600 mg IV q 8 h if anaerobic organisms are suspected.[3]

5. Intravitreal antibiotics (e.g., amikacin 0.4 mg in 0.1 mL or ceftriaxone 2 mg in 0.1 ml and vancomycin 1.0 mg in 0.1 mL; clindamycin 1 mg in 0.1–0.2 mL may be used in place of vancomycin) at the time of vitrectomy.

6. Topical cycloplegic (e.g., atropine 1%) 3–4 times per day.

Steroids are usually started topically, subconjunctivally, and intravitreally, because fungus is not usually suspected in acute-onset postoperative endophthalmitis.

7. Topical steroid (e.g., prednisolone acetate 1%) 6 times per day.

8. Subconjunctival steroid (e.g., triamcinolone 40 mg) at the time of vitrectomy and sometimes daily. Appendix 7 explains the technique.

9. Intravitreal steroid (e.g. dexamethasone 0.4 mg) at the time of vitrectomy at the discretion of the surgeon.

❖ **Note** *Antibiotic and steroid therapy are usually withheld until* after *the vitrectomy is performed, unless a prolonged delay before surgery is expected.*

Follow-up
1. Monitor the clinical course every 4–8 hours.

2. The antibiotic regimen is refined according to the patient's response to treatment and to the culture and sensitivity results. If a patient is getting worse or an identified organism is found to be resistant to the intravitreal antibiotics injected, an additional intravitreal injection of one antibiotic can be given 48 hours after the initial injection.

3. If the patient is responding well to treatment, topical fortified antibiotics may be slowly tapered after 48 hours and then switched to regular strength. IV antibiotics are maintained for 6–10 days, depending on the ocular status, and then comparable oral antibiotics are substituted for a total 14-day course. Patients are usually discharged from the hospital after IV antibiotics are discontinued. Close outpatient follow-up is warranted.

❖ **Note** *Some physicians administer a systemic steroid (e.g., prednisone 60–100 mg po daily) once the responsible organism has been treated appropriately for 24 hours. This regimen is maintained for 7–10 days and then tapered. We do not generally do this.*

---

[3]Systemic antibiotic doses may need to be reduced in patients with renal disease. Check gentamicin peak and trough levels one-half hour before and after the fifth dose, and follow the blood urea nitrogen and creatinine levels every other day. Adjust the doses accordingly.

Delayed-Onset (A Week to a Month or More after Surgery)

Symptoms

Insidious decreased vision, increasing redness and pain.

Critical Signs

Reduced visual acuity, anterior-chamber and vitreous inflammation, vitreous abscesses, hypopyon; clumps of exudate in the anterior chamber, on the iris surface, or along the pupillary border.

Other Signs

Corneal infiltrate and edema; may have a surgical bleb.

Etiology/Organisms

- Fungi (*Aspergillus, Candida, Cephalosporium,* and *Penicillium* species; others)
- *Proprionibacterium acnes* (Recurrent, granulomatous anterior uveitis, often with a hypopyon, but with minimal conjunctival injection and pain. A white plaque or opacities on the posterior lens capsule may be evident. There is only a transient response to steroids.)
- Other bacteria   [Related to a filtering bleb (often streptococci), vitreous wick, or partial suppression with antibiotics during or after surgery.)

Differential Diagnosis

See Postoperative Uveitis, Section 13.9.

Work-up

1. Complete ocular history and examination.
2. Vitrectomy for smears (Gram's, Giemsa, and methenamine-silver) and cultures [blood, chocolate, Sabouraud's, thioglycolate, and a solid media for anaerobic culture (e.g., *Brucella* or blood agar); *P. acnes* will be missed unless proper anaerobic cultures are obtained]. Intravitreal antibiotics are given as described in the following section.
3. CBC with differential, serum electrolytes, liver function studies.

Treatment

1. Initially treat as acute postoperative endophthalmitis, as described previously, but do *not* start steroids.
2. If a fungal infection is suspected or an intraoperative smear is consistent with fungus, administer intravitreal amphotericin B, 5–10 μg at the time of vitrectomy.
3. Broad-spectrum antifungal therapy is delayed until a fungus is positively identified in a direct smear or culture. Antifungal therapy consists of:
   a. Topical natamycin (5% suspension) q 1 h.

b. Flucytosine 37.5 mg/kg po q 6 h.

c. Amphotericin B 0.25–0.3 mg/kg/day IV initially (in test doses of 1 mg), then increase the dose slowly to 0.75–1.0 mg/kg/day IV in divided doses.

d. Consider miconazole 10 mg in 1 mL subconjunctivally.

e. A therapeutic vitrectomy should be performed if it was not done with the initial cultures.

Antifungal therapy is modified in accordance with sensitivity testing, clinical course, and tolerance to antifungal agents.

4. Removal of the lens and capsular remnants may be required for diagnosis and treatment of *P. acnes. P. acnes* may be sensitive to intravitreal penicillin, cefoxitin, clindamycin, or vancomycin.

Follow-up

Dependent on the organism. In general, follow-up is as described previously for acute postoperative endophthalmitis. Repeat CBC, serum electrolytes, and liver function tests 2 times per week during treatment for fungal endophthalmitis.

13.11 TRAUMATIC ENDOPHTHALMITIS

This condition constitutes an emergency. If suspected, prompt action is required.

Symptoms and Signs

Same as "Acute Postoperative Endophthalmitis," Section 13.10.

❖ **Note** *Patients with* Bacillus *endophthalmitis may develop a high fever, leukocytosis, proptosis, a corneal abscess in the form of a ring, and rapid visual deterioration.*

Organisms

Bacillus species, *Staphylococcus epidermidis,* gram-negative species, fungi, *Streptococcus* species, others. A mixed flora may be present.

Differential Diagnosis

• Sterile inflammatory response from a retained intraocular foreign body or blood in the vitreous

• Sterile inflammation as a result of surgical complications

- Phacoanaphylactic endophthalmitis   (A sterile autoimmune inflammatory reaction as a result of exposed lens protein. See Section 13.14.)

Work-up

Same as for "Acute Postoperative Endophthalmitis," Section 13.10. An orbital CT scan (axial and coronal views) and ultrasound are also performed to rule out an intraocular foreign body.

Treatment

1. Hospitalization.
2. Management for a ruptured globe or penetrating ocular injury if present (see Section 3.15).
3. Topical fortified gentamicin or tobramycin q 1 h and fortified cefazolin or fortified vancomycin q 1 h, alternating every one-half hour. See Appendix 10, which describes fortified drop preparation.
4. Subconjunctival gentamicin 40 mg and subconjunctival clindamycin 34 mg. Can be repeated daily as needed. (See Appendix 7 for the technique.)
5. Systemic antibiotics (e.g., gentamicin 2.0 mg/kg IV load followed by 1.0 mg/kg IV q 8 h and clindamycin 600 mg IV q 8 h with or without cefazolin 500–1000 mg IV q 8 h.[4]
6. Intravitreal antibiotics (amikacin 0.4 mg in 0.1 mL or ceftriaxone 2 mg in 0.1 mL and vancomycin 1 mg in 0.1 mL or clindamycin 1 mg in 0.1 mL). These may be repeated every 48–72 hours, as needed.
7. A surgical vitrectomy is performed as soon as the condition is highly suspected.

❖ **Notes**

1. *Antibiotics are usually withheld until after the vitrectomy is performed unless a prolonged delay until surgery is expected.*
2. *Steroids should not be given initially, because a fungal etiology cannot be ruled out. If cultures are negative for fungi, topical, subconjunctival, and perhaps systemic steroids may be started (e.g., topical prednisolone acetate 1% 6 times per day and subconjunctival dexamethasone 4 mg with or without predisone 40–80 mg po daily).*

Follow-up

Same as for "Postoperative Endophthalmitis," Section 13.10. The specific antibiotics and the frequency of their administration should be modified in accordance with the patient's response to tretment, as well as the culture and sensitivity results.

---

[4]Drug doses may need to be reduced in children and patients with renal disease. Check gentamicin peak and trough levels one-half hour before and after the fifth dose, and follow the blood urea nitrogen and creatinine levels.

13.12 ENDOGENOUS BACTERIAL ENDOPHTHALMITIS

Symptoms

Decreased vision in an acutely ill (e.g., septic) patient, an immunocompromised host, or an IV drug abuser. No history of recent intraocular surgery.

Critical Signs

Vitreous cells and debris, anterior-chamber cell and flare, or a hypopyon in a high-risk patient.

Other Signs

Iris microabscess, absent red fundus reflex, retinal inflammatory infiltrates, flame-shaped retinal hemorrhages with or without white centers, corneal edema, eyelid edema, chemosis, conjunctival injection. Panophthalmitis [orbital involvement (proptosis, restricted ocular motility) and endophthalmitis] may develop.

Etiology

Bacillus cereus (especially in IV drug abusers), streptococci, *Neisseria meningitidis, Staphylococcus aureus, Haemophilus influenzae,* others).

Differential Diagnosis

- Endogenous fungal endophthalmitis   (May see fluffy, white vitreous opacities. Fungi grow on cultures. See "Candida Retinitis/Uveitis/Endophthalmitis," Section 13.13.)
- Retinochoroidal infection (e.g., toxoplasmosis and toxocariasis)   (Yellow or white retinochoroidal lesion present.)
- Noninfectious posterior uveitis (e.g., sarcoidosis, pars planitis)   (May have a known history of uveitis. Unlikely to coincidentally get the first episode during sepsis.)
- Neoplastic conditions [e.g., reticulum cell sarcoma (usually older than 50–55 years of age), retinoblastoma (usually in the first few years of life)]

Work-up

1. History: Duration of symptoms? Underlying disease or infections? IV drug abuse? Immunocompromised?
2. Complete ocular examination, including a dilated fundus examination.
3. B-scan ultrasound to determine the extent of posterior segment ocular involvement if it cannot be determined on clinical examination.
4. Complete medical work-up by an infectious disease expert.

5. Cultures of blood, urine, and all indwelling catheters and IV lines, as well as Gram's stain of any discharge. A lumbar puncture is indicated when meningeal signs are present.
6. Vitrectomy with intraocular antibiotics (e.g., amikacin 0.4 mg in 0.1 mL or ceftriaxone 2 mg in 0.1 mL and vancomycin 1 mg in 0.1 mL; clindamycin 1 mg in 0.1 mL may be used in place of vancomycin): The timing of this procedure is controversial. We perform it as soon as possible. Other physicians initially perform aqueous and vitreous aspirations when the systemic cultures are negative and the organism remains unknown.

Treatment

(In conjunction with a medical internist.)

1. Hospitalize the patient.
2. Broad-spectrum antibiotics are started after appropriate smears and cultures are obtained. Antibiotic choices vary according to the suspected source of septic infection (e.g., gastrointestinal tract, genitourinary tract) and are determined by an infectious disease expert. Dosages recommended for meningitis and severe infections are used.

❖ **Note** *IV drug abusers are given an aminoglycoside and clindamycin to eradicate* Bacillus cereus.

3. Topical cycloplegic (e.g., atropine 1% tid).
4. Topical steroid (e.g., prednisolone acetate 1% q 1–6 h, depending on the degree of anterior-segment inflammation).
5. Periocular antibiotics (e.g., subconjunctival or subtenons injections) are sometimes used. See Appendix 7 for injection techniques.

Follow-up

Daily in the hospital. Peak and trough levels for many antibiotic agents are examined every few days. Blood urea nitrogen and creatinine levels are monitored during aminoglycoside therapy. The antibiotic regimen is guided by the culture and sensitivity results, as well as the patient's clinical response to treatment. IV antibiotics are maintained for at least 2 weeks and until the condition has resolved.

13.13 CANDIDA RETINITIS/UVEITIS/ ENDOPHTHALMITIS

Symptoms

Decreased vision, floaters, pain, often bilateral. Patients typically are IV drug abusers, immunocompromised hosts (e.g., as a result of cancer, immunosuppressive agents, AIDS, long-term antibiotics, or systemic steroids) or possess a long-term indwelling catheter (e.g., for hyperalimentation or hemodialysis).

Critical Signs

Multifocal, yellow-white, fluffy retinal lesions from one to several disc diameters in size. With time, the lesions increase in size, spread into the vitreous, and appear as "cotton balls."

Other Signs

Vitreous cells and haze, vitreous abscesses, retinal hemorrhages with or without pale centers (pale centers indicate Roth's spots), aqueous cells and flare, hypopyon. Retinal detachment may develop.

Differential Diagnosis

The following should be considered in immunocompromised hosts.

- Cytomegalovirus (CMV) retinitis   (Minimal-to-mild vitreous reaction, more retinal hemorrhage, tends to concentrate along vessels; consider strongly in AIDS patients. See Section 14.1.)
- Toxoplasmosis   (Yellow-white lesion confined to the retina. An adjacent chorioretinal scar may or may not be present. Vitreous cells and debris are common, but vitreous abscesses or "cotton balls" are not. See Section 13.3.)
- Others (e.g., herpes simplex; *Mycobacterium avium-intracellulare; Nocardia, Aspergillus,* and *Cryptococcus* species; coccidiomycosis)

Work-up

1. History: Medications? Medical problems? IV drug abuse? Other risk factors for AIDS?
2. Search the skin for scars from IV drug injection.
3. Complete ocular examination, including a dilated retinal evaluation.
4. Blood, urine, and catheter site (if present) cultures for *Candida* species; these often need to be repeated several times and may be negative despite ocular candidiasis.
5. Diagnostic (and therapeutic) vitrectomy is indicated when a significant amount of vitreous involvement is present. Cultures and smears are taken at the time of vitrectomy to confirm the diagnosis and to evaluate the organisms' sensitivity to antifungal agents. Amphotericin B 5 μg in 0.1 mL is injected into the central vitreous cavity at the conclusion of the procedure.
6. Baseline CBC, blood urea nitrogen, creatinine, and liver function tests.

Treatment

1. Hospitalize all unreliable patients, systemically ill patients, or those with moderate-to-severe vitreous involvement.

2. An infectious-disease specialist or internist familiar with antifungal therapy should be consulted.
3. Fluconazole 200–400 mg po q day.
4. In resistant cases, amphotericin B may be administered. For the first few days, amphotericin B 1 mg IV is given 5 times per day, then larger doses totaling 20 mg/day are administered. Therapy is discontinued when a total dose of 1000 mg has been given. Patients with endophthalmitis can be given up to 1 mg/kg/day for several weeks, not to exceed a total dose of 2 g.
5. Topical cycloplegic agent (e.g., atropine 1% tid).
6. See "Inflammatory Open-Angle Glaucoma," Section 10.4, for intraocular pressure (IOP) control. Note, however, that steroids are generally contraindicated in candidiasis.

Follow-up

Patients are seen daily. Visual acuity, IOP, and the degree of anterior-chamber and vitreous inflammation are assessed. Serum blood urea nitrogen levels, creatinine levels, and CBC are repeated a few times per week. Liver function tests are repeated periodically. Serum levels of antifungal agents are followed, and dosages are adjusted accordingly.

❖ **Note** *Systemic antifungal agents may not be necessary if no systemic disease is uncovered.*

13.14 PHACOANAPHYLACTIC ENDOPHTHALMITIS

Definition

A sterile autoimmune inflammatory reaction to exposed lens protein. It usually occurs 1 day to a few weeks following surgical, traumatic, or spontaneous disruption of the lens capsule.

Symptoms

Pain, photophobia, red eye, decreased vision.

Critical Signs

A greater anterior-chamber inflammatory reaction than is typically seen after a surgical procedure (more cells and flare; sometimes, a hypopyon and mutton-fat keratic precipitates). Lens material may be seen in the anterior chamber.

Other Signs
Eyelid edema, chemosis, increased intraocular pressure (IOP), posterior synechiae.

Differential Diagnosis
See "Postoperative Uveitis," Section 13.9.

Work-up
See "Postoperative Uveitis," Section 13.9, for a generalized uveitis work-up in a postoperative patient.

1. History: Recent ocular surgery or trauma?
2. Complete ocular examination: Look for lens particles in the anterior chamber, measure the IOP, and search for any inflammatory reaction in the vitreous. The red fundus reflex should be assessed during a dilated retinal examination.
3. If infectious endophthalmitis cannot be ruled out, cultures are obtained and antibiotics started (see "Postoperative Endophthalmitis," Section 13.10).
4. B-scan ultrasound to help in diagnosis and follow-up.

Treatment
1. Topical steroids (e.g., prednisolone acetate 1%) q 1–2 h.
2. Subconjunctival steroids (e.g., methylprednisolone 40 mg). See Appendix 7 for the technique.
3. If the IOP is elevated, see "Inflammatory Open-Angle Glaucoma," Section 10.4, and "Steroid-Response Glaucoma," Section 10.5, for management.

If severe:

4. Systemic steroids (e.g., prednisone 80–100 mg po daily) and an antacid or histamine H_2 blocker (e.g., ranitidine 150 mg po bid).
5. After the inflammation has subsided, surgery may be indicated to remove residual lens material and capsule.

Follow-up
Every 1–7 days, depending on the severity of the condition (some patients may need to be hospitalized).

• Check the IOP: Watch for glaucoma.
• Assess the degree of inflammation. Taper the steroids slowly as the inflammation subsides.

13.15 SYMPATHETIC OPHTHALMIA

Symptoms

Bilateral eye pain, photophobia, decreased vision (near vision is often affected before distance vision), red eye. A history of penetrating trauma or intraocular surgery to one eye (usually 4–8 weeks prior, but the range is from 5 days to 66 years, with 90% occurring within 1 year) may be elicited.

Critical Signs

Bilateral severe anterior-chamber reaction with large mutton-fat keratic precipitates, small depigmented nodules at the level of the retinal pigment epithelium (Dalen-Fuchs' nodules), and thickening of the uveal tract. Signs of previous injury or surgery in one eye are usually present, including indications of previous laser therapy or cryotherapy.

Other Signs

Nodular infiltration of the iris, peripheral anterior synechiae, neovascularization of the iris, occlusion and seclusion of the pupil, cataract, exudative retinal detachment, papillitis. The earliest sign may be loss of accommodation or a mild anterior or posterior uveitis in the uninjured eye.

Differential Diagnosis

- Vogt-Koyanagi-Harada (VKH) syndrome (Similar signs, but often no history of ocular trauma or surgery. Other symptoms and signs may include headache, nausea, vomiting, fever, malaise, vertigo, bizarre behavior, focal neurologic symptoms, alopecia, vitiligo, or poliosis. Darkly pigmented persons, especially Asians, are more commonly affected. See Section 13.7.)
- Phacoanaphylactic endophthalmitis (Severe anterior-chamber reaction from injury to the lens capsule, usually from trauma or surgery. No posterior uveitis is present. See Section 13.14.)
- Sarcoidosis (May cause a granulomatous panuveitis with exudates over retinal veins or white clumps in the anterior vitreous inferiorly. Concomitant pulmonary disease is common. See Section 13.4.)
- Syphilis (Granulomatous panuveitis may be accompanied by interstitial keratitis, dilated capillary nests on the iris, or a diffuse pigmentary retinopathy. Positive FTA-ABS. See Section 14.2.)

Work-up

1. History: Any prior eye surgery or injury? Venereal disease? Difficulty breathing?
2. Complete ophthalmic examination, including a dilated retinal examination.

3. CBC, RPR, FTA-ABS, with or without angiotensin converting enzyme (ACE) level if sarcoidosis is a serious consideration.
4. Chest x-ray to rule out sarcoidosis.
5. Fluorescein angiography and/or B-scan ultrasonography to help confirm the diagnosis.

Treatment

1. Prevention: Enucleation of a blind, traumatized eye before a sympathetic reaction can develop (usually considered within 7–14 days of the trauma). If sympathetic ophthalmia develops, enucleation may still be beneficial, regardless of the time period since the trauma.

Inflammation is controlled with steroids; the dose depends on the severity of the inflammation. In moderate-to-severe cases, the following regimen can be used initially. Steroids are tapered slowly as the condition improves.

2. Topical steroids (e.g., prednisolone acetate 1% q 1–2 h).
3. Periocular steroids (e.g., subconjunctival dexamethasone 4–5 mg, 2–3 times per week). See Appendix 7 for the administration technique.
4. Systemic steroids [e.g., prednisone 60–80 mg po daily and an antacid or histamine H_2 blocker (e.g., ranitidine 150 mg po bid)].
5. Cycloplegic (e.g., scopolamine 0.25% tid).
6. If steroids are ineffective or contraindicated, an immunosuppressive agent (e.g., methotrexate or cyclosporin) may be tried, usually in conjunction with a medical consultant.

Follow-up

Every 1–7 days initially, to monitor the effectiveness of therapy. As the condition improves, the follow-up interval may be extended to every 3–4 weeks. Intraocular pressure must be monitored closely. Steroids should be maintained for 3–6 months after all signs of inflammation have resolved. Because of the possibility of recurrence, periodic checkups are important.

Systemic Disorders

14.1 Acquired Immunodeficiency Syndrome (AIDS)

Risk Groups

Homosexual or bisexual men, IV drug abusers, hemophiliacs and transfusion recipients, sexual partners of persons with AIDS or at risk for AIDS, prostitutes and their sexual partners, infants born to mothers with AIDS.

Laboratory Diagnosis

1. Serum enzyme-linked immunosorbent assay (ELISA) for human immunodeficiency virus (HIV) antibody (sensitive, but not very specific).
2. Western blot if ELISA is positive (the Western blot is very rarely falsely positive).

OCULAR COMPLICATIONS

External Disease

Herpes Zoster Ophthalmicus

May be the initial clinical manifestation of HIV infection.

Signs
Vesicular lesions of the face in a trigeminal-nerve distribution; may be associated with almost any eye abnormality, in both the anterior and posterior segment. See "Herpes Zoster Virus," Section 4.16.

The Wills Eye Manual: Office and Emergency Room Diagnosis and Treatment of Eye Diseases, Second Edition, edited by R. Douglas Cullom, Jr., M.D., and Benjamin Chang, M.D. © 1994 J. B. Lippincott Company.

❖ **Note** *A variety of associated necrotizing retinopathies have been described, including an acute retinal necrosis–like syndrome that may be rapidly progressive, leading to rhegmatogenous retinal detachments (RRDs).*

Treatment
1. Acyclovir 30 mg/kg/day IV in 3 divided doses for 7–10 days. (For patients with a creatinine level >2 mg/dL, the dosage is reduced to 20 mg/kg/day in 2 divided doses.) An oral maintenance dose (600–800 mg 5 times per day) may be required to prevent reactivation of infection.
2. When intraocular inflammation is present, a topical cycloplegic (e.g., scopolamine 0.25% tid) and a topical steroid (e.g., prednisolone acetate 1% q 1–2 h) are given.
3. Bacitracin ointment to the skin lesions bid.

- Cimetidine 400 mg po bid is controversial in prophylaxis against postherpetic neuralgia. We generally do not prescribe cimetidine.
- Patients probably should not receive oral steroids because of the risk of further immunosuppression and extension of the infection.

Kaposi's Sarcoma

Signs
Bright-red subconjunctival lesion most commonly located in the inferior cul-de-sac. It may be mistaken for a localized subconjunctival hemorrhage. Eyelid lesions are purple-red, nontender nodules and can have associated edema, trichiasis, or entropion formation. Orbital lesions with associated periorbital edema occur rarely.

Treatment
1. Vinblastine and vincristine have each had some success in causing remission of Kaposi's sarcoma.
2. Local treatment by excision, cryotherapy, or irradiation may be performed for single lesions.

Posterior-Segment Disease

Noninfectious Retinopathy ("AIDS Retinopathy")

The following are common retinal abnormalities seen in patients with AIDS. They are nonspecific and not diagnostic of AIDS. Cotton-wool spots (most common), flame-shaped hemorrhages, dot hemorrhages, Roth's spots (white-centered hemorrhages), microaneurysms and microvascular abnormalities. An ischemic maculopathy (decreased visual acuity, retinal edema, and macular star formation) occasionally can be seen.

Treatment

The guidelines are not well established. There may be a role for focal laser therapy in the presence of macular edema.

Cytomegalovirus (CMV) Retinopathy

Most common ocular infection in patients with AIDS, with a prevalence of about 25%.

Symptoms

Painless, decreased vision in one or both eyes.

Critical Signs

Multiple distinct areas of white, granular retinal opacification with irregular feathered borders, often mixed with retinal hemorrhages. The necrotic areas usually initiate along the major vascular arcades in the posterior pole and enlarge and coalesce with time.

Other Signs

The eye is typically white and quiet with little to no aqueous or vitreous cells. Atrophy and pigment dispersion result once the active process resolves. Optic neuritis, exudative retinal detachment, or cystoid macular edema may develop. RRDs (late complication) occur in about 25% of patients with CMV retinitis.

Work-up

1. History and complete ocular examination, including dilated fundus examination.
2. Fluorescein angiography may be helpful in the fundus evaluation.
3. Refer the patient to an internist for a systemic CMV work-up (e.g., urine for CMV and repeat complement fixation and neutralization titers).

Treatment

Ganciclovir and foscarnet appear equally effective in halting the progression of CMV retinitis. Treatment of choice is based primarily on the toxicity profile. (Foscarnet may offer a survival advantage in patients with normal renal function.)

GANCICLOVIR

- Induction with 5 mg/kg IV q 12 h for 14 days, then a maintenance IV dose of 5 mg/kg/day (or 6 mg/kg/day for 5 of 7 days).
- The dosage may need to be reduced in the presence of renal disease.
- Main side-effect is myelosuppression.
- Check complete blood count (CBC) with differential and platelet count

2–3 times per week during induction, then weekly thereafter. Discontinue if absolute neutrophil count is <500 or platelet count is <10,000.

- Zidovidine (AZT) doses may need adjustment. (The use of hematopoietic growth factors such as regramostim or filgrastim allow for simultaneous full-dose AZT and ganciclovir.)
- Intravitreal ganciclovir can be used as an alternative to systemic treatment.

FOSCARNET

- Induction with 60 mg/kg IV q 8 h for 14 days, then a maintenance IV dose of 90–120 mg/kg/day. (Hydrate with 1 L of normal saline, if possible.)
- Renal toxicity is the main adverse effect. (Alterations in calcium and magnesium balance with secondary seizures have been reported.)
- Check serum creatinine, calcium, magnesium, and hemoglobin 2–3 times per week initially, then weekly thereafter.
- Adjust dosage for renal function and discontinue if serum creatinine is >2.8 mg/dL (resume once serum creatinine is <2.0 mg/dL).

Toxoplasmosis

Symptoms
Decreased vision, floaters, photophobia, pain, red eye.

Critical Signs
Hazy yellow-white retinochoroidal lesions accompanied by vitreous cells and debris. Hemorrhage is minimal when the infection is newly acquired; an old retinochoroidal scar is typically not observed. The lesions may be single or multifocal, discrete or diffuse, and unilateral or bilateral. Recurrences frequently occur at the edge of an old scar or as a satellite lesion.

Work-up
1. Complete ocular examination with special emphasis on the neuro-ophthalmic aspects.
2. Referral to an internist for a complete medical work-up (emphasize the need to watch for CNS toxoplasmosis).

❖ **Note** *Toxoplasmosis antibody titers may be unreliable.*

Treatment
Not well established. See "Toxoplasmosis," Section 13.3, for drug dosages.

1. Pyrimethamine plus sulfadiazine, clindamycin, or tetracycline (or an equivalent).
2. Topical steroid (e.g., prednisolone acetate 1% q 1–6 h; the dosage depends on the degree of anterior-segment inflammation).

3. Topical cycloplegic (e.g., scopolamine 0.25% tid) in the presence of anterior-segment inflammation.

❖ **Notes**

1. *Maintenance therapy may be required to prevent recurrence of the disease. Clindamycin should probably not be used for this purpose.*
2. *Systemic steroids may allow for advancement of infection, and their role in ocular toxoplasmosis in AIDS is uncertain.*

Candida Retinitis

See Section 13.13.

Pneumocystis carinii choroidopathy

Relatively rare ocular manifestation of AIDS.

Symptoms

Mild decrease in visual acuity; may be asymptomatic.

Critical Signs

Multifocal, yellow, round, deep choroidal lesions about one-half to two disc diameters in size, located in the posterior pole. Typically, no retinal vascular changes or vitritis.

Work-up

1. History of *P. carinii* pneumonia and associated treatment (e.g., aerosolized pentamidine).
2. Complete dilated ocular examination.
3. Refer the patient to an internist for complete medical evaluation and management consultation.

Treatment

IV trimethoprim/sulfamethoxazole or IV pentamidine.

Others

Herpes simplex virus. *Mycobacterium tuberculosis* or *Mycobacterium avium-intracellulare, Cryptococcus neoformans, Histoplasma capsulatum,* herpes zoster, *Aspergillus* species, and *Nocardia* species are all rarely seen.

Neuro-ophthalmic Manifestations

Cranial-nerve palsies, pupillary abnormalities, brain stem ocular motility defects, ischemic or infectious optic neuritis, visual field defects, and visual hallucinations may occur as a result of CNS infection (e.g., toxoplasmosis) or tumor (optic-nerve swelling may also be observed in these cases). There is an increased incidence of neurosyphilis in the AIDS population, suggesting the need for lumbar puncture in all patients with syphilis and a positive HIV titer (see "Acquired Syphilis," Section 14.2).

TREATMENT FOR AIDS

Antiretroviral treatment with AZT has been shown to decrease mortality and the frequency of opportunistic infections. Dideoxycitidine (investigational) is an alternative antiretroviral agent without bone-marrow toxicity. Hematopoietic growth factors or colony-stimulating factors like regramostim (Prokine) or filgrastim (Neupogen) can be used to treat myelosuppression.

REFERENCES

Studies of Ocular Complications of AIDS Research Group. Mortality in patients with the acquired immunodeficiency syndrome treated with either foscarnet or ganciclovir for cytomegalovirus retinitis. *N Engl J Med* 326:213, 1992.

14.2 ACQUIRED SYPHILIS

Systemic Signs

STAGES

Primary Chancre (ulcerated, painless lesion), regional lymphadenopathy.

Secondary Skin or mucous membrane lesions, generalized lymphadenopathy, constitutional symptoms (e.g., sore throat, fever), other less common but more severe abnormalities including symptomatic or asymptomatic meningitis.

Latent No clinical manifestations.

Tertiary Cardiovascular disease (e.g., aortitis), central nervous system disease (e.g., meningovascular disease, general paresis, tabes dorsalis).

Ocular Signs

Primary A chancre may occur on the eyelid or conjunctiva.

Secondary or tertiary Uveitis, optic neuritis, active chorioretinitis, retinitis, retinal vasculitis, conjunctivitis, dacryoadenitis, dacryocystitis, episcleritis, scleritis, monocular interstitial keratitis, others.

Tertiary Optic atrophy, old chorioretinitis, interstitial keratitis, chronic iritis, Argyll-Robertson pupil (will not react to light, but will accommodate; see Section 11.3), and other signs seen in secondary disease.

❖ **Note** *Patchy hyperemia of the iris with the development of fleshy, pink nodules near the iris sphincter is pathognomonic of syphilis.*

Differential Diagnosis

See "Anterior Uveitis," Section 13.1, and "Posterior Uveitis," Section 13.2.

Work-up

See Sections 13.1 and 13.2 for a nonspecific uveitis work-up.

1. Complete ophthalmic examination, including pupillary evaluation, slit-lamp examination, and dilated fundus examination.
2. VDRL or RPR reflects the activity of the disease and is important in following the patient's response to treatment. Used for screening, but many false-negatives can occur in early primary, latent, or late syphilis. Not as specific as FTA-ABS or MHA-TP.
3. FTA-ABS or MHA-TP are very sensitive and specific in all stages of syphilis. Once reactive, these tests do not revert back to normal and therefore cannot be used to assess the patient's response to treatment.
4. HIV serology: Should be offered to patients with sexually transmitted diseases.
5. Lumbar puncture (LP). The indications are controversial. We consider LP in the following situations:
   a. Positive FTA-ABS and neurologic or neuro-ophthalmologic signs, papillitis, active chorioretinitis, or anterior or posterior uveitis.
   b. Patients who are HIV-positive as well as FTA-ABS-positive.
   c. Treatment failures.
   d. Patients to be treated with a nonpenicillin regimen (as a baseline).
   e. Patients with untreated syphilis of unknown duration or longer than 1-year duration.

Treatment Indications

A. FTA-ABS-negative: No treatment indicated. Patient probably does not have syphilis. Consider retesting if clinical circumstances are compelling.

B. FTA-ABS-positive and VDRL-negative
   • If appropriate past treatment *cannot* be documented, treatment is indicated.
   • If appropriate past treatment *can* be documented, treatment is not indicated.

C. FTA-ABS-positive and VDRL-positive: A VDRL titer of 1:8 or greater (e.g., 1:64) is expected to decline at least fourfold within 1 year of appropriate treatment, and should revert to negative (or at least to 1:4 or less) within 1 year in primary syphilis, 2 years in secondary syphilis, and 5 years in tertiary syphilis. A VDRL of <1:8 (e.g., 1:4) often does *not* drop fourfold. Therefore, the following recommendations are made:

- If appropriate past treatment *cannot* be documented, treatment is indicated.
- If appropriate past treatment *can* be documented, and . . .
  A previous VDRL titer greater than or equal to four times the current titer can be documented, no treatment is indicated (unless 5 years have passed and the titer is still >1:4).
  A previous VDRL titer was ≥1:8 and did not drop fourfold, treatment is indicated.
  The previous VDRL titer was <1:8, treatment is not indicated, unless the current titer has *risen* fourfold.
  A previous VDRL is unavailable, treatment is not required unless treatment was more than several years prior and the VDRL is still >1:4.

❖ **Note** *If active syphilitic signs (e.g., active chorioretinitis, papillitis) are present despite appropriate past treatment (regardless of the VDRL titer), LP and treatment may be needed.*

❖ **Note** *Patients with concurrent HIV and active syphilis may have negative serologies (FTA, RPR) because of their immunocompromised state. These patients manifest aggressive, recalcitrant syphilis disease. They should be treated with neurosyphilis dosages, usually over longer treatment periods. Consultation with an infectious-disease specialist is recommended.*

Treatment

A. *Neurosyphilis* [positive FTA-ABS in the serum and either cell count >5 WBC/mm^3, protein >45 mg/dL, or positive cerebrospinal fluid (CSF)-VDRL on LP]: IV aqueous crystalline penicillin (PCN) G 2–4 million U q 4 h for 10–14 days, followed by benzathine PCN 2.4 million U IM weekly for 3 weeks (1.2 million U in each buttock).

B. *Syphilis with abnormal ocular but normal CSF findings:* Benzathine PCN 2.4 million U IM weekly for 3 weeks.

❖ **Notes**

1. *Treatment for possible chlamydia infection with tetracycline 250 mg po qid, doxycycline 100 mg po bid, or erythromycin 250 mg po qid for 2–3 weeks is typically indicated.*

2. *Therapy for PCN-allergic patients is not well established. Tetracycline 500 mg po qid for 30 days is used by some for both late syphilis and neurosyphilis, but better CSF penetration may be obtained with doxycycline (200 mg po bid for 30 days) or a third-generation cephalosporin.*
3. *If anterior-segment inflammation is present, treatment with a cycloplegic (e.g., cyclopentolate 2% tid) and topical steroid (e.g., prednisolone acetate 1% qid) may be beneficial.*

Follow-up

A. *Neurosyphilis:* Repeat LP every 6 months for 2 years, less if the cell count returns to normal sooner. The cell count should fall to a normal level within this time period, and the CSF VDRL titer should drop fourfold (these changes typically occur within 6–12 months). An elevated CSF protein falls more slowly. If these indices do not fall as expected, retreatment may be indicated.

B. *Other forms of syphilis:* Repeat the VDRL titer at 3 and 6 months after treatment.

If a VDRL titer of 1:8 or more does not decline fourfold within 6 months, if the VDRL titer rises fourfold at any point, or if clinical symptoms or signs of syphilis persist or recur, LP and retreatment are indicated.

If a pretreatment VDRL titer is less than 1:8, retreatment is only indicated when the titer rises during follow-up or when symptoms or signs of syphilis recur.

See "Congenital Syphilis," Section 14.3, for additional information.

14.3 CONGENITAL SYPHILIS

Presenting Ocular Signs

Any of the following may be present.

Interstitial keratitis (IK)   Usually presents acutely in the first or second decade of life with cellular infiltration and superficial and deep vascularization of the cornea (corneal "salmon patch"). Both eyes eventually become affected. As the inflammation resolves, the cornea may thin, opacify, or exhibit blood vessels containing no blood within their lumens (ghost vessels).

Anterior uveitis   Cells and flare in the anterior chamber.

Chorioretinitis   Typically appears as a salt-and-pepper fundus (pigmented areas interspersed among atrophic white areas).

Optic atrophy   A pale optic nerve.

Systemic Signs

Widely spaced, peg-shaped teeth (Hutchinson's teeth), frontal bossing, depressed nasal bridge (saddle nose), nerve deafness, recurrent arthropathy, linear scars at the angles of the mouth, mental retardation, others.

Differential Diagnosis

- Other congenital infections [toxoplasmosis, rubella, CMV, herpes simplex or zoster virus, rubeola (measles)]   (Specific serological titers will usually be positive; RPR and FTA-ABS will usually be negative.)

Work-up

1. History: Maternal syphilis? Medical problems since birth (persistent runny nose, rash, deafness, scars on the skin, others)? Previous treatment for syphilis?
2. Complete ocular examination, including a pupillary assessment, a slit-lamp examination if possible, and a dilated fundus examination (in interstitial keratitis, the fundus may not be well visualized).
3. B-scan ultrasound should be considered when no fundus view is obtained to rule out a retinal detachment and mass lesion.
4. Blood tests: RPR (or VDRL) and FTA-ABS (or MHA-TP)[1]; consider viral and toxoplasma titers when the diagnosis is uncertain.
5. Consider darkfield examination of scrapings from skin lesions, if available.
6. LP for routine studies including a VDRL is indicated in all cases of active disease or in cases of inactive disease not previously treated.

Treatment

See "Acquired Syphilis," Section 14.2, for treatment indications.

1. Systemic antibiotic (one of the following):
   a. Aqueous crystalline PCN G 50,000 U/kg/day IM or IV in 2 divided doses for 10–14 days.
   b. Aqueous procaine PCN G 50,000 U/kg IM daily for 10–14 days.
   c. For PCN-allergic patients: Erythromycin 50 mg/kg/day po in 4 divided doses for 2 weeks.
2. In the presence of acute IK or anterior-chamber inflammation, a topical steroid (prednisolone acetate 1% 4–8 times per day) and a cycloplegic (e.g., scopolamine 0.25% tid) should be used.
3. Intraocular pressure control (e.g., if >30 mm Hg, consider levobunolol 0.25–0.5% bid or timolol 0.25–0.5% bid and/or acetazolamide 5 mg/kg po q 6 h).

---

[1]Both the RPR (or VDRL) and FTA-ABS (or MHA-TP) can be positive in a syphilis-free infant born to a mother with the disease. The RPR usually converts back to negative by 3 months of age in a disease-free child; the FTA-ABS is usually found to be negative by 6 months of age. A positive IgM-FTA-ABS in an infant suggests active disease.

Follow-up

Patients are seen daily until their systemic therapy is completed, then in 1–2 weeks. When the LP is abnormal (e.g., positive CSF VDRL, white blood cell count >5 WBC/mm³ or protein >45 mg/dL), follow-up is as described for neurosyphilis (see "Acquired Syphilis," Section 14.2). Otherwise, follow-up is as described for other forms of acquired syphilis (see Section 14.2). The FTA-ABS typically remains reactive despite treatment.

14.4 LYME DISEASE

Symptoms

Decreased vision, double vision, pain, photophobia, facial weakness. Patients may also complain of headache, malaise, fatigue, fever, chills, palpitations, or muscle or joint pains. A history of a tick bite within the previous few months can often be elicited.

Ocular Signs

Optic neuritis; vitritis; iritis; choroiditis; exudative retinal detachment; third-, fourth-, or sixth-cranial-nerve palsy, bilateral optic-nerve swelling; conjunctivitis; episcleritis; exposure keratopathy; stromal keratitis; other rare abnormalities, including orbital inflammatory pseudotumor.

Critical Systemic Signs

One or more flat erythematous or "bull's-eye" skin lesions, which enlarge in all directions (erythema chronica migrans); unilateral or bilateral facial-nerve palsies; arthritis. The skin lesions and arthritis may be transient and migratory. These findings may not be present at the time the ocular signs develop. A high serum antibody titer against the causative agent, *Borrelia burgdorferi,* is often, but not always present.

Other Systemic Signs

Meningitis, peripheral radiculoneuropathy, synovitis, joint effusions, cardiac abnormalities, and/or a low false-positive FTA-ABS titer

Differential Diagnosis

- Syphilis (High positive FTA-ABS titer may produce a low false positive antibody titer against *B. burgdorferi.* No history of a tick bite. May have interstitial keratitis, patchy iris hyperemia, a salt-and-pepper chorioretinitis, or pigmented "bone spicules" on fundus examination.)

- Others (Rickettsial infections, acute rheumatic fever, juvenile rheumatoid arthritis.)

Work-up

1. History: Prior tick bite, skin rash, Bell's palsy, joint or muscle pains, flulike illness? Meningeal symptoms?
2. Complete systemic (especially neurological) and ocular examinations.
3. Serum antibody levels against *B. burgdorferi*, using an immunofluorescence assay or ELISA. (These tests are sometimes negative despite the presence of Lyme disease because of a long period of latency to response.)
4. Serum RPR and FTA-ABS.
5. Consider lumbar puncture when meningitis is suspected or neurologic signs or symptoms are present.

Treatment

Current recommendations vary, but include one of the following:

ADULTS

First choice Tetracycline 250 mg po qid or doxycycline 100 mg po bid for 21–28 days.

Second choice Amoxicillin 500 mg po qid (and probenecid 500 mg) for 21–28 days.

Third choice Erythromycin 250 mg po qid for 21–28 days.

CHILDREN

First choice Penicillin 50 mg/kg/day po in 4 divided doses (not <1 g/day or >2 g/day) for 21–28 days.

Second choice Erythromycin 30 mg/kg/day po in 3–4 divided doses for 21–28 days.

PATIENTS WITH NEURO-OPHTHALMIC SIGNS OR RECURRENT OR RESISTANT INFECTION

Ceftriaxone 1 g IV q 12 h or 2 g IV q 24 h for 14–21 days
or
Cefotaxime 3 g IV q 12 h for 14–21 days
and
Aqueous crystalline PCN G 2–4 million U IV q 4 h for 10 days.

Follow-up
Daily, until improvement is demonstrated.

REFERENCES

Sigal LH. Current recommendations for the treatment of Lyme disease. *Drugs* 45(5):683, 1992.
Winterkorn JM. Lyme disease: Neurologic and ophthalmic manifestations. *Surv Ophthalmol* 35(3):191, 1990.
Lesser RL, Kornmehl EW, Pachner AR, et al. Neuro-ophthalmic manifestations of Lyme disease. *Ophthalmology* 97(6):699, 1990.

14.5 CHICKEN POX

Symptoms
Facial rash, red eye, foreign-body sensation.

Ocular Signs

Early   Acute conjunctivitis with vesicles or papules at the limbus, eyelid margin, or on the conjunctiva. Pseudodendritic corneal epithelial lesions, stromal keratitis, anterior uveitis, optic neuritis, retinitis, and ophthalmoplegia occur rarely.

Late (weeks to months after the outbreak)   Immune stromal or neurotrophic keratitis may occur.

Treatment

A. *Conjunctival involvement:* Cool compresses and erythromycin ointment to the eye and periorbital lesions tid.
B. *Corneal epithelial lesions:* Same as for conjunctival involvement.
C. *Stromal keratitis with uveitis:* Topical steroid (e.g., prednisolone acetate 1% qid), cycloplegic (e.g., atropine 1% bid), and erythromycin ointment qhs.
D. *Neurotrophic keratitis:* See "Neurotrophic Keratopathy," Section 4.5.

❖ **Note** *Do not give aspirin to these children because of the possible risk of Reye's syndrome. Immunocompromised children with chicken pox may require IV acyclovir.*

Follow-up
Follow-up in 1–7 days, depending on the severity of ocular disease. Taper the topical steroids slowly. Watch for stromal or neurotrophic keratitis weeks to months after the chicken pox resolves.

14.6 DIABETES MELLITUS

Diabetic Retinopathy

Signs

Mild nonproliferative   Dot and blot hemorrhages, microaneurysms, and hard exudates, generally most prominent in the posterior pole. Nearly always bilateral.

Moderate-to-severe nonproliferative   Cotton-wool spots, venous beading and loops, intraretinal microvascular abnormalities (IRMA), and widespread capillary nonperfusion (seen on fluorescein angiography) plus findings in mild nonproliferative disease.

Proliferative   Neovascularization within 1 disc diameter of or involving the optic disc (NVD), retina (NVE), or iris (NVI), fibrous tissue along the posterior surface of the vitreous and adherent to the retina, retinal detachment, vitreous hemorrhage. The findings in mild and moderate-to-severe nonproliferative disease are sometimes present. Usually bilateral. Almost always in the posterior pole.

❖ **Note** *Macular edema may be present in any of the above stages.*

Differential Diagnosis

NONPROLIFERATIVE

- Central retinal vein occlusion (CRVO)   (Optic-disc swelling is present, veins are more tortuous, hard exudates are usually absent, hemorrhages are more prominent, and it is generally unilateral and of more sudden onset. See Section 12.3.)
- Branch retinal vein occlusion (BRVO)   [The hemorrhages are distributed along the course of a vein, and do *not* extend across the horizontal raphé (midline). See Section 12.4.]
- Ocular ischemic syndrome   (The hemorrhages are larger and mostly in the midperiphery; exudate is absent. See Section 12.7.)
- Hypertensive retinopathy   (The hemorrhages are more commonly flame-shaped and rarely abundant, microaneurysms occur less frequently, and the retinal arterioles are narrowed. See Section 12.5.)
- Radiation retinopathy   (Microaneurysms are rarely present. Follows radiation therapy to the eye or adnexal structures such as the brain, sinus, or nasopharynx, when the eye is irradiated inadvertently. May develop anytime after the radiation therapy, but occurs most commonly within a few years. Generally, 3000 rads are necessary, but it has been noted to occur with 1500 rads.)

PROLIFERATIVE

- Neovascular complications of BRVO, CRVO, or central retinal artery occlusion   (History of one of these events. See previous discussion.)
- Sickle-cell retinopathy   (Retinal neovascularization occurs peripherally, generally not in the macula. "Sea-fans" of retinal neovascularization are present. See Section 12.23.)
- Embolization from IV drug abuse (e.g., talc retinopathy)   (History of IV drug abuse, peripheral retinal neovascularization, may see particles of talc in macular vessels.)
- Sarcoidosis   [May have uveitis, exudates around veins ("candle-wax drippings") or systemic findings. See Section 13.4.]
- Ocular ischemic syndrome   (Generally accompanied by pain; mild anterior-chamber reaction; corneal edema; episcleral vascular congestion; a mid-dilated, poorly reactive pupil; iris neovascularization; and pulsations of the central retinal artery induced by light digital pressure. See Section 12.7.)

Work-up

1. Examine the iris carefully for neovascularization. (Check the angle with gonioscopy, especially if intraocular pressure is elevated.)
2. Dilated fundus examination using a 90- or 60-diopter or fundus contact lens with a slit lamp to obtain a stereoscopic view of the posterior pole. Rule out neovascularization and macular edema. Use indirect ophthalmoscopy to examine the retinal periphery.
3. Fasting blood sugar and, if necessary, a glucose tolerance test, if the diagnosis is not established.
4. Check the blood pressure.
5. Consider fluorescein angiography to determine areas of perfusion abnormalities, foveal ischemia, microaneurysms, and clinically indistinguishable neovascularization.
6. Consider blood tests for hyperlipidemia if extensive exudate is present.

Treatment

INDICATIONS

A. Focal or grid laser treatment should be considered when any of the following forms of macular edema are present (clinically significant macular edema; Fig. 14.1).
   1. Retinal thickening within 500 μ (one third of disc diameter) of the center of the macula.
   2. Hard exudates within 500 μ of the center of the macula, if associated with thickening of the adjacent retina.

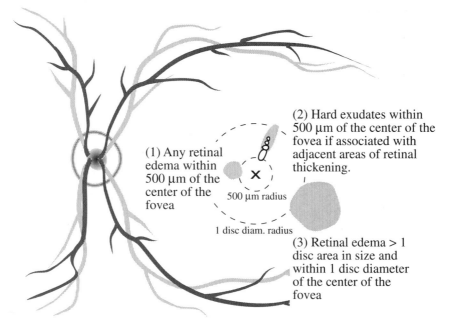

(1) Any retinal edema within 500 µm of the center of the fovea

500 µm radius

(2) Hard exudates within 500 µm of the center of the fovea if associated with adjacent areas of retinal thickening.

1 disc diam. radius

(3) Retinal edema > 1 disc area in size and within 1 disc diameter of the center of the fovea

Figure 14.1
Clinically significant macular edema in diabetic retinopathy that warrants grid-pattern photoco-agulation.

3. Retinal thickening greater than 1 disc area in size, part of which is within 1 disc diameter of the center of the macula.

❖ **Note** *Patients with enlarged foveal avascular zones on fluorescein angiography are treated lightly, away from the regions of foveal ischemia, if they are treated at all. Patients with extensive, frank foveal ischemia are not good candidates for treatment.*

B. Panretinal photocoagulation (laser) is indicated for any one of the following conditions (high-risk characteristics; Fig. 14.2).
   1. NVD greater than one fourth to one third of the disc area in size.
   2. Any degree of NVD when associated with preretinal or vitreous hemor-rhage.
   3. NVE greater than one half of the disc area in size when associated with a preretinal or vitreous hemorrhage.
   4. NVI.

❖ **Note** *Some physicians treat NVE or any degree of NVD without preretinal or vitreous hemorrhage.*

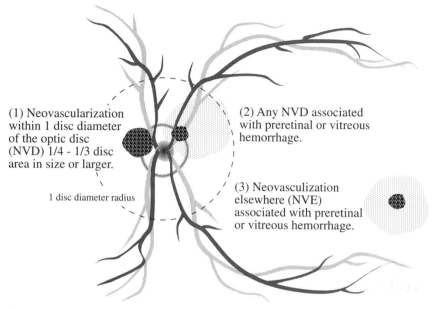

(1) Neovascularization within 1 disc diameter of the optic disc (NVD) 1/4 - 1/3 disc area in size or larger.

1 disc diameter radius

(2) Any NVD associated with preretinal or vitreous hemorrhage.

(3) Neovasculization elsewhere (NVE) associated with preretinal or vitreous hemorrhage.

Figure 14.2
High-risk characteristics for visual loss in proliferative diabetic retinopathy that warrants panretinal photocoagulation.

(If the ocular media are too hazy for an adequate fundus view, yet one of the above conditions is met, peripheral retinal cryotherapy may be indicated, if there is no vitreous traction. Pars plana vitrectomy and endolaser therapy with or without lensectomy and posterior-chamber intraocular lens is another alternative.)

C. Vitrectomy may be indicated for any one of the following conditions.
   1. Dense vitreous hemorrhage causing decreased vision, especially when present for several months.
   2. Traction retinal detachment involving and progressing within the macula.
   3. Macular epiretinal membranes or recent onset displacement of the macula.
   4. Severe retinal neovascularization and fibrous proliferation that are unresponsive to laser photocoagulation.

 Note *Juvenile type 1 diabetics are known to have more aggressive proliferative diabetic retinopathy and therefore may benefit from earlier vitrectomy and laser photocoagulation. B-scan ultrasonography, a visual evoked potential, or both may be required to rule out tractional detachment of the macula in eyes with dense vitreous hemorrhage obscuring a fundus view.*

Follow-up

Diabetes without retinopathy   Dilated fundus examination yearly.

Mild nonproliferative diabetic retinopathy   Dilated fundus examination every 6 months.

Moderate to severe nonproliferative retinopathy   Dilated fundus examination every 2–4 months.

Proliferative retinopathy not meeting treatment criteria   Dilated fundus examination every 1–3 months.

See Section 14.8 for pregnancy-related follow-up diabetics.

Neuro-ophthalmic Problems

Cranial-Nerve Abnormalities

An isolated third-, fourth-, or sixth-cranial-nerve palsy, often associated with pain in or around the eye, may result from diabetic microvascular disease. Only very rarely are two nerves involved simultaneously. Typically, third-nerve involvement spares the pupil (i.e., it does not become dilated). A diabetic cranial-nerve paralysis usually resolves within 3 months. No treatment is indicated.

Acute Disc Edema

Benign disc edema may occur in one or both eyes of a diabetic, most commonly with mild visual loss. It generally resolves after several weeks. There is no correlation with the severity of diabetic retinopathy. Telangiectasia of disc vessels may accompany the disc edema, simulating neovascularization. This entity is more common in juvenile-onset diabetics. No treatment is indicated, and resolution usually occurs in 6–8 weeks.

Idiopathic anterior ischemic optic neuropathy may also occur in diabetics. Usually, it is associated with more dramatic visual loss (manifested as decrease in acuity and visual field loss).

Glaucoma

Primary Open-Angle Glaucoma

Diabetics are at an increased risk for this form of glaucoma. When treating with a topical beta-blocker, additional care must be exercised in monitoring for side effects. A diabetic being treated with a beta-blocker may not experience the warning symptoms of hypoglycemia (e.g., sweating, shaking, nightmares, restlessness), and may, therefore, remain hypoglycemic for a dangerously long period of time without correcting the situation.

Neovascular Glaucoma

As discussed previously, neovascularization of the iris and glaucoma are complications of diabetes, and panretinal photocoagulation is indicated as soon as possible.

Miscellaneous

Refractive Changes

Acute hyperglycemia may produce a sudden hyperopic or myopic shift, causing bilateral blurred vision. Glasses should not be prescribed until the patient's blood sugar has been stable for several months.

Cataract

Diabetics are at an increased risk of cataract, especially posterior subcapsular cataracts.

Mucormycosis

A rare life-threatening orbital infection by mucormycosis can occur in diabetics, particularly those with ketoacidosis. Any diabetic or compromised host with the appearance of orbital cellulitis (eyelid edema, proptosis, external ophthalmoplegia, and fever) should be further examined for necrosis of the skin, nasal mucosa, or palate. An emergency CT scan of the sinuses, orbit, and brain should be performed to aid in diagnosis. A biopsy should be obtained from any necrotic tissue as well as the nasopharynx and paranasal sinuses if this condition is suspected. Treat with amphotericin B. See "Cavernous Sinus/Superior Orbital Fissure Syndrome," Section 11.9.

REFERENCES

The Diabetic Retinopathy Vitrectomy Study Research Group. Early vitrectomy for proliferative diabetic retinopathy in eyes with useful vision: Results of a randomized trial—diabetic retinopathy vitrectomy study report 3. *Ophthalmology* 95:1307, 1988.

The Diabetic Retinopathy Study Research Group. Photocoagulation treatment of proliferative diabetic retinopathy. The second report of diabetic retinopathy study findings. *Ophthalmology* 85:82, 1978.

The Early Treatment Diabetic Retinopathy Research Study Group; Photocoagulation for diabetic macular edema. ETDRS Report #1. *Arch Ophthalmol* 103:1796, 1985.

The Early Treatment Diabetic Retinopathy Research Study Group. Early photocoagulation for diabetic retinopathy. ETDRS Report #9. *Ophthalmology* 98(Suppl):766, 1991.

14.7 ALBINISM

Symptoms
Decreased vision and photophobia.

Signs
Nystagmus, iris transillumination defects, visible choroidal vasculature, absent foveal pit, absence of macular hyperpigmentation, failure of the retinal vessels to wreathe the fovea, pink reflex through an undilated pupil.

Types
I. Oculocutaneous: Hair, skin, and eye affected.
   A. Tyrosinase-positive: Some pigment as adults.
   B. Tyrosinase-negative: No pigment, ever.
II. Ocular: Decreased ocular pigment only. Skin may be lighter than that of siblings, but appears normal.

❖ **Note** *The only reliable ocular finding (always present) is foveal hypoplasia.*

Associated Disorders
- Hermansky-Pudlak syndrome   (An autosomal recessive bleeding disorder secondary to platelet dysfunction. There is a high incidence in patients of Puerto-Rican descent.)
- Chédiak-Higashi syndrome   (An autosomal recessive disorder affecting white blood cell function, causing a high susceptibility to infection and a predisposition for a lymphoma-like condition.)

Work-up
1. History: Early bruisability? Frequent nosebleeds? Prolonged bleeding after dental work? Frequent infections?
2. Family history.
3. External examination (check hair and skin color).
4. Complete ocular examination including a slit-lamp evaluation (nystagmus, iris color, and iris transillumination) and a dilated fundus examination.
5. Obtain a bleeding time if the patient is planning to undergo surgery. Some physicians feel a bleeding time should be obtained in all albinos. If the Hermansky-Pudlak syndrome is suspected, bleeding time, platelet aggregation studies, and platelet electron microscopy are indicated.
6. If the Chédiak-Higashi syndrome is suspected, polymorphonuclear leukocyte function should be evaluated by a hematologist.

Treatment

There is currently no effective treatment for albinism, but the following may be helpful:

1. Tinted eyeglasses may reduce photophobia.
2. Low-vision aides may be helpful in adults.
3. Genetic counseling.

❖ **Notes**

1. *Albinos with strabismus rarely achieve binocularity after strabismus surgery, possibly because of a lack of the necessary neuronal connections.*
2. *Albinos do poorly after retinal detachment repair because of nystagmus and inherently weak retinal pigment epithelium-retinal adhesions.*
3. *Patients with the Hermansky-Pudlak syndrome may require platelet transfusion prior to surgery.*

14.8 PREGNANCY

Many ocular problems can arise as a result of pregnancy. Below are listed some of the complaints that induce pregnant women to seek eye care and some of the disorders that should be considered in pregnancy.

Blurred or Decreased Vision

Change in Refractive Error

(Visual acuity decreased with current glasses, but can be improved to normal status with a new refraction or a pin hole. No other findings on examination.)

The patient's change in refraction is probably the result of a shift in fluid, hormonal status, or both and will most likely revert back to normal after delivery. Some of this change is attributable to the increased corneal thickness and secondary change in corneal refractive index during pregnancy. A transient loss of accommodation may also occur. Unless the patient has a strong desire (e.g., occupational need) to change her glasses prescription, it is best to wait until several weeks postpartum before giving a new prescription.

Preeclamptic/Eclamptic Hypertensive Retinopathy

(Occurs after 20 weeks of gestation. Same clinical findings as hypertensive retinopathy of other etiologies: Focal or generalized narrowing of the arterioles, flame-shaped hemorrhages, cotton-wool spots; disc swelling may or may not be present. An exudative retinal detachment can occur. Bilateral occipital lobe infarction and cortical blindness rarely can occur.)

The severity of retinal changes correlates with the risk of fetal mortality and possibly with the risk of damage to the mother's kidneys. If severe retinopathy is present and progressing, strong consideration should be made with regard to terminating the pregnancy. Sometimes the clinical findings (e.g., exudative retinal detachment) resolve with blood pressure control. (See Section 12.5.)

Central Serous Choriodopathy

(Localized detachment of the sensory retina from the underlying pigment epithelium by clear serous fluid in the macular area. The margins of the detachment are sloping and merge gradually into attached retina. No blood is present.)

With rare exception, observation is the treatment of choice, with most cases resolving postpartum. A more hyperopic correction may be provided as a temporary visual aid. Focal laser therapy is rarely needed. (See Section 12.8.)

Retinal Detachment

Usually exudative, resolving a few weeks after delivery. The visual prognosis is generally good, and no treatment is indicated. The pregnancy does not have to be terminated if preeclampsia/eclampsia can be ruled out. (See Section 12.19.)

Diabetic Retinopathy

Visual loss from diabetes may occur in patients who had diabetes prior to gestation. The following are our recommendations for management.

A. Gestational diabetes: Not at risk for retinopathy. No treatment or retinal follow-up is required.
B. No retinopathy or only minimal background retinopathy prior to pregnancy: The vast majority of patients do not experience progression, and few of those patients who do have any visual impairment. Baseline examination in the first trimester and a repeat examination in the third trimester. No treatment is needed.
C. Background retinopathy (microaneurysms, dot and blot hemorrhages, hard exudates): Up to 50% of patients may experience progression, with many regressing postpartum. Examination every trimester. No treatment is needed.
D. Preproliferative retinopathy (cotton-wool spots, venous beading and loops, intraretinal microvascular abnormalities): Up to 50% may experience progression, with some showing regression postpartum. Examine every month. No treatment is indicated.

E. Proliferative retinopathy (during any stage of pregnancy; neovascularization of the disc, retina or iris): Laser panretinal photocoagulation as per current treatment recommendations. In earlier stages, more aggressive institution of therapy is important in pregnant women because proliferative diabetes tends to progress rapidly. This is not an indication to terminate pregnancy. (See Section 14.6.) Examine monthly.

❖ **Note** *Active proliferative retinopathy at the time of labor may indicate a need for cesarean section because Valsalva's maneuver at the time of delivery may cause vitreous hemorrhage.*

Headache

Pituitary Adenoma

Pituitary adenomas may enlarge during pregnancy, producing a visual field disturbance (classically a bitemporal hemianopsia) or headache. Because subclinical pituitary adenomas may produce amenorrhea, women who underwent treatment to induce ovulation should be examined with a high index of suspicion.

A possible cause of pituitary adenoma enlargement during pregnancy is pituitary apoplexy, a potentially life-threatening event. Therefore, any woman with a diagnosis of pituitary adenoma who presents with a headache or a new visual field defect should receive an MRI with or without LP to rule out subarachnoid hemorrhage from the tumor. Women with growing pituitary adenomas (especially those with evidence of subarachnoid blood on imaging) should be delivered by cesarean section to avoid the risk of apoplexy during the delivery. Postpartum hemorrhage or shock can cause an infarction of the pituitary gland leading to hypopituitarism (Sheehan's syndrome).

Pseudotumor Cerebri

Recent reports suggest the incidence of this entity is not increased in pregnant women relative to age-matched controls. Headache, papilledema, a normal CT scan of the head, and a high opening pressure on LP with a normal spinal fluid composition confirm the diagnosis. Treatment may be difficult, because many of the medications generally used to treat this entity are contraindicated in pregnant women. The visual outcome of pregnant women with this entity is no different than that of nonpregnant women with this disorder. (See Section 11.14.)

Preeclamptic/Eclamptic Hypertensive Disease

As discussed previously. Refer to the obstetrician for blood pressure control.

Migraine Headache

Usually worse during pregnancy and immediately postpartum. (See Section 15.4.)

Meningioma of Pregnancy

Very aggressive growth pattern. Difficult to treat.

Others

For example, cortical vein thrombosis.

❖ **Note** *All pregnant women complaining of a headache should have their blood pressure, visual fields, and fundus checked (particularly looking for papilledema). As mentioned above, MRI with or without LP is often required if a hemorrhage or cortical venous thrombosis is suspected.*

Difficulty Wearing Contact Lenses

Corneal Changes

Physiological changes in the cornea may hinder contact lens wear. As corneal sensitivity is also known to decrease during pregnancy (possibly increasing the risk of infection), discontinuation of contact lenses is often advisable.

REFERENCE

Sunness JS. The pregnant woman's eye. *Surv Ophthalmol* 32:219, 1988.

14.9 STEVENS-JOHNSON SYNDROME
(ERYTHEMA MULTIFORME MAJOR)

Symptoms
　　Acute onset of fever, rash, red eye, often with generalized malaise and arthralgias.

Critical Signs
　　"Target" lesions on the skin (red-centered vesicles surrounded by a pale ring surrounded by a red ring), hemorrhagic crusting of the lips, bilateral conjunctivitis.

Other Signs
　　Skin vesicles, bullae, and maculopapular lesions concentrated on the hands and feet; ruptured bullae of the mouth; ulcerative stomatitis. Corneal neovascu-

larization; scarring of the conjunctiva, cornea, or both; dry eyes; symblepharon; eyelid deformities; corneal ulcers; corneal perforation; and/or endophthalmitis may develop. Patients may appear toxic. The mortality rate is 10–33%.

Etiology

May be precipitated by many agents, including any of the following:

- Drugs (e.g., sulfonamides, barbiturates, chlorpropamide, thiazide diuretics, phenytoin, salicylates, tetracycline, codeine, penicillins)
- Infectious agents (e.g., various bacteria, viruses, and fungi, especially herpes and mycoplasma)

Differential Diagnosis

- Ocular cicatricial pemphigoid   (Slowly progressive scarring of the conjunctiva with symblepharon formation, forniceal shortening, and dry eye. Mucous membrane vesicles or ruptured or formed bullae are evident. See Section 5.9.)

Work-up

1. History: Attempt to determine the precipitating factor.
2. Slit-lamp examination: Be certain to evert the eyelids and examine the fornices.
3. Conjunctival and corneal scrapings for stains and cultures if infection is suspected (see "Infectious Corneal Infiltrate/Ulcer," Section 4.12).
4. Electrolyte profile, complete blood count (CBC).

Treatment

1. Hospitalize the patient.
2. Treat the precipitating factor (e.g., remove the antibiotic, treat the infection).
3. Topical steroid (e.g., prednisolone acetate 1% 4–8 times per day, depending on the severity of the anterior-segment inflammation).
4. Systemic steroids (e.g., prednisone 80–100 mg po daily; controversial) and a histamine H_2 blocker (e.g., ranitidine 150 mg po bid). See medical glossary for a systemic steroid work-up.
5. Topical antibiotic (e.g., erythromycin or bacitracin ointment 2–3 times per day).—
6. Artificial tears (e g , Refresh drops q 1–2 h) prn and punctal occlusion as needed. Moisture chambers or tarsorrhaphy may be necessary.
7. Cycloplegic (e.g., atropine 1% tid).
8. Break symblepharon with a glass rod bid after instilling a topical anesthetic (e.g., proparacaine).

9. Supportive systemic care (e.g., hydration, local mouth and skin care, systemic antibiotics) prn.

Follow-up

- Examine the patient daily in the hospital, watching for the development of an infectious ulcer or elevated intraocular pressure. When the acute phase has resolved, weekly outpatient follow-ups are initiated, watching for long-term ocular complications.
- Steroid and antibiotic treatment are maintained for 48 hours after the eye is healed, then tapered.
- Artificial tears and lubricating ointment may need to be maintained indefinitely if the conjunctiva has been severely scarred.
- If trichiasis develops, cryotherapy or surgical repair may be indicated.
- Consider a keratoprosthesis in a scarred, end-stage eye with visual potential.

14.10 VITAMIN A DEFICIENCY

Symptoms

Dry eye, foreign-body sensation, ocular pain, night blindness, severe loss of vision. Gradual onset in most cases.

Critical Signs

Patients often appear malnourished or are victims of a process causing defective vitamin A absorption or utilization. Bilateral conjunctival and corneal dryness with lack of normal luster, Bitot's spot (paralimbal silvery white dots in a triangular patch), and a decreased tear-film break-up time are typical.

Other Signs

Sterile corneal ulceration with a sharp delineation between normal and abnormal stroma; corneal perforation or secondary bacterial infection may occur. There may be loss of pigment in the retinal periphery.

Etiology

Primary   Dietary lack of vitamin A (usually from malnutrition or an extreme dietary habit—relatively uncommon in developed countries).

Secondary   Vitamin A deficiency in the presence of an adequate dietary intake, often from cystic fibrosis in children and young adults, chronic pancreatitis, postgastrectomy surgery, inflammatory bowel disease, intestinal bypass surgery for obesity, chronic liver disease, abetalipoproteinemia (Bassen-Kornzweig syndrome), others.

Differential Diagnosis

See "Dry-Eye Syndrome," Section 4.2.

Work-up

1. History: Malnutrition? Poor or extreme diet? Gastrointestinal or liver disease? Previous surgery?
2. Complete ophthalmic examination: Be certain to test eyelid closure, inspect the eyelid margins, and pull down the lower eyelids to examine the inferior fornices.
3. Serum vitamin A level before treatment is initiated (typically <20–80 μg/dL).
4. Consider impression cytology of the conjunctiva if available.
5. Dark-adaptation electroretinogram (may be more sensitive than the serum vitamin A level, which may not fall until the body's reserves are depleted).
6. If a corneal ulcer exists and appears infected, scrapings for stains and cultures are obtained (see "Infectious Corneal Infiltrate/Ulcer," Section 4.12).

Treatment

1. Vitamin A replacement therapy: Vitamin A palmitate in oil 200,000 IU (60,000 μg) po daily for 2 days (an additional dose is usually given 1 to 4 weeks later to "top up" liver reserves).
   - One-half dose for children under 1 year of age and for pregnant women.
   - If unable to utilize the oral route (e.g., due to gastroenteritis) the equivalent dose is given intramuscularly in the water-dispersible form.
2. Intensive ocular lubrication with artificial tears (e.g., Refresh drops) q 15–60 minutes and artificial tear ointment (e.g., Refresh PM) qhs.
3. Topical vitamin A ointment 2–4 times per day may be of some benefit.
4. Treatment of malnutrition if present.
5. Consider supplementing the patient's diet with zinc.
6. Consider a penetrating keratoplasty or keratoprosthesis for corneal scars in eyes with potentially good vision.

Follow-up

Determined by the clinical presentation and response to treatment. Some patients need to be admitted to the hospital, while others can be followed every several days to weeks.

14.11 NEUROFIBROMATOSIS
(VON RECKLINGHAUSEN'S SYNDROME)

Criteria for Diagnosis

Type I—Two or more of the following:

- Six or more café-au-lait macules whose greatest diameter is >5 mm in prepubertal patients and >15 mm in postpubertal patients.
- Two or more neurofibromas of any type or one plexiform neurofibroma.
- Intertriginous freckling.
- Optic-nerve glioma.
- Two or more Lisch's nodules (iris hamartomas).
- Distinctive osseous lesion (e.g., sphenoid dysplasia or thinning of long-bone cortex).
- Parent, sibling, or child of the patient has the diagnosis.

Type II—One of the following:

- Bilateral acoustic-nerve masses (diagnosed by CT or MRI).
- Parent, sibling, or child of the patient has type II neurofibromatosis and either unilateral acoustic-nerve mass or any two of the following: neurofibroma, meningioma, glioma, schwannoma, or juvenile posterior subcapsular cataract.

Other Ocular Signs

Neurofibromas or plexiform neuromas of the eyelid and conjunctiva, glaucoma, pulsating proptosis (absence of the greater wing of the sphenoid bone with a herniated encephalocele), prominent corneal nerves, astrocytoma of the retina, myelinated nerve fibers, diffuse uveal thickening, choroidal nevi and melanomas, optic-nerve meningiomas, orbital neurofibromas, schwannomas.

Other Systemic Signs

Intracranial astrocytomas (gliomas), pituitary tumors, other cranial or spinal nerve schwannomas (with potential for malignant degeneration), mental deficiencies, pheochromocytoma, gastrointestinal and genitourinary malignancies (including Wilms' tumor).

❖ **Note** *The presence of Lisch's nodules is a highly sensitive and specific sign for type I neurofibromatosis. Moreover, Lisch's nodules often precede the development of cutaneous neurofibromas. (These iris nodules are highly unusual in type II neurofibromatosis.)*

Inheritance

Autosomal dominant with incomplete penetrance (type I, chromosome 17; type II, chromosome 22).

Work-up

1. Family history: Examination of family members is important.
2. Complete general and ophthalmic examinations.
3. CBC, electrolytes.
4. CT scan (axial and coronal views) or MRI of the orbit and brain.
5. IQ and psychological testing.
6. Electroencephalogram.
7. Audiography.
8. Urine tests for levels of epinephrine and norepinephrine.

Treatment

1. Depends on findings.
2. Genetic counseling.
3. Psychological support and counseling.

Follow-up

Every 6–12 months in the absence of a disorder requiring therapy.

REFERENCES

Lubs MLE, Bauer MS, Formas ME, Djokic B. Lisch nodules in neurofibromatosis type I. *N Engl J Med* 324:1264, 1991.
Martuza RL, Eldridge R. Neurofibromatosis 2. *N Engl J Med* 318:684, 1988.

14.12 TUBEROUS SCLEROSIS
(BOURNEVILLE'S SYNDROME)

Ocular Signs

Astrocytic harmartoma of the retina or optic disc (a white, semitransparent or mulberry-appearing tumor in the superficial retina that may undergo calcification with age; no prominent feeder vessels, no associated retinal detachment.)

Critical Systemic Signs

Adenoma sebaceum (yellow-red papules in a butterfly distribution on the upper cheeks, apparent in the prepubertal years), astrocytic harmartomas of the brain with seizures and/or subnormal intelligence or mental retardation.

Other Systemic Signs

Subungal angiofibromas (yellow-red papules around and beneath the nails of the fingers or toes); shagreen patches; ash-leaf sign (depigmented macules on the skin); café-au-lait spots; renal angiomyolipoma; cardiac rhabdomyoma; pleural cysts causing spontaneous pneumothorax; cystic bone lesions; harmartomas of the liver, thyroid, pancreas, or testes.

Inheritance

Autosomal dominant with incomplete penetrance.

Differential Diagnosis

- Retinoblastoma   (Flat or elevated white retinal tumor which has prominent feeder vessels; may be bilateral and/or multifocal. Vitreous seeding, retinal detachment, pseudohypopyon, iris neovascularization, or vitreous hemorrhage may be present. No systemic signs, initially.)

Work-up

1. Family history: Examination of the family members is important.
2. Complete general physical and ophthalmic examinations.
3. CBC, electrolytes.
4. CT scan (axial and coronal views) or MRI of the brain.
5. Electroencephalogram.
6. Echocardiogram.
7. Chest x-ray.
8. Abdominal CT scan.

Treatment

1. Retinal astrocytomas generally require no treatment.
2. Genetic counseling.

Follow-up

Yearly in the absence of a disorder requiring therapy.

14.13 STURGE-WEBER SYNDROME
(ENCEPHALOFACIAL CAVERNOUS HEMANGIOMATOSIS)

Ocular Signs

Diffuse choroidal hemangioma ("tomato catsup" fundus—the lesion obscures all detail of the choroidal vasculature and produces a uniform red fundus background; best appreciated when compared to the other eye), unilateral glaucoma (facial hemangioma of the upper eyelid increases the risk of glaucoma), iris heterochromia, blood in Schlemm's canal (seen on gonioscopy), secondary serous retinal detachment, secondary retinal pigment epithelial alterations (retinitis pigmentosa–like picture).

Critical Systemic Sign

Port-wine stain or nevus flammeus (facial hemangioma along the first and second divisions of the trigeminal nerve).

Other Signs

Subnormal intelligence or mental retardation, Jacksonian-type seizures, peripheral arteriovenous communications, facial hemihypertrophy ipsilateral to nevus flammeus, leptomeningeal angiomatosis, cerebral calcifications.

Inheritance

Sporadic.

Work-up

1. Complete general and ophthalmic examinations.
2. CT scan (axial and coronal views) or MRI of the brain.
3. Electroencephalogram.

Treatment

1. Treat glaucoma if present: First-line drugs are aqueous suppressants (e.g., timolol or levobunolol and/or methazolamide); pilocarpine and epinephrine compounds are less effective because of high episcleral venous pressure. See "Primary Open-Angle Glaucoma," Section 10.1.
2. Consider treating serous retinal detachments that are large or threaten or involve the macula (laser photocoagulation is often used, but the success rate is low).
3. Anticonvulsants for epilepsy.

Follow-up

Every 6 months, watch carefully for glaucoma or a serous retinal detachment.

- If glaucoma is present, closer follow-up may be required.
- If skin involvement is only in the mandibular area, the risk of glaucoma is much lower, and the interval for follow-up may be extended to 1 year.

14.14 VON HIPPEL-LINDAU SYNDROME
(RETINOCEREBELLAR CAPILLARY HEMANGIOMATOSIS)

Critical Ocular Signs

Retinal capillary hemangioma (small, yellow-red tumor with a tortuous dilated feeder artery and a draining vein), sometimes associated with subretinal exudations, a retinal detachment, or both.

Other Signs

Cerebellar hemangioblastoma, hypernephroma, pheochromocytoma, renal cysts, pancreatic cysts, epididymal cysts, syringomyelia.

Inheritance

Autosomal dominant with incomplete penetrance.

Differential Diagnosis

- Racemose hemangiomatosis   (No definable tumor present; large, dilated, tortuous vessels form arteriovenous communications.)
- Coats' disease   (Characteristic aneurysmal dilatation of blood vessels is found with prominent subretinal exudate. No identifiable tumor is present.)

Work-up

(Indicated when multiple or bilateral retinal capillary hemangiomas are discovered, or when a unilateral retinal capillary hemangioma is found along with characteristic systemic findings or a positive family history.)

❖ **Note** *Some physicians work-up all patients with retinal capillary hemangiomas.*

1. Family history and examination of family members.
2. Complete general physical and ophthalmic examinations.
3. CBC, electrolytes.
4. MRI of the brain (visualizes the posterior fossa better than CT scan).
5. Urine tests for levels of epinephrine and norepinephrine.
6. Abdominal CT scan.
7. Fluorescein angiogram if treatment of the retinal capillary hemangioma is planned.

Treatment

1. Photocoagulation or cryotherapy of a retinal hemangioma is often indicated if it is affecting or threatening vision.
2. Genetic counseling.
3. Systemic therapy, depending on findings.

Follow-up

Every 3–6 months, depending on the retinal condition.

14.15 WYBURN-MASON SYNDROME
(RACEMOSE HEMANGIOMATOSIS)

Ocular Signs

Enormously dilated, tortuous retinal vessels with arteriovenous communications. No distinct mass or subretinal exudate is present. Rarely, proptosis from a racemose hemangioma of the orbit is present.

Systemic Signs

Midbrain racemose hemangiomas, seizures, hemiparesis, mental changes, and ipsilateral pterygoid fossa, mandible, and maxillary hemangiomas. Intracranial hemorrhage from a midbrain hemangioma can occur.

Inheritance

Sporadic.

Differential Diagnosis

- Retinal capillary hemangioma (A distinct mass is present, sometimes with subretinal exudate.)

Work-up

1. Complete general and ophthalmic examinations.
2. MRI of the brain.
3. Electroencephalogram.

Treatment
1. No treatment is required for the retinal lesions. The condition is congenital and does not progress.
2. Warn the patient of the risk of massive hemorrhage with ipsilateral dental and facial surgery.

Follow-up
Yearly.

14.16 ATAXIA TELANGIECTASIA
(LOUIS-BAR SYNDROME)

Ocular Signs
Dilated conjunctival vessels, strabismus, impaired convergence, nystagmus, oculomotor apraxia.

Critical Systemic Signs
Cerebellar ataxia that becomes apparent after the child learns to walk; cutaneous telangiectasias in a butterfly distribution on the face, on the antecubital and popliteal fossa, behind the ears, or at the base of neck during the first decade of life. Recurrent sinopulmonary infections as a result of IgA deficiency and impaired T-cell function can occur.

Other Systemic Signs
Leukemia or lymphoma (often leading to death in childhood or early adulthood), mental retardation, seborrheic dermatitis, pigmentary changes of the skin, testicular or ovarian atrophy, hypoplastic or atrophic thymus.

Inheritance
Autosomal recessive.

Work-up
1. Family history (examination of the family members often aides in the diagnosis).
2. Complete general and ophthalmic examinations.
3. CBC.
4. Chest x-ray.
5. MRI of the brain.

Treatment
1. Systemic treatment, depending on findings.
2. Genetic counseling.

Follow-up

Patients need close medical follow-up. Routine eye examinations should be performed every 1–2 years.

GENERAL OPHTHALMIC PROBLEMS

15.1 ACQUIRED CATARACT

Symptoms

Slowly progressive visual loss or blurring, usually over months to years, affecting one or both eyes. Glare, particularly from oncoming headlights while driving at night, and reduced color perception may occur. The particular symptoms are based on the location and density of the opacity.

Critical Sign

Opacification of the normally clear lens (see the respective types, following).

Other Signs

The retina often appears indistinct on funduscopic examination, and the dilated red reflex may be dim on retinoscopy. The patient may be found to be more myopic than he or she was previously. A cataract alone does not cause a relative afferent pupillary defect.

Types of Cataracts

A. Nuclear   (Yellow or brown discoloration of the central part of the lens on slit-lamp examination. Typically blurs distance vision more than near vision.)

B. Posterior subcapsular   (Opacities appear near the posterior aspect of the lens, often forming a plaque. They are best seen in retroillumination against a red fundus reflex. Glare and difficulty reading are common complaints. May be associated with ocular inflammation, prolonged steroid use, diabe-

The Wills Eye Manual: Office and Emergency Room Diagnosis and Treatment of Eye Diseases, Second Edition, edited by R. Douglas Cullom, Jr., M.D., and Benjamin Chang, M.D. © 1994 J. B. Lippincott Company.

tes, trauma, or radiation. Classically occurs in patients younger than 50 years of age.)

C. Cortical   (Radial or spokelike opacities in the lens periphery that expand to involve the anterior and posterior lens. Often asymptomatic until the changes develop centrally.)

❖ **Note** *A mature cataract is defined as anterior cortical changes sufficiently dense to totally obscure the view of the posterior lens and posterior segment of the eye.*

Etiology

- Age-related
- Trauma   (Ocular or head contusion, others.)
- Toxic   [Steroids, anticholinesterases, antipsychotics (e.g., phenothiazines), others.]
- Intraocular inflammation (e.g., uveitis)
- Radiation
- Intraocular tumor   (A ciliary body malignant melanoma may produce a sector cortical cataract.)
- Degenerative ocular disease (e.g., retinitis pigmentosa)
- Systemic disease:
  A. Diabetes   (The juvenile form is characterized by white "snowflake" opacities in the anterior and posterior subcapsular locations. It often progresses rapidly. Adults develop age-related cataracts as described previously, but at an earlier age.)
  B. Hypocalcemia   (Small, white, iridescent cortical changes, usually seen in the presence of tetany.)
  C. Wilson's disease   (Red-brown pigment-colored deposition in the cortex beneath the anterior capsule (a "sunflower" cataract). Seen with a corneal Kayser-Fleischer ring.)
  D. Myotonic dystrophy   (Multicolored opacities cause a "Christmas-tree cataract" behind the anterior capsule.)
  E. Others (e.g., Down's syndrome, atopic dermatitis)

Work-up

Determine the etiology, whether the cataract is responsible for the decreased vision, and whether surgical removal would improve vision.

1. History: Medications? Systemic diseases? Trauma? Ocular disease or poor vision in youth or young adulthood (before the cataract)?
2. Complete ocular examination, including distance and near vision, pupillary examination, and refraction. A dilated slit-lamp examination using both direct and retroillumination techniques is usually required to properly view

the cataract. Fundus examination, concentrating on the macula, is essential in ruling out other causes of decreased vision.

3. B-scan ultrasound when the fundus is obscured by a dense cataract to rule out posterior-segment pathology.
4. The potential acuity meter or laser interferometry can be used to estimate the visual potential when cataract extraction is being considered in an eye with age-related macular degeneration changes.

❖ **Note** *Laser interferometry and the potential acuity meter often overestimate the eye's visual potential in the presence of macular holes or macular pigment epithelial detachments. Interferometry also makes an overprediction of results in cases of amblyopia. Near vision is often the most accurate manner of evaluating macular function if the cataract is not too dense.*

5. When surgery is planned, keratometry readings and an A-scan ultrasound measurement of axial length are required for determining the power of the desired intraocular lens. An evaluation of the corneal endothelium, usually done at the slit lamp but occasionally requiring an endothelial cell count, is also needed.

Treatment
1. Cataract surgery may be performed for the following reasons:
   a. To improve visual function in patients with symptomatic visual disability.
   b. As surgical therapy of ocular disease (e.g., lens-related glaucoma or uveitis).
   c. To facilitate management of ocular disease (e.g., to monitor or treat diabetic retinopathy or glaucoma).
2. Correct any refractive error if the patient declines cataract surgery.
3. A trial of mydriasis (e.g., scopolamine 0.25% daily) may be used successfully in some patients if the patient opts not to have the cataract removed.

Follow-up
Unless there is a secondary complication from the cataract (e.g., glaucoma; quite rare), a cataract itself does not require urgent action. Patients who decline surgical removal are reexamined yearly, sooner if there is a symptomatic decrease in visual acuity.

If congenital, see "Congenital Cataract," Section 9.7.

15.2 SUBLUXED OR DISLOCATED LENS

Subluxation   Partial disruption of the zonular fibers; the lens is decentered but remains partially in the pupillary aperture.

Dislocation   Complete disruption of the zonular fibers; the lens is displaced out of the pupillary aperture.

Symptoms

Decreased vision, double vision that persists when covering one eye (monocular diplopia).

Critical Signs

Decentered or displaced lens, iridodonesis (quivering of the iris), phakodonesis (quivering of the lens).

Other Signs

Marked astigmatism, cataract, angle-closure glaucoma as a result of pupillary block, acquired high myopia, vitreous in the anterior chamber, asymmetry of the anterior chamber.

Etiology

- Trauma   [Most common cause. Results in subluxation if more than 25% of the zonular fibers are ruptured. Need to rule out a predisposing condition (see other etiologies). Can be associated with syphilis.]
- Marfan's syndrome   (Cardiomyopathy, aortic aneurysm, tall stature with long extremities and kyphoscoliosis. Typically, bilateral lens subluxation superiorly and temporally. Patients are at increased risk for a retinal detachment. Often autosomal dominant.)
- Homocystinuria   [Frequent mental retardation, skeletal deformities, resembles Marfan's syndrome in stature, high incidence of thromboembolic events (particularly with general anesthesia). Patients with a mild clinical course may be undiagnosed prior to occurrence of lens subluxation. Typically, bilateral lens subluxation inferiorly and nasally. Increased risk of retinal detachment. Autosomal recessive.)
- Weill-Marchesani syndrome   [Short fingers and short stature, seizures, microspherophakia (small, round lens), myopia, no mental retardation. Often autosomal recessive.]
- Others   (Acquired syphilis, congenital ectopia lentis, aniridia, Ehlers-Danlos syndrome, Crouzon's disease, hyperlysinemia, sulfite-oxidase deficiency, high myopia, chronic inflammations, hypermature cataract, others.)

Work-up

1. History: Family history of the disorders listed above? Trauma? Systemic illness (e.g., syphilis, seizures)?
2. Complete ocular examination: At the slit lamp, note whether the condition is unilateral or bilateral and determine the direction of the displaced lens.
3. Systemic examination: Evaluate stature, extremities, hands, and fingers; often in conjunction with an internist.

4. RPR and FTA-ABS, even if there is a history of trauma.
5. Sodium nitroprusside test or urine chromatography to rule out homocystinuria.
6. Echocardiogram to rule out Marfan's syndrome.

Treatment
I. Lens dislocated into the anterior chamber
  A. Dilate the pupil, place the patient on his or her back, and replace the lens into the posterior chamber by head manipulation. It may be necessary to indent the cornea after topical anesthesia (e.g., proparacaine) with a Zeiss's gonioprism or a cotton swab to reposition the lens. After the lens is repositioned in the posterior chamber, constrict the pupil with chronic pilocarpine 0.5–1% qid, and perform a peripheral laser iridectomy.
    or
  B. Surgically remove the lens (usually performed if the lens is a cataract, if treatment described in "A" fails, if the patient develops recurrent dislocations, or if the patient cannot be trusted to take the pilocarpine).
II. Lens dislocated into the vitreous
  A. Lens capsule intact, patient asymptomatic, no signs of inflammation: Observe.
  B. Lens capsule broken, patient asymptomatic, eye inflamed: Lensectomy either through the pars plana or using a limbal approach.
III. Subluxation
  A. Asymptomatic: Observe.
  B. High uncorrectable astigmatism or monocular diplopia: Surgical removal of the lens.
  C. Symptomatic cataract: Options include surgical removal of the lens, mydriasis (e.g., scopolamine 0.25% daily) and aphakic correction, pupillary constriction (e.g., pilocarpine 4% gel qhs) and phakic correction, or a large optical iridectomy (away from the lens).
IV. Pupillary block: Treatment is identical to that for aphakic pupillary block (see "Postoperative Glaucoma," Section 10.15).

- If Marfans syndrome is present: Refer the patient to a cardiologist for an annual echocardiogram and management of any cardiac-related abnormalities. Prophylactic systemic antibiotics are required if the patient undergoes surgery (or a dental procedure), to prevent endocarditis.
- If homocystinuria is present:
  1. Pyridoxine 50–1000 mg po daily.
  2. Reduce dietary methionine.
  3. Avoid surgery if possible because of the risk of thromboembolic complications. If surgical intervention is necessary, anticoagulant therapy is indicated.

Follow-up

Depends on the etiology, degree of subluxation or dislocation, and symptoms.

15.3 HEADACHE

Most headaches are not dangerous nor ominous symptoms; however, they can be symptoms of a life- or vision-threatening problem. Below are listed accompanying signs and symptoms that may indicate a life- or vision-threatening headache and some of the specific signs and symptoms of various headaches.

Warning Symptoms and Signs of a Serious Disorder
- Scalp tenderness, weight loss, pain with chewing, muscle pains, or malaise in patients at least 55 years of age (giant cell arteritis).
- Optic-nerve swelling
- Fever
- Altered mentation or behavior
- Stiff neck
- Neurologic signs
- Decreased vision
- Subhyaloid (preretinal) hemorrhages on fundus examination

Less Alarming But Suspicious Symptoms and Signs
- Onset in a previously headache-free individual
- A different, more severe headache than the usual headache
- A headache that is *always* in the same location
- A headache that awakens the person from sleep
- A headache that does not respond to pain medications that previously relieved it
- Nausea and vomiting, particularly projectile vomiting

Etiology

LIFE- OR VISION-THREATENING

- Giant cell arteritis (GCA)   (Age ≥55 years, weight loss, fever, malaise, anorexia, muscle aches, scalp tenderness, pain on chewing, palpable tender nodule or cordlike pulseless area along the temporal artery, or decreased vision. May have high ESR. See Section 11.16.)
- Acute angle-closure glaucoma   [Decreased vision, red and painful eye, cloudy cornea, fixed mid-dilated pupil, high intraocular pressure (IOP). See Section 10.10.]

- Ocular ischemic syndrome (Periorbital eye pain, midperipheral retinal hemorrhages, dilated retinal veins, neovascularization of the iris, disc, or retina, spontaneous or easily inducible retinal arterial pulsations. See Section 12.7.)
- Malignant hypertension (Marked elevation of blood pressure, often accompanied by retinal cotton-wool spots, hemorrhages, and when severe, optic-nerve swelling. Headaches typically are occipital in location.)
- Increased intracranial pressure (May have papilledema, loss of venous pulsations[1] in the disc vessels, or a sixth-cranial-nerve palsy. See Section 11.13.)
- Infectious central nervous system disorder (meningitis or brain abscess) (Fever, stiff neck, mental status changes, photophobia, neurological signs.)
- Structural abnormality of the brain (tumor, aneurysm, arteriovenous malformation) (Mental status change, signs of increased intracranial pressure, or neurologic signs during, and often after, the headache episode.)
- Subarachnoid hemorrhage (Extremely severe headache, stiff neck, mental status change; rarely, subhyaloid hemorrhages seen on fundus examination, usually from a ruptured aneurysm.)
- Epidural or subdural hematoma (Follows head trauma; altered level of consciousness; may produce anisocoria.)

OTHERS

- Migraine (See Section 15.4.)
- Cluster (See Section 15.5.)
- Tension
- Herpes zoster virus [Headache or pain may precede the herpetic vesicles (see Section 4.16).]
- Sinus disease

❖ **Note** *A "sinus" headache can be a serious headache in diabetics and immunocompromised hosts because mucormycosis may be responsible (see Section 11.9).*

- Tolosa-Hunt syndrome (See "Cavernous Sinus Superior Orbital Fissure Syndrome," Section 11.9.)
- Cervical spine disease
- Temporomandibular joint syndrome
- Dental disease
- Trigeminal neuralgia (tic douloureux)

---

[1]The presence of spontaneous venous pulsations indicates normal intracranial pressure at that moment; however, the absence of pulsations has little significance. A significant number of normal individuals do not have spontaneous venous pulsations.

- Anterior uveitis   (See Section 13.1.)
- Following spinal tap
- Paget's disease
- Depression/psychogenic
- Convergence insufficiency   (See Section 15.6.)
- Accommodative spasm   (See Section 15.7.)

Work-up

1. History: Ask about the location, intensity, frequency, possible precipitating factors, and time of day of the headaches. Determine the patient's age of onset, what relieves the headaches, and whether there are any associated signs or symptoms. Specifically, ask about the serious or suspicious symptoms and signs listed above: trauma, medications and birth-control pills, family history of migraine, and whether the patient experienced motion sickness or cyclic vomiting as a child.
2. Complete ocular examination, including pupillary, motility, and visual field evaluation; intraocular pressure measurement, optic-disc and venous pulsation assessment, and a dilated retinal examination. Manifest and cycloplegic refractions may be helpful.
3. Neurologic examination (check neck flexibility and other meningeal signs).
4. Palpate the temporal arteries in potential GCA cases (to see if they are swollen, hard, and tender).
5. Temperature and blood pressure.
6. Immediate ESR with or without temporal artery biopsy when giant cell arteritis is suspected (see Section 11.16).
7. CT scan (axial and coronal views) or MRI of the brain when an intracranial abnormality is suspected.
8. Carotid noninvasive flow studies when ocular ischemic syndrome is suspected.
9. Lumbar puncture (in the hospital) is obtained in suspected cases of meningitis or subarachnoid hemorrhage.
10. Refer the patient to a neurologist; ear, nose, and throat specialist; internist; or family doctor, as indicated.

Treatment/Follow-up

See individual sections.

15.4 MIGRAINE

Symptoms

Typically unilateral (although it may occur behind both eyes or across the entire front of the head), throbbing or boring head pain accompanied by nausea, vomiting, mood changes, fatigue, or photophobia. Visual disturbances, including flashing (zig-zagging) lights, blurred vision, or a visual field defect lasting 15–50 minutes, may precede the migraine. The migraine is often preceded by an aura (a sensation of an impending migraine). Neurological deficits may occur. A positive family history is common, as is a history of car sickness or cyclic vomiting as a child. Migraine in children may present as recurrent abdominal pain and malaise. Of these patients, 60–70% are female.

❖ **Note** *The majority of unilateral migraine headaches at some point change sides of the head. Patients who* always *have a headache on the same side of the head may have a more serious headache disorder.*

Signs

Usually none. Complicated migraines may have a permanent neurological or ocular deficit (see the following discussion).

Classification

Definitions and classifications vary.

I. *Common migraine* (80%) Nausea, vomiting, fatigue, and mood changes are associated with this variant.

II. *Classical migraine* (10%) The headache is *preceded* by a 15- to 50-minute visual disturbance or transient focal neurological change. See "Complicated migraine" for specific types of visual and neurological defects.

III. *Visual migraine without headache (acephalgic migraine)* The patient experiences the visual aura of a classical migraine without the subsequent headache. Some of these patients have and some have not had migraine headaches in the past.

IV. *Complicated migraine* A subset of migraine in which neurological deficits outlast the headache. Rarely, a deficit may be permanent.

   A. Cerebral: A neurological deficit involving the motor, sensory, or visual systems. Onset can be at the height of a migraine headache, but more commonly, it follows the headache. Examples include focal motor deficits, speech disorders, and paresthesias of the extremities, face, tongue, or lips. "Hemiplegic migraine" consists of total paralysis or weakness on one side of the body.

   B. Ophthalmoplegic: Ipsilateral paralysis of one or more extraocular muscles, usually occurring during a migraine attack in childhood. The ophthalmoplegia usually occurs as the headache is resolving.

   C. Retinal: Sudden monocular visual loss in a migraine patient. Light flashes and headache do not usually occur.

   D. Basilar artery migraine: Mimics vertebrobasilar artery insufficiency with bilateral blurring or blindness, vertigo, gait disturbances, formed hallucinations, and dysarthria in a patient with migraine.

Associations or Precipitating Factors

Birth-control or other hormonal pills, puberty, pregnancy, menopause, foods containing tyramine or phenylalanine (e.g., aged cheeses, wines, chocolate), nitrates or nitrites, monosodium glutamate, alcohol, fatigue, emotional stress, refractive errors, or bright lights.

Differential Diagnosis

See "Headache," Section 15.3.

Work-up

See Section 15.3 for a general headache work-up.

1. History: May establish the diagnosis.
2. Ocular and neurologic examinations, including refraction.
3. CT scan or MRI of the head is indicated for:
   a. Atypical migraines (e.g., migraines that are always on the same side of the head, those that begin in middle age in a person with no family history nor a history of car sickness or cyclic vomiting as a child, or those with an unusual sequence, such as visual disturbances persisting into or occurring after the headache phase).
   b. Complicated migraines.

Treatment

1. Avoid agents that precipitate the headaches (e.g., stop using birth-control pills; avoid alcohol and any foods that may precipitate attacks; reduce stress).
2. Correct any significant refractive error.
3. Medications to be used at the onset of the headache (the earlier the better) in patients with infrequent headaches:
   a. Initial therapy: Aspirin or nonsteroidal antiinflammatory agents (e.g., tolfenamic acid 200 mg q 3 h, naproxen sodium 750 mg in one dose).
   b. More potent therapy (when initial therapy fails):
      Ergotamine[2] 2.0 mg in one dose.
      Dihydroergotamine 4.0 mg in one dose.

For prolonged attacks lasting longer than 24 hours, some physicians recommend systemic steroids.

❖ **Note** *Morphinomimetic drugs should be avoided.*

---

[2]Contraindicated in elderly patients or those with cardiovascular, cerebrovascular, renal, or hepatic disease, and pregnant patients. Muscle weakness and pain or even cardiac ischemic pain can occur.

4. Prophylactic medication to be used in patients with frequent or severe headache attacks (e.g., two or more headaches per month) or those with neurological changes:

Propranolol (e.g., Inderal)[3] 10–80 mg po daily in divided doses initially; slowly increase the dose by 10–20 mg every 2–3 days until the desired effect is obtained (can go up to 160–240 mg/day). Metoprolol may have fewer side-effects for asthmatics and diabetics (100 mg in 1 slow-release tablet per day).

Amitriptyline (e.g., Elavil)[4] 25–200 mg po qhs (start at a low dose and increase the dose by 25 mg every 1–2 weeks if needed).

Calcium channel blockers (e.g., flunarizine 5–10 mg daily); we rarely use these.

5. Antinausea medication as needed for an acute episode (e.g., prochlorperazine 25 mg rectally bid).

Follow-up

Patients are generally reevaluated in 4–6 weeks to assess the efficacy of the therapy.

15.5 CLUSTER HEADACHE

Symptoms

Typically unilateral, very painful, periorbital, frontal, or temporal headache associated with ipsilateral tearing, rhinorrhea, sweating, nasal stuffiness, and/or a droopy eyelid. Usually lasts for minutes to hours. Typically recurs once or twice daily for several weeks, followed by a headache-free interval of months to years. The cycle can then repeat itself. Predominantly affects men.

Signs

Ipsilateral conjunctival injection, facial flush, or Horner's syndrome (third-order neuron etiology) may be present. Ptosis may become permanent.

---

[3]Do not give to patients with asthma, congestive heart failure, bradycardia, or hypotension. Do *not* discontinue this drug suddenly; it must be tapered slowly.

[4]Do not give to patients taking a monoamine oxidase inhibitor or patients with narrow anterior-chamber angles or benign prostatic hypertrophy.

Precipitating Factors
Alcohol, nitroglycerin.

Differential Diagnosis
- Migraine headache   (Positive family history of migraines or a history of car sickness or cyclic vomiting in many cases. The associated symptoms listed previously are typically absent. See Section 15.4.)
- Chronic paroxysmal hemicrania (several attacks per day with a dramatic response to oral indomethacin).
- Others   (See "Headache," Section 15.3.)

Work-up
1. History and complete ocular examination.
2. Neurologic examination, particularly a cranial-nerve evaluation.
3. Consider an hydroxyamphetamine (e.g., Paredrine) test if Horner's syndrome accompanies a suspected cluster headache to confirm a third-order neuron etiology (see Section 11.2).
4. Obtain a CT scan (axial and coronal views) or MRI of the brain when the history is atypical or a neurologic abnormality other than a third-order neuron Horner's syndrome is found.

Treatment
1. No treatment is necessary if the headache is mild.
2. No alcoholic beverages or cigarette smoking during a cluster cycle.
3. Abortive therapy for acute attack:
   - Oxygen 5–8 l/min via face mask for 10 minutes at onset of attack. Relieves pain in 70% of adults.
   - Ergotamine—inhalation is the fastest way to reach therapeutic blood levels (Medihaler, 3 puffs 5 minutes apart).
   - Dihydroergotamine IM or IV (1.0 mg IM in one dose).
   - Corticosteroids (e.g., dexamethasone 8.0 mg IV in one dose).
4. When headaches are moderate to severe and are unrelieved by nonprescription medication, one of the following drugs may be an effective prophylactic agent during cluster periods:
   - Calcium channel blockers (e.g., verapamil 360–480 mg po per day in divided doses).
   - Ergotamine 1.0–2.0 mg po daily.
   - Methysergide 2 mg po tid with meals. Do not use for longer than 3–4 months because of the significant risk of retroperitoneal fibrosis. Methysergide is not recommended in patients with coronary artery or peripheral vascular disease, thrombophlebitis, hypertension, pregnancy, or hepatic or renal disease.
   - Oral steroids (e.g., prednisone 40–80 mg po for 1 week, tapering rapidly over an additional week if possible) and an antiulcer agent (e.g., ranitid-

ine 150 mg po bid). See medical glossary (prednisone) for steroid work-up.

- Lithium 600–900 mg po daily is administered in conjunction with the patient's medical doctor. Baseline renal (blood urea nitrogen, creatinine, urine electrolytes) and thyroid function tests (T3, T4, TSH) are obtained. Lithium intoxication may occur in patients using indomethacin, tetracycline, or methyldopa.

Some physicians administer an ergotamine inhaler (9 mg/mL, containing 0.36 mg per inhalation) 1 inhalation q 5 minutes for 3 inhalations (maximum every 12–24 hours) or ergotamine 2 mg sublingual q 30 minutes for 3 times (maximum in 24 hours) to be started at the onset of an attack. Ergotamine pills may be used in prophylaxis. Ergotamine has the same contraindications as methysergide. We do not use ergotamine as a first-line agent.

If necessary, an acute, severe attack can be treated with IV diazepam.

Follow-up

Patients started on systemic steroids are seen within a few days and then every several weeks to evaluate the effects of treatment and monitor intraocular pressure. Patients on methysergide or lithium are reevaluated in 7–10 days. Plasma lithium levels are monitored in patients taking this agent.

15.6 CONVERGENCE INSUFFICIENCY (CI)

Symptoms

Eye discomfort, headache, sleepiness, or blurred vision from reading or doing near work. It is most common in teenagers and young adults, but may be seen in presbyopes.

Critical Sign

An inability to maintain fusion at near as a result of a reduced amplitude of fusional convergence power (see Work-up).

Other Signs

A distant near point of convergence, an exophoria greater at near than at distance, and a reduced amplitude of accommodation.

Etiology

Fatigue or illness, drugs, uveitis, Adie's tonic pupil, glasses inducing a base-out prism effect. Often idiopathic.

Differential Diagnosis

(Other causes of eyestrain with reading.)

- Uncorrected refractive error (especially hyperopia and astigmatism)
- Accommodative insufficiency (AI)   (Symptoms develop after 20–40 minutes of reading, same age group as CI, but these patients have normal fusional capacities. When a 4-diopter base-in prism is placed in front of the eye while reading, the print is noted to blur in patients with AI, but become clearer in those with CI. Patients with AI usually benefit from reading glasses; those with CI do not.)

Work-up

1. Manifest (without cycloplegia) refraction.
2. Determine the near point of convergence: Ask the patient to focus on an accommodative target (e.g., the eraser of a pencil) and to inform you when double vision develops as you bring the target toward him or her; a normal near point of convergence is <6–8 cm.
3. Check for exodeviations or esodeviations at distance and near using the cover tests (see Appendix 2) or the Maddox rod test.
4. Measure the patient's fusional ability at near: Have the patient focus on an accommodative target at his or her reading distance. With a prism bar, slowly increase the amount of base-out prism in front of one eye until the patient notes double vision (the break point), then slowly reduce the amount of base-out prism until a single image is again noted (the recovery point). A low break point (i.e., 10–15 prism diopters) and/or a low recovery point is consistent with convergence insufficiency.
5. Place a 4-diopter base-in prism in front of one eye while the patient is reading and determine whether the print becomes clearer or more blurred to rule out accommodative insufficiency.
6. Cycloplegic refraction (performed after the previous tests and measurements).

❖ **Note** *The above tests are performed with the patient's spectacle correction in place (if glasses are worn for near work).*

Treatment

1. Correct any refractive error (hyperopia should be slightly undercorrected, while myopia should be fully corrected).
2. Near-point exercises (e.g., pencil push-ups): The patient is taught to focus on the eraser of a pencil while slowly moving it from arm's length toward the face. The patient must concentrate on maintaining one image of the eraser. When double vision results, the maneuver is repeated. An attempt is made to draw the pencil in closer each time while maintaining single vision. The exercise is repeated 15 times, 5 times per day.

3. Near-point exercises with base-out prisms (for patients whose near point of convergence is satisfactory or for those who have mastered pencil push-ups without a prism): Pencil push-ups as described previously are performed while the patient additionally holds a 6-diopter base-out prism in front of one eye.
4. Encourage use of good lighting and time for relaxation between periods of concentrated close work.
5. For older patients, or those whose condition shows no improvement despite near-point exercises, reading glasses with base-in prism can be useful.

Follow-up
This is not an urgent condition. Patients are reexamined in 1 month.

15.7 ACCOMMODATIVE SPASM

Symptoms
Bilateral blurred distance vision or fluctuating vision, headache, and eyestrain while reading. Typically, patients are teenagers who are under stress.

Critical Signs
Cycloplegic refraction reveals substantially less myopia (or more hyperopia) than was originally found when the refraction was performed without cycloplegia (the manifest refraction). Manifest myopia may be as high as 10 diopters.

Other Signs
Abnormally close near point of focus, miosis, a normal amplitude of accommodation that may appear low.

Etiology
Inability to relax the ciliary muscles. Accommodative spasm is involuntary and is associated with stressful situations or functional neuroses. Fatigue and prolonged reading may also precipitate episodes.

Differential Diagnosis
- Uncorrected hyperopia   (Patients accept plus lenses during the manifest refraction.)
- Other causes of pseudomyopia   [Hyperglycemia, medication induced (e.g., sulfa drugs), forward displacement of the lens.]

Work-up

1. Complete ophthalmic examination, including an initial manifest refraction. The manifest refraction may be highly variable, but it is important to determine the least amount of minus power or the most amount of plus power that provides clear distance vision.
2. Cycloplegic refraction.

Treatment

1. True refractive errors should be corrected. If a significant amount of esophoria at near is present, additional plus power (e.g., + 2.50 diopters) in reading glasses or bifocal form may be helpful for close work.
2. Gentle counseling of the patient and parents to provide a more relaxed atmosphere and avoid stressful situations is important.
3. Cycloplegics, including atropine, have been used to break the spasm, but are rarely needed except in the most resistant cases.

Follow-up

Reevaluate in several weeks. The physician should also be available for additional consultative support.

15.8 HYPOTONY

Symptoms

May be asymptomatic or complain of mild-to-severe pain. Vision may be reduced.

Critical Signs

Low IOP, usually <6 mm Hg.

Other Signs

Corneal folds, aqueous cell and flare, shallow anterior chamber, retinal edema, chorioretinal folds, choroidal detachment, the appearance of optic-disc swelling.

Etiology

• Postsurgical   [Wound leak, cyclodialysis cleft (disinsertion of the ciliary body from the sclera at the scleral spur), perforation of the sclera from a superior rectus bridle suture or retrobulbar injection, iridocyclitis, retinal or choroidal detachment, others.]
• Posttraumatic   (Same causes as postsurgical.)

- Pharmacological   (Usually from a carbonic anhydrase inhibitor or topical beta-blocker.)
- Systemic (bilateral hypotony)   [Conditions that cause blood hypertonicity (e.g., dehydration, uremia, exacerbation of diabetes), myotonic dystrophy, others.)
- Vascular occlusive disease (e.g., ocular ischemic syndrome, giant cell arteritis, central retinal vein or artery occlusion   Usually a mild hypotony.)

Work-up

1. History: Recent ocular surgery or trauma? Other systemic symptoms (nausea, vomiting, twitching, drowsiness, polyuria)? History of renal disease, diabetes, or myotonic dystrophy? Medications?
2. Complete ocular examination, including a slit-lamp evaluation of surgical or traumatic ocular wounds (check for poor wound apposition), intraocular pressure (IOP) check, gonioscopy of the anterior-chamber angle to rule out a cyclodialysis cleft, and indirect ophthalmoscopy to rule out a retinal and/or choroidal detachment and look for signs of a scleral perforation.
3. Seidel's test to rule out a wound leak (see Appendix 4).

❖ **Note** *A wound leak may drain under the conjunctiva, producing a filtering bleb. Seidel's test will then be negative.*

4. B-scan ultrasound when the fundus cannot be seen clinically.
5. Blood tests in bilateral cases: Glucose, blood urea nitrogen, and creatinine.

Treatment

Repair the underlying disorder.

WOUND LEAK

- Large wound leaks: Suture the wound closed.
- Small wound leaks: Can be sutured closed or can be patched with a pressure dressing and an antibiotic ointment (e.g., erythromycin) for 1 night to allow the wound to close spontaneously. A carbonic anhydrase inhibitor and a nonselective topical beta-blocker (e.g., acetazolamide 500 mg sequel po and a drop of levobunolol 0.5% or timolol 0.5%) are usually given if patching is to be employed.

❖ **Note** *Occasionally, cyanoacrylate glue is applied to small wound leaks and covered with a bandage contact lens.*

- Wound leaks under a conjunctival flap (only repaired if the hypotony is affecting vision or producing a secondary ocular complication such as a flat anterior chamber or endophthalmitis): Consider cryotherapy or argon laser therapy after painting the conjunctiva with methylene blue or rose bengal.

CYCLODIALYSIS CLEFT

Reattach the ciliary body to the sclera by suturing, cryotherapy, laser photoco-agulation or diathermy.

SCLERAL PERFORATION

The site may be closed by suturing or cryotherapy.

IRIDOCYCLITIS

Topical steroid (e.g., prednisolone acetate 1% q 1–6 h) and a topical cycloplegic (e.g., scopolamine 0.25% tid).

RETINAL DETACHMENT

Surgical repair.

CHOROIDAL DETACHMENT

(See also Section 12.21.)
Treated as iridocyclitis. Surgical drainage of the choroidal effusion along with reformation of the eye and anterior chamber is indicated for any of the following:

1. Retinal apposition ("kissing" choroidal detachments).
2. Lens-corneal touch.
3. A flat or persistently shallow anterior chamber accompanied by a failing filtering bleb or an inflamed eye.

PHARMACOLOGICAL

Reduce or discontinue the IOP-lowering medication.

SYSTEMIC DISORDER

Refer to an internist.

❖ **Note** *In myotonic dystrophy, the hypotony is rarely severe enough to produce deleterious effects, and treatment of hypotony, from an ocular standpoint, is unnecessary.*

Follow-up

If vision is good, the anterior chamber is well formed, and there is no wound leak, retinal detachment, or kissing choroidal detachments, then the low IOP poses no immediate problem, and treatment and follow-up are not urgent. Fixed retinal folds in the macula may develop from long-standing hypotony.

15.9 BLIND, PAINFUL EYE

A patient with a nonseeing eye and unsalvageable vision may develop mild-to-severe pain in it for a variety of reasons. The etiology, work-up, and treatment are discussed below.

Causes of Pain
- Corneal decompensation   (Fluorescein-staining defect on slit-lamp examination.)
- Uveitis   (Anterior-chamber or vitreal white blood cells. If the cornea is opaque, the cells may not be seen.)
- Extremely high intraocular pressure (IOP)   (May result from neovascular glaucoma and angle closure, uveitis, or intraocular tumor-related glaucoma. IOP may be difficult to measure if the corneal surface is irregular.)

Work-up
1. History: Determine the etiology and duration of the blindness.
2. Ocular examination: Stain the cornea with fluorescein to detect an epithelial defect and measure the IOP. If the cornea is not opaque, look for neovascularization of the iris and angle by gonioscopy, and inspect the anterior chamber for cells and flare. Attempt a dilated retinal examination to rule out an intraocular tumor.
3. B-scan ultrasound of the posterior segment is required to rule out an intraocular tumor when the fundus cannot be adequately visualized.

Treatment
A. Sterile corneal decompensation (if it appears infected, see "Infectious Corneal Infiltrate/Ulcer," Section 4.12)
   1. Antibiotic ointment (e.g., erythromycin), cycloplegic (e.g., atropine 1%) and a pressure patch for 24–48 hours.
   2. Lubricating ointment (e.g., Refresh PM) qhs (after the patch is removed) for weeks to months (or even permanently).
   3. Consider teaching the patient to patch his or her own eye nightly.
   4. Consider a tarsorrhaphy in refractile cases.
B. Uveitis
   1. Cycloplegic (e.g., atropine 1% tid).
   2. Topical steroid (e.g., prednisolone acetate 1% q 1–6 h).
C. Markedly elevated IOP
   1. Treat uveitis if it is present or if the cornea is opaque and its presence cannot be ruled out.
   2. Topical beta-blocker (e.g., levobunolol 0.5% bid or timolol 0.5% bid) with or without an epinephrine compound (e.g. dipivefrin 0.1% bid).

Carbonic anhydrase inhibitors are effective, but their potential systemic side-effects may not warrant their use for pain relief; miotics may increase ocular irritation.

3. If the IOP remains markedly elevated and is thought to be responsible for the pain, a cyclodestructive procedure (e.g., YAG laser cyclophoto-coagulation or cyclocryotherapy) may be attempted.

4. If pain persists despite the previously described treatment, a retrobulbar alcohol block may be given. *Technique:* 2–3 mL of lidocaine is adminis-tered in the retrobulbar region. The needle is then held in place while the syringe of lidocaine is replaced with a 1-cc syringe containing 95%–100% alcohol (some physicians use 50% alcohol). The contents of the alcohol syringe are then injected into the retrobulbar space through the needle. The syringes are again switched, so a small amount of lidocaine can rinse out the remaining alcohol. The retrobulbar needle is then withdrawn. Patients are warned that transient eyelid droop or swelling, limitation of eye movement, or anesthesia may result.

D. Cause of pain unknown
  1. Cycloplegic (e.g., atropine 1% tid).
  2. Topical steroid (e.g., prednisolone acetate 1% q 1–6 h).

• When the above treatment fails to relieve the pain, enucleation is offered to the patient.
• The patient should wear protective glasses (e.g., polycarbonate lens) at all times to prevent injury to the contralateral eye.

Follow-up
Depends on the degree of pain and the clinical abnormalities present. Once the pain resolves, patients are reexamined every 6–12 months.

DILATING DROPS
(Mydriatic and Cycloplegic Agents)

Drops	Approximate Maximum Effect	Approximate Duration of Action
MYDRIATIC		
Phenylephrine 2.5, 10%	20 minutes	3 hours
CYCLOPLEGIC/MYDRIATIC		
Tropicamide 0.5, 1%	20–30 minutes	3–6 hours
Cyclopentolate 0.5, 1, 2%	20–45 minutes	24 hours
Homatropine 2, 5%	20–90 minutes	2–3 days
Scopolamine 0.25%	20–45 minutes	4–7 days
Atropine 0.5, 1, 2%	30–40 minutes	1–2 weeks

The usual regimen for a dilated examination is:

Adults   Phenylephrine 2.5% and tropicamide 1%. Repeat these drops in 15–30 minutes if the eye is not dilated.

Children   Phenylephrine 2.5%, tropicamide 1%, and cyclopentolate 1–2%. Repeat these drops in 25–35 minutes if the eye is not dilated.

Infants   Phenylephrine 2.5% and tropicamide 0.5%. Homatropine 2% or cyclopentolate 0.5% (generally reserved for infants older than 1–2 months of age) may also be used. The drops can be repeated in 35–45 minutes if the eye is not dilated.

445

❖ **Notes**

1. *Dilating drops are contraindicated in most types of angle-closure glaucoma and in eyes with severely narrow anterior-chamber angles.*

2. *Dilating drops tend to be less effective at the same concentration in darkly pigmented eyes.*

COVER/UNCOVER AND ALTERNATE COVER TESTS

Cover/Uncover Test

Differentiates a phoria (the eyes are straight when fixating on a target, but misaligned when tired or not focusing) from a tropia (the eyes are misaligned at all times).

Requirements

Full range of ocular motility, vision adequate to see the target of fixation, foveal fixation in each eye, attention, and patient cooperation. This test should be performed before the alternate cover test.

1. The patient is asked to fixate on an accommodative target at distance (e.g., a letter on the vision chart).
2. Cover one of the patient's eyes while observing the uncovered eye. A refixation movement of the uncovered eye suggests the presence of a tropia.
3. Remove the cover. A phoria is identified by refixation of the eye now being uncovered while the contralateral eye maintains its position and fixation.
4. Repeat the procedure, covering the opposite eye.

❖ **Note** *A tropia may be unilateral, the same eye may be always turned in or out, or it may alternate between eyes. In an alternating tropia, the contralateral eye is sometimes deviated after the cover/uncover test.*

5. The patient is asked to fixate on an accommodative target at near. Both eyes are tested at near in the manner described previously.

❖ **Note** *An esodeviation is detected by a refixation movement temporally (the eye being observed turns away from the nose). An exodeviation is detected* *by a refixation movement nasally (the eye being observed turns toward the nose). A hyperdeviation is detected by a refixation movement inferiorly.*

Alternate Cover Test (Prism and Cover Test)

Measures the total deviation: phoria combined with tropia.

Requirements

Same as for the cover/uncover test.

1. The patient is asked to fixate on an accommodative target at distance.
2. An occluder is held over one eye for a few seconds, then quickly switched to the other eye. As the occluder alternately covers each eye for a few seconds, the eye being uncovered may be noted to swing into position to refixate on the target. Such eye movement indicates the presence of a deviation.
3. To measure the deviation, prisms are placed in front of one eye until eye movement ceases as the cover is alternated from eye to eye. The base of the prism is placed in the direction of eye movement. The strength of the weakest prism that eliminates eye movement during the alternate cover test is the amount of the deviation.
4. Measurements may be done for any direction of gaze by turning the patient's head away from the target while asking him or her to maintain fixation on it (i.e., right gaze is measured by turning the patient's head toward his or her left shoulder and asking the patient to look at the target).
5. In general, measurements are taken in the straight-ahead position (both at distance and near), in right gaze, left gaze, down-gaze (the chin is tilted up while the patient focuses on the target), up-gaze (the chin is tilted down while the patient focuses on the target), and with the patient's head tilted toward his or her left shoulder and then toward his or her right shoulder. Measurements are taken both with and without glasses in the straight-ahead position.

AMSLER'S GRID

Used to test macular function or to detect a central or paracentral scotoma.

1. Have the patient wear his or her glasses and occlude the left eye while an Amsler's grid is held approximately 12 inches in front of the right eye (Fig. A.1).
2. The patient is asked what is in the center of the page. Failure to see the central dot may indicate a central scotoma.
3. Have the patient fixate on the central dot (or the center of the page if he or she cannot see the dot) and ask if all four corners of the diagram are visible. Are any of the boxes missing?
4. Again, while staring at the central dot, the patient is asked if all of the lines are straight and continuous or if some are distorted and broken.
5. The patient is asked to outline any missing or distorted areas on the grid with a pencil.
6. Repeat the procedure, covering the right eye and testing the left.

❖ **Notes**
   1. *It is very important to monitor the patient's eye for movement away from the central dot.*
   2. *A red Amsler's grid may define more subtle defects.*

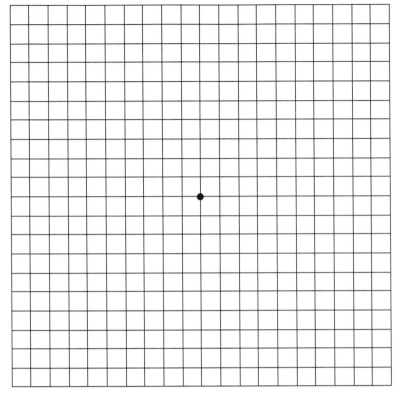

Figure A.1
Amsler's grid.

SEIDEL'S TEST TO DETECT
A WOUND LEAK

Concentrated fluorescein dye (from a moistened fluorescein strip) is applied directly over the potential site of perforation while observing the site with the slit lamp (using the white light; Fig. A.2). If a perforation and leak exist, the fluorescein dye will be diluted by the aqueous and will appear as a green (dilute) stream within the dark-orange (concentrated) dye. The stream of aqueous may also be seen with the blue light of the slit lamp.

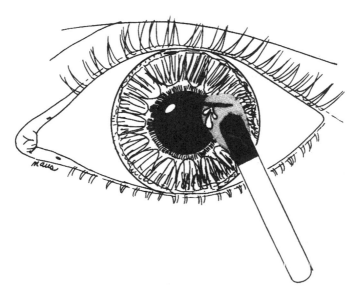

Figure A.2
Seidel's test.

FORCED DUCTION TEST AND ACTIVE FORCE GENERATION TEST

Forced Duction Test

This test distinguishes restrictive causes of decreased ocular motility from other motility disorders. One technique is the following:

1. Place a drop of topical anesthetic (e.g., proparacaine) into the eye.
2. Place a cotton-tipped applicator soaked with cocaine 10% on the muscle to be grasped (i.e., the muscle away from the "paretic" field) for about 1 minute.
3. The anesthetized muscle is grasped firmly with toothed forceps (e.g., Graefe's fixation forceps) and the eye is rotated in the "paretic" direction (Fig. A.3). If there is resistance to passive rotation of the eye, a restrictive disorder is diagnosed.

Active Force Generation Test

The patient is asked to look in the "paretic" direction while a sterile cotton swab is held just beneath the limbus on that same side. The amount of force generated by the "paretic" muscle is compared with that generated in the normal contralateral eye.

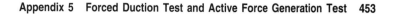

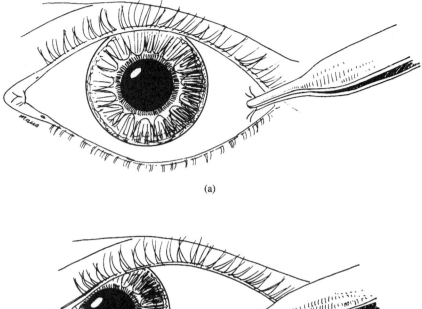

(a)

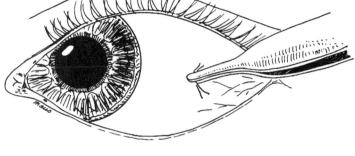

(b)

Figure A.3
Forced ductions. In the case illustrated, the left eye could not look inward. (a) The lateral rectus muscle is grasped with forceps. (b) The eye can be moved in the paretic direction (inward in this case) without resistance, ruling out a restrictive muscle condition.

TECHNIQUE FOR DIAGNOSTIC PROBING AND IRRIGATION OF THE LACRIMAL SYSTEM

1. Anesthetize the eye with a drop of topical anesthetic (e.g., proparacaine) and hold a cotton-tipped applicator soaked in the topical anesthetic on the involved punctum for several minutes.
2. Dilate the punctum with a punctum dilator.
3. Gently insert a small Bowman's probe into the punctum 2 mm vertically, and then 8 mm horizontally, toward the nose (Fig. A.4). Pull the involved eyelid laterally while slowly moving the probe horizontally to facilitate the procedure and to avoid creating a false passageway.
4. In the presence of an eyelid laceration, a torn canaliculus may be diagnosed by the appearance of the probe in the site of the eyelid laceration.
5. Irrigation of the lacrimal system is performed after removing the probe and inserting an irrigation canula in the same manner in which the probe was inserted. Five to 10 mL of saline is gently pushed into the system. Leakage through a torn eyelid also diagnoses a severed canaliculus. Resistance to injection of the saline, ballooning of the lacrimal sac, or leakage of the saline out of either punctum may be the result of a lacrimal-system obstruction. A patent lacrimal system usually drains into the throat quite readily, and the arrival of saline there may be noted by the patient.

❖ **Note** *If solely evaluating the patency of the lacrimal system, and not ruling out a laceration, the system can be irrigated as described previously, right after punctum dilatation.*

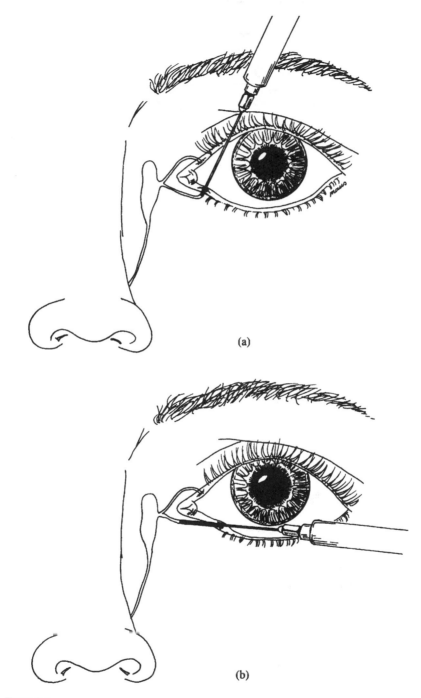

Figure A.4
Diagnostic probing of the lacrimal system. (a) After punctum dilatation, the probe or irrigation needle is directed inferiorly for 2 mm. (b) The instrument is rotated horizontally, and with the eyelid stretched laterally, is inserted toward the nose.

TECHNIQUE FOR SUBTENONS AND SUNCONJUNCTIVAL INJECTIONS

Technique for Subtenons Injection

1. Topical anesthesia is applied to the area to be injected (e.g., topical proparacaine and/or a cotton-tipped applicator soaked in proparacaine held on the area for 1–2 minutes). If subtenons steroids are to be injected, then 0.1 mL of lidocaine may be injected in the same manner as described next, several minutes before the steroids. The inferotemporal quadrant is usually the easiest location for injection.
2. With the aperture of a 25-gauge, ⅝-inch needle facing the sclera, the bulbar conjunctiva is penetrated 2–3 mm from the fornix, avoiding the conjunctival blood vessels (Fig. A.5).
3. As the needle is inserted, lateral motions of the needle are made to ensure that the needle has not penetrated the sclera (at which point lateral motion would be inhibited).
4. The curvature of the eyeball is followed, attempting to place the aperture of the needle near the posterior sclera.
5. When the needle has been pushed in to the hilt, the stopper of the syringe is pulled back to ensure against intravascular penetration.
6. The contents of the syringe are injected, and the needle is removed.

Technique for Subconjunctival Injection

1. Topical anesthesia is applied as described previously.
2. Forceps are used to tent the conjunctiva, allowing the tip of a 25-gauge, ⅜-inch needle to penetrate the subconjunctival space. The needle is placed several millimeters below the limbus at the 4- or 8-o'clock position, with the aperture facing the sclera and the needle pointed inferiorly toward the fornix (Fig. A.6).

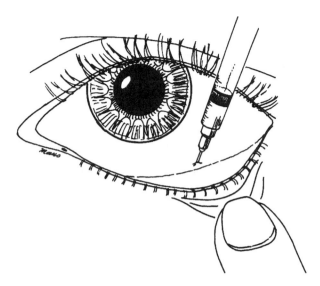

Figure A.5
Subtenons injection. The needle is placed 2–3 mm from the fornix, through conjunctiva and tenon's capsule. If possible, angle the injection so the syringe does not lie over the cornea.

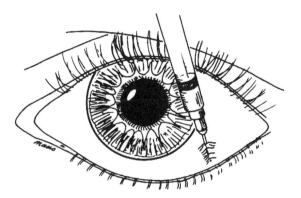

Figure A.6
Subconjunctival injection. The tip of the needle is placed into the subconjunctival space.

3. When the entire tip of the needle is beneath the conjunctiva, the stopper of the syringe is withdrawn to ensure against intravascular penetration.
4. The contests of the syringe are injected, and the needle is removed.

❖ **Note** *An eyelid speculum may be helpful in keeping the eyelids open during these procedures.*

VITREOUS EXAMINATION FOR CELLS

1. Best performed in a completely darkened room with the patient's pupil widely dilated.
2. *Anterior vitreous*   Use the high-power magnification of the slit lamp, reduce the beam height to less than the pupil diameter, and narrow the beam width to focus through the pupil. Set the illumination to the brightest setting. Move the slit lamp forward with the joy stick, angling the beam of light until the anterior vitreous can be seen posterior to the lens. By moving the joy stick, several optical sections can be sampled. Patients are sometimes asked to move their eyes from left to right, facilitating the recognition of vitreous cells as they float by.
3. *Middle and posterior vitreous*   Using a Hruby (first choice), fundus contact, or 60-diopter lens, the slit beam is initially focused on the disc. The joy stick is then used to slowly pull the slit lamp away from the eye, refocusing the light on the posterior vitreous. Again, patients may be asked to look toward their left and right and then to resume primary position to produce movement of cells and to facilitate their recognition.

MAKING FORTIFIED TOPICAL ANTIBIOTICS

Fortified Tobramycin (or Gentamicin)

With a syringe, inject 2 mL of tobramycin 40 mg/mL directly into a 5-mL bottle of tobramycin 0.3% ophthalmic solution (e.g., Tobrex). This gives a 7-mL solution of fortified tobramycin (approximately 15 mg/mL). Refrigerate. Expires after 14 days.

Fortified Cefazolin

Add enough sterile water (without preservative) to 500 mg of cefazolin dry powder to form 10 mL of solution. This provides a strength of 50 mg/mL. Refrigerate. Expires after 7 days.

Fortified Vancomycin

Add enough sterile water (without preservative) to 500 mg of vancomycin dry power to form 10 mL of solution. This provides a strength of 50 mg/mL. To achieve a 25 mg/mL concentration, take 5 mL of 50 mg/mL solution and add 5 cc sterile water. Refrigerate. Expires after 4 days.

Fortified Bacitracin

Add enough sterile water (without preservative) to 50,000 U bacitracin dry power to form 5 mL of solution. This provides a strength of 10,000 U/mL. Refrigerate. Expires after 7 days.

TETANUS PROPHYLAXIS

History of Tetanus Immunization (doses)	Clean Minor Wounds		All Other Wounds	
	Tetanus Toxoid	*Immune Globulin*	*Tetanus Toxoid*	*Immune Globulin*
Uncertain	Yes	No	Yes	Yes
0–1	Yes	No	Yes	Yes
2	Yes	No	Yes	No*
3 or more	No†	No	No‡	No

Dose of tetanus toxoid is 0.5 mL IM.

*Unless wound is more than 24 hours old.
†Unless more than 10 years since last dose.
‡Unless more than 5 years since last dose.

From U.S. Public Health Service, Advisory Committee on Immunization Practices. Morbidity and Mortality Weekly Report, Supplement. vol. 21, no. 25, June 24, 1972. Atlanta, Centers for Disease Control.

ANGLE CLASSIFICATION

Spaeth's Classification (See Fig. A.7)

Iris Insertion

    A. *Above Schwalbe's line*   Schwalbe's line is not visible.

    B. *Below Schwalbe's line*   Schwalbe's line is visible, but the trabeculum is not.

    C. *Scleral spur*   Part of the scleral spur is visible. Usually seen in patients of African or Asian descent.

    D. *Deep*   The anterior ciliary body is visible. Usually seen in Caucasian patients.

    E. *Extremely deep*   An unusually large part of the ciliary body is visible.

Indentation gonioscopy may be necessary to differentiate false opposition of the iris against structures in the iridocorneal angle (letters put in parentheses; see Fig. A.7) from the true iris insertion (letters without parentheses; see Fig. A.7).

Curvature of the Peripheral Iris

    R. *Regular*   Slight anterior bowing of the iris.

    S. *Steep*   Steep convex curvature of the iris (increased risk of developing angle-closure glaucoma).

    Q. *Queer*   Marked posterior concavity of the peripheral iris (may be seen in patients with high myopia or lens subluxation).

Angular Approach

The subjective measure of the angle between Schwalbe's line and the peripheral one third of the iris.

For example, on initial gonioscopy (without indentation) of a (B)C30R angle, Schwalbe's line, but not the trabeculum, is visible; yet on indentation, the scleral spur comes into view. The angle formed by Schwalbe's line and the peripheral

462

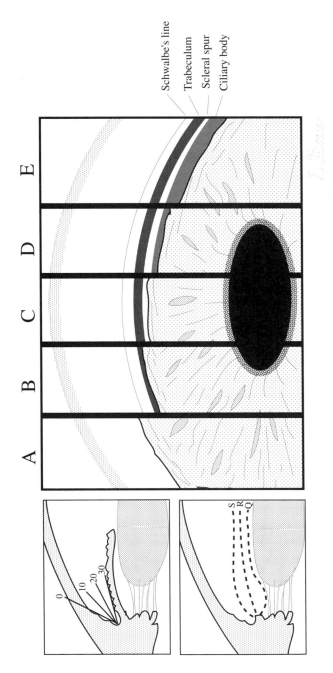

Schwalbe's line
Trabeculum
Scleral spur
Ciliary body

Figure A.7
Spaeth's classification of the anterior-chamber angle.

one third of the iris is subjectively measured to be 30 degrees, and there is a normal degree of anterior bowing to the iris.

Angle Occluded

A or B iris insertion

Angle Potentially Occludable

C or D iris insertion (without indentation), R iris curvature, angle 5 degrees or less.

C or D iris insertion (without indentation), S iris curvature, angle 20 degrees or less.

Shaffer's Classification (See Fig. A.8)

Grade 0 The angle is closed.

Grade 1 Extremely narrow angle (10 degrees). Only Schwalbe's line, and perhaps also the top of the trabeculum, can be visualized. Closure is probable.

Grade 2 Moderately narrow angle (20 degrees). Only the trabeculum can be seen. Closure is possible.

Grade 3 Moderately open angle (20–35 degrees). The scleral spur can be seen. Closure is not possible.

Grade 4 Angle wide open (35–45 degrees). The ciliary body can be visualized with ease. Closure is not possible.

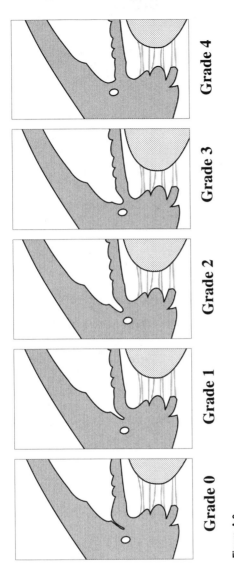

Grade 0   Grade 1   Grade 2   Grade 3   Grade 4

Figure A.8
Shaffer's classification for grading of the anterior-chamber angle.

464

DRUG GLOSSARY
Contraindications and Side Effects

The following is a list of drugs commonly used in ophthalmology along with some of their contraindications and side-effects that have clinical importance. Most of these drugs should not be used in pregnant or breast-feeding women, in infants, in those with significant renal or hepatic disease, or in patients in whom an allergy to the drug is suspected or known (therefore, these contraindications are not listed separately for each drug, and should be investigated further if therapy is desired for a patient who is under one of these circumstances).

Acetazolamide (e.g., Diamox) Contraindicated in patients with sulfa allergy, metabolic acidosis, adrenal insufficiency, and a history of kidney stones (a relative contraindication). Be careful in patients using another diuretic, a systemic steroid, or digoxin, because their potassium level may be lowered to a dangerous level. Side-effects: Blood dyscrasias, kidney stones, others.

Aminocaproic acid (e.g., Amicar) Contraindicated in patients with an intravascular clotting disorder. Side-effects: Hypotension (particularly postural), nausea, vomiting, others.

Atropine (topical) Contraindicated in most angle-closure situations, infants, albinos, and Down's syndrome patients. Use cautiously in pediatric patients as the margin for toxicity is low. Side-effects: Urinary retention, tachycardia, delirium, others.
Treatment of anticholinergic (e.g., atropine) overdose Physostigmine 1–4 mg IV, repeating 0.5–1.0 mg IV q 15 minutes until the symptoms improve.

Carbachol (topical) See **Pilocarpine.**

Carbogen (95% O$_2$, 5% CO$_2$) Contraindicated in patients with pulmonary disease or an electrolyte disorder.

Clindamycin Side-effects: Pseudomembranous colitis, others

Cocaine (topical) Contraindicated with compromised cardiovascular or cerebrovascular status.

Cyclopentolate (topical) See **Atropine.**

Dipivefrin (e.g., Propine; topical) See **Epinephrine.**

Doxycycline See **Tetracycline.**

Echothiophate iodide (e.g., Phospholine Iodide; topical) See **Pilocarpine.** Patients (or parents) are told that succinylcholine should never be given for general anesthesia (the combination of the two drugs can be lethal).

Treatment of anticholinesterase overdose Atropine 2 mg IV q 5 minutes until relief of symptoms or pralidoxime 25 mg/kg IV in 500 mL of 5% D5W over 2 hours (do *not* use in overdose of neostigmine and physostigmine).

Epinephrine (topical) Contraindicated in patients with severe cardiovascular disease. Side-effects: Macular edema in aphakic patients, conjunctival reaction, precipitation of narrow-angle glaucoma, others. Allergic conjunctivitis is common.

Fluorometholone (topical) See **Prednisolone acetate.**

Gentamicin Side-effects: Nephrotoxicity, ototoxicity, neuromuscular blockade (myasthenialike syndrome), others.

Homatropine (topical) See **Atropine.**

Isosorbide See **Mannitol.**

Ketoconazole Side-effects: Hepatotoxicity (patients are told to return immediately if anorexia, nausea and vomiting, dark urine, pale stools, or jaundice is noted), others.

Levobunolol (e.g., Betagan; topical) See **Timolol.**

Mannitol Contraindicated in patients with hypotension, cardiovascular compromise, or concomitant administration of another osmotic agent. Side-effects: Congestive heart failure, subarachnoid or subdural hemorrhage, mental confusion, others.

Methazolamide (e.g., Neptazane) See **Acetazolamide.**

Neomycin (topical) Side-effects: Superficial punctate keratitis and allergic conjunctivitis are common.

Phenylephrine (e.g., Neo-Synephrine; topical) Contraindicated in patients with significant cardiac disease, sympathetic denervation (i.e., those on monoamine oxidase inhibitors and diabetics with neuropathy), most angle-closure glaucomas, and in the presence of occludable anterior-chamber angles.

Pilocarpine (topical) Side-effects: Exacerbates iritis, can precipitate or exacerbate angle-closure glaucoma when used in high concentrations (usually 4–6% or greater), retinal detachment (with especially high concentrations or other strong miotic agents such as echothiophate), brow ache, others.

Prednisolone acetate (topical) Often contraindicated in patients with herpes simplex or fungal keratitis. Side-effects: Increased intraocular pressure, cataract, increased susceptibility to infectious organisms, others.

Prednisone Contraindicated in patients with peptic ulcer disease, tuberculosis, active infection, psychosis, or pregnancy. Work-up includes complete blood count, glucose tolerance test, pregnancy test, PPD, anergy panel, chest x-ray, stool guaiac test. Side-effects: Hyperglycemia, hypokalemia, hypertension, peptic ulcer, increased intraocular pressure, cataract, pseudotumor cerebri, mental status changes, aseptic necrosis of bone, osteoporosis, decreased wound healing, growth suppression in children, fluid retention, others.

Proparacaine (topical) Side-effects: Corneal epithelial erosions and ulcers with repeated and prolonged use.

Scopolamine (topical) See **Atropine.**

Steroids See **Prednisone.**

Sulfacetamide (topical) Side-effects: Stevens-Johnson syndrome, bone-marrow suppression, others.

Sulfadiazine See **Sulfacetamide.**

Tetracycline   Contraindicated in children younger than 8 years of age (tooth discoloration). Side-effects: Gastrointestinal upset, pseudotumor cerebri, hepatotoxicity, skin sensitivity to sunlight (patients are told upon starting the drug to avoid sunlight if possible), others.

Timolol (e.g., Timoptic; topical)   Contraindicated in patients with asthma or other breathing problems, bradycardia (the patient's pulse is checked before administering a beta-blocker), arrhythmias, congestive heart failure, hypotension, others.

Tobramycin   See **Gentamicin.**

Tropicamide (topical)   See **Atropine.**

Vancomycin   Side-effects: Nephrotoxicity, ototoxicity, others.

GENERAL GLOSSARY

Accommodation an increase in the refractive power of the natural lens of the eye; it is generally employed while doing near work (e.g., reading).

Amaurosis fugax monocular blurring of vision developing completely by 30 seconds and lasting from 10 minutes to 2 hours. It may be associated with visible emboli in the retinal vessels.

Amblyopia a unilateral or bilateral reduction of best-corrected central visual acuity in the absence of a visible organic lesion corresponding to the degree of visual loss.

Anisocoria a difference in size between the two pupils.

Anisometropia a difference in refractive error between the two eyes (e.g., one eye may be farsighted and one nearsighted, one eye may be relatively normal and the other very nearsighted).

Anterior chamber the space in the eye bordered anteriorly by the cornea and posteriorly by the iris and the pupil.

Applanation tonometer an instrument that measures intraocular pressure.

Astigmatism the refracting power of the eye is not the same in all meridians (e.g., more hyperopic vertically than horizontally).

Bulbar conjunctiva a freely movable tissue which forms the most superficial covering of the globe from the limbus to the fornices.

Buphthalmos distention of the globe in response to elevated intraocular pressure; seen in patients with congenital glaucoma.

Chemosis edema of the conjunctiva.

Coloboma congenital absence of any eye structure.

Conjunctivitis inflammation of the conjunctiva.

Cotton-wool spot a superficial retinal infarction appearing as a fluffy white lesion, sometimes obscuring retinal vessels.

Crowding phenomenon individual letters can be read better than a whole line; most commonly seen in amblyopic patients.

Cycloplegic anything that causes paralysis of the ciliary muscle and therefore paralysis of accommodation.

Descemet's membrane an inner (posterior) corneal layer.

Diplopia double vision.

Ectopia lentis dislocated lens.

Ectropion iridis (ectropion uveae)   eversion of the iris at the pupillary rim such that the pigmented posterior aspect of the iris is visualized.

Enophthalmos   a measurable depression of the globe within the bony orbit.

Enucleation   removal of the eye.

Episcleritis   inflammation of the external surface of the sclera (beneath the bulbar conjunctiva).

Esophoria   the eyes are aligned during binocular vision, but have a latent tendency to cross (e.g., while not focusing).

Esotropia   ocular misalignment in which the nonfixating eye is turned inward ("cross-eyed").

Exenteration   removal of the eye and orbital contents.

Exophoria   the eyes are aligned during binocular vision, but have a latent tendency to turn away from one another.

Exophthalmos   a measurable protrusion of the globe from the bony orbit.

Exotropia   ocular misalignment in which the nonfixating eye is turned outward ("wall-eyed").

Flare   increased protein in the anterior-chamber fluid, permitting visualization of the slit-lamp beam.

Floaters   visual perception of dots or spots which may seem to "swim" or shift location when the position of gaze is shifted.

Fluorescein angiography   a diagnostic test utilizing intravenously injected fluorescein to highlight vascular abnormalities in the eye, most commonly in the fundus.

Fovea   an area of the retina corresponding to central vision, approximately 1.5 mm in diameter, located temporal and slightly inferior to the center of the optic disc.

Foveola   the center of the fovea, 0.5 mm in diameter.

Ghost vessels   corneal stromal blood vessels containing no blood.

Gonioscopy   examination of the anterior-chamber angle structures of the eye, including the trabecular meshwork.

Guttata (corneal)   dropletlike excrescences on the posterior surface of Descemet's membrane.

Hard exudates   deep retinal lipid, often glistening yellow in appearance.

Heterochromia   a difference in coloration, especially between the two irides in a given patient.

Hyperopia (farsightedness)   a condition in which the eye is too short or the refractive power too weak to bring objects at distance or near into clear focus (without the use of accommodation).

Hyphema   blood in the anterior chamber; when layering or clotting of the blood is present, the term *hyphema* is used; when only suspended red blood cells are present, the term *microhyphema* is employed.

Hypopyon   layering of white blood cells inferiorly in the anterior chamber.

Hypotony   abnormally low intraocular pressure, usually below 6 mm Hg.

Indirect ophthalmoscopy   the use of a relatively large lens located between the patient and the observer, in combination with a light source, to view the fundus.

Intraretinal microvascular abnormalities   dilated, often telangiectatic, retinal capillaries that act as shunts between arterioles and venules.

Iritis (anterior uveitis, iridocyclitis, cyclitis)   inflammation of the iris, ciliary body, or both.

Keratic precipitates   cellular aggregates that form on the corneal endothelium, often inferiorly, in a base-down triangular pattern.

Krukenberg's spindle a narrow, vertically oriented band of pigment located along the central corneal endothelium.

Leukocoria a grossly visible white pupil.

Macula an area 3–4 disc diameters in size centered at the posterior part of the retina.

Meibomianitis inflamed, inspissated oil glands along the eyelid margins, reflecting inflammation of the meibomian glands.

Microphthalmia a congenitally small, disorganized eye.

Miosis constriction of the pupil.

Mydriasis dilatation of the pupil.

Myopia (nearsightedness) a condition in which the eye is too long or the refractive power too great to bring objects at a distance clearly into focus.

Nanophthalmos a congenitally small but otherwise normal eye.

Neovascularization growth of abnormal new blood vessels.

Nystagmus rhythmic oscillations or tremors of the eyes that occur independently of normal movements.

Ophthalmoplegia paralysis of the extraocular muscles.

Optic neuritis inflammation of the optic nerve.

Ora serrata the most peripheral portion of the retina.

Oscillopsia the perception that the environment is moving back and forth.

Palpebral conjunctiva the most superficial covering of the underside of the eyelids from the fornices to the eyelid margins.

Papilledema optic-disc swelling produced by increased intracranial pressure.

Peripapillary surrounding the optic disc.

Peripheral anterior synechiae adhesions between the peripheral iris and anterior-chamber angle or peripheral cornea.

Peripheral iridectomy removal of a portion of the peripheral iris.

Phoria the eyes remain well aligned under conditions of normal binocular vision but have a latent tendency to become misaligned (e.g., when not focusing).

Photophobia ocular pain on exposure to light.

Photopsia a sensation of instantaneous flashes of light; most commonly indicative of retinal traction.

Polycoria presence of many openings in the iris.

Posterior synechiae adhesions between the iris and the anterior lens capsule, most commonly at the pupillary border.

Proptosis protrusion of the globe from the bony orbit.

Pseudohypopon a layered collection of noninflammatory cells in the anterior chamber, usually associated with neoplastic conditions.

Ptosis (blepharoptosis) drooping of the upper eyelid.

Punctum the opening of the tear drainage system in the eyelid margin.

Pupillary block aqueous humor is prevented from flowing from the posterior chamber into the anterior chamber between the iris and lens.

Radial keratotomy a surgical technique in which radial incisions are made into the superficial cornea in an effort to change the corneal topography and therefore the patient's refractive error.

Relative afferent pupillary defect a decreased pupillary constriction to light in one eye as compared with the other eye, using the swinging-flashlight test.

Retinitis inflammation of the retina.

Retinoscopy a technique by which the reflex from a streak of light shined on the retina is used to estimate the refractive error of the eye.

Rhegmatogenous retinal detachment   detachment of the retina as a result of a retinal break (hole).

Scleral depression   a technique by which indentation of the peripheral retina is combined with indirect ophthalmoscopy in order to view the peripheral retina.

Scleritis   inflammation of the sclera.

Scotoma   an area of loss of sensitivity in the visual field.

Staphyloma   an outpouching of the sclera that involves the uvea.

Strabismus   ocular misalignment.

Tarsorrhaphy   a surgical technique by which the margins of the upper and lower eyelids of an eye are joined together, either partially or completely.

Trabeculectomy   a surgical technique used to improve aqueous outflow in glaucoma patients.

Tropia   ocular misalignment.

Vitritis   inflammation of the vitreous.

BIBLIOGRAPHY

American Academy of Ophthalmology. Basic and Clinical Science Course. Volumes 1–11, 1992–1993. San Francisco: American Academy of Ophthalmology, 1993.

Benson WE. Retinal Detachment: Diagnosis and Management. 2nd ed. Philadelphia: JB Lippincott, 1988.

Benson WE, Brown GC, Tasman W, eds. Diabetes and Its Ocular Complications. Philadelphia: WB Saunders, 1988.

Burde RM, Savino PJ, Trobe JD, eds. Clinical Decisions in Neuro-ophthalmology, 2nd ed. St. Louis: CV Mosby, 1992.

Cohen E. Contact lenses and external disease. *Int Ophthalmol Clin* 26:1, 1988.

Deutsch TA, Feller DB, eds. Paton and Goldberg's Management of Ocular Injuries. 2nd ed. Philadelphia: WB Saunders, 1985.

Gass, JDM. Stereoscopic Atlas of Macular Diseases: Diagnosis and Treatment. 3rd ed. St. Louis: CV Mosby, 1987.

Kanski, JJ. Uveitis: A Colour Manual of Diagnosis and Treatment. London: Butterworths, 1987.

Kaufman HE, Barron BA, McDonald MB, Waltman SST, eds. The Cornea. New York: Churchill Livingstone, 1988.

Reynolds LA, Closson RG, eds. Extemporaneous Ophthalmic Preparations. Vancouver, WA: Applied Therapeutics, Inc., 1993.

Roy FH. Ocular Differential Diagnosis. 5th ed. Philadelphia: Lea & Febiger, 1992.

Shields JA. Diagnosis and Management of Intraocular Tumors. St. Louis: CV Mosby, 1983.

Shields JA and Shields CL. Intraocular Tumors: A Text and Atlas. Philadelphia: WB Saunders, 1992.

Shields JA. Diagnosis and Management of Orbital Tumors. Philadelphia: WB Saunders, 1989.

Shields MB. Textbook of Glaucoma. 3rd ed. Baltimore: Williams & Wilkins, 1991.

Smolin G, Thoft RA, eds. The Cornea: Scientific Foundations and Clinical Practice. Boston: Little, Brown, 1987.

Spoor TC, Nesi GA, eds. Management of Ocular, Orbital and Adnexal Trauma. New York: Raven Press, 1988.

Tasman W, Jaeger EA, eds. Duane's Clinical Ophthalmology. rev. ed. Philadelphia: J.B. Lippincott, 1993.

Walsh TJ. Neuro-ophthalmology: Clinical Signs and Symptoms, 3rd ed. Philadelphia: Lea & Febiger, 1991.

INDEX

Page numbers in boldface type indicate major discussions; page numbers followed by f indicate figures.